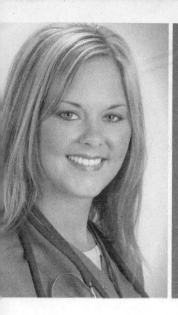

"I immediately went to my nurse manager after I failed the NCLEX® and she referred me to ATI. I was able to discover the areas I was weak in, and focused on those areas in the review modules and online assessments.

I was much more prepared the second time around!"

Terim Richards
Nursing student

Danielle Platt
Nurse Manager • Children's Mercy Hospital • Kansas City, MO

"The year our hospital did not use the ATI program, we experienced a 15% decrease in the NCLEX® pass rates. We reinstated the ATI program the following year and had a 90% success rate."

"As a manager, I have witnessed graduate nurses fail the NCLEX® and the devastating effects it has on their morale. Once the nurses started using ATI, it was amazing to see the confidence they had in themselves and their ability to go forward and take the NCLEX® exam."

Mary Moss
Associate Dean of Nursing - Service and Health Division • Mid-State Technical College • Wisconsin Rapids, WI

"I like that ATI lets students know what to expect from the NCLEX®, helps them plan their study time and tells them what to do in the days and weeks before the exam. It is different from most of the NCLEX® review books on the market."

Editor

Jeanne Wissmann, PhD, RN, CNE
Director Nursing Curriculum and Educational Services
Assessment Technologies Institute®, LLC

Associate Editors

Audrey Knippa, MS, MPH, RN, CNE
Curriculum Project Coordinator

Kristen M. Lawler, MBA
Director of Development

Brant L. Stacy, BS Journalism
Product Developer

Important Notice to the Reader of this Publication

Preface

Overview

The overall goal of this Assessment Technologies Institute®, LLC (ATI) Content Mastery Series module is to provide nursing students with an additional resource for the focused review of "Pharmacology for Nursing Care" content relevant to NCLEX® preparation and entry level nursing practice. Content within this review module is provided in a key point plus rationale format in order to focus recall and application of relevant content. Unit and chapter selections are reflective of the relevant pharmacological categories and content explanations of the NCLEX® test plan, the ATI "Pharmacology for Nursing Care" assessment test plans, and standard nursing curricular content. Each chapter begins with an overview of some of the topic-relevant nursing activities outlined by the NCLEX® test plan in an effort to guide the learner's review and application of chapter content.

Contributors

ATI would like to extend appreciation to the nurse educators and nurse specialists who contributed chapters for this review module. The name of each contributor is noted in the chapter byline. We would also like to thank those talented individuals who reviewed, edited, and developed this module. In the summer and fall of 2005, two focus groups of committed nurse educators gave invaluable input and feedback regarding the format and purposes of review modules. Their input and ideas were instrumental to the development of this review module and we are very appreciative. Additionally, we would like to recognize and extend appreciation to the multiple nursing students and educators who have contacted us in the past year with comments and ideas regarding the content of this review module. And finally, we want to recognize and express appreciation to all of the contributors, reviewers, production developers, and editors of previous editions of this Content Mastery Series module.

Suggestions for Effective Utilization

Δ   Understanding the organizational framework of this review module will facilitate focused review. Unit 1 presents the foundation for medication administration. The medications in units 2 to 12 are organized into groups that affect similar body systems and/or disorders. Within Units 2 to 12 are the major classifications of medications with identified prototypes. Keep in mind that just as there may be more than one classification used for a specific disorder there may also be more than one medication identified as a prototype. Often the identified prototype may be the first medication developed in a classification, which may or may not be a "commonly prescribed" medication in health care today. A prototype serves as a learning tool. What is learned about one prototype can be applied to all medications within a classification and the learner only has to recognize and learn those few aspects of a medication that might differ from the prototype.

Δ   Some suggested uses of this review module include:

•   As a review of NCLEX® relevant pharmacology content in developing and assessing your readiness for NCLEX®.

•   As a focused review resource based on the results of an ATI "Pharmacology" or "Comprehensive Predictor" assessment. "Topics to Review" identified upon completion of these assessments can be used to focus your efforts to a review of content within specific chapter(s) of this review module. For example, an identified "Topic to Review" of "Side effects of anti-inflammatory medications: Aspirin" suggests that a review of Unit 4 "Medications for Pain and Inflammation" and completion of the application exercises at the end of the chapter would be helpful.

Δ   To foster long-term recall and development of an ability to apply knowledge to a variety of situations, learners are encouraged to take a comprehensive approach to topic review. Using this review module along with other resources (class notes, course textbooks, nursing reference texts, instructors, ATI DVD series):

•   Consider an exploration of major classifications of medications, prototype medications within a major classification, therapeutic uses, and nursing interventions related to the risk of side effects and/or interactions. Address such questions as:

◊ What are the major classifications of medications and the prototype(s) within a classification that are used to treat various disorders (e.g., infections, cardiovascular, neurological, digestive, endocrine, reproductive, and respiratory disorders)?

◊ What is the pharmacological action of each prototype medication? What are some major therapeutic uses?

◊ What are the major side/adverse effects for each major classification of medications/specific prototype medications? What are important nursing interventions to take because of the associated major side/adverse effects?

◊ What are the nursing interventions for a client experiencing an allergic reaction to a medication?

◊ What are the possible interactions between a prototype drug and other medications/foods? What are important nursing interventions to take because of the possibility of a particular medication/food interaction?

◊ How do you evaluate and monitor the effectiveness of a prototype medication? What client findings provide evidence of therapeutic effects?

◊ What are general nursing interventions for safe administration of a particular medication? What assessments are appropriate prior to administration? In what circumstances should a specific prototype medication be held?

• Consider some synthesizing learning activities, such as addressing questions like these:

◊ What are similarities and differences within medication classifications?

◊ What are the different classifications that can be used to treat one specific disorder?

◊ What are the different conditions that one medication can be used for?

◊ What are high risk medications?

Δ Complete application exercises at the end of each chapter after a review of the topic. Answer questions fully and note rationales for answers. Complete exercises initially without looking for the answers within the chapter or consulting the answer key. Use these exercises as an opportunity to assess your readiness to apply knowledge. When reviewing the answer key, in addition to identifying the correct answer, examine why you missed or answered correctly each item – was it related to ability to recall?, recognition of a common testing principle?, or perhaps attention to key words?

Feedback

All feedback is welcome – suggestions for improvement, reports of mistakes (small or large), and testimonials of effectiveness. Please address feedback to: comments@atitesting.com

Table of Contents

Unit 3 Medications Affecting the Immune System

Unit 4 Medications for Pain and Inflammation

Unit 5 Medications Affecting the Nervous System

Unit 6 Medications Affecting the Cardiovascular System

Unit 9 Medications Affecting Fluid, Electrolytes, Minerals, and/or the Renal System

Unit 10 Medications Affecting the Digestive System and Nutrition

Unit 11 Medications Affecting the Endocrine System

Unit 12 Medications Affecting Reproduction

Unit 1   Basic Pharmacologic Principles & Safe Administration of Medications

Chapter 1:   Basic Pharmacologic Principles
                  Contributor: Judith A. Harris, MSN, RNC

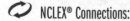 **NCLEX® Connections:**

> **Learning Objective**: Review and apply knowledge within "**Basic Pharmacologic Principles**" in readiness for performance of the following nursing activities as outlined by the NCLEX® test plans:
>
> Δ   Apply knowledge of basic pharmacologic principles, such as pharmacokinetics and pharmacodynamics in understanding and interpreting medication orders, in safely administering medications, in monitoring side/adverse effects, and in evaluating medication effectiveness.

 Key Points

- Δ   **Pharmacokinetics** refers to the movement of medication molecules in the body, including **absorption**, **distribution**, **metabolism**, and **excretion** of medications.

  - •   **Absorption** – the movement of a medication from its site of administration (e.g., GI tract, muscle, skin, or subcutaneous tissue) to the bloodstream. The most common routes of administration are enteral (through the GI tract) and parenteral (by injection). Each of these routes will have a unique pattern of absorption.

    - ◊   **Rate** of medication absorption determines how soon the medication will take effect.

    - ◊   **Amount** of medication absorbed determines its intensity.

    - ◊   **Route** of administration affects the rate and amount of absorption.

Routes and Absorption		
Route	**Barriers to Absorption**	**Absorption Pattern**
Oral	• Medications must pass through the layer of epithelial cells that line the GI tract.	• Varies greatly due to the following variables: ◊ Stability and solubility of the medication ◊ Gastric intestinal pH and emptying time ◊ Presence of food in the gut ◊ Other medications currently being administered ◊ Forms of medications (e.g., enteric coated pills, liquids).

Intramuscular (Subcutaneous – almost identical)	• The capillary wall has large spaces between cells; therefore, there is no significant barrier.	• Absorption may be rapid or slow depending on the following variables:
		◊ Water solubility of the medication:
		  ° Highly soluble medications will be absorbed in 10 to 30 min.
		  ° Poorly soluble medications will be absorbed slower.
		• Site of injection blood flow – sites with high blood flow will have rapid absorption. Sites with low blood flow will have slow absorption.

Intravenous	• No barriers	• Instantaneous – administered directly into blood. • Complete – all of it reaches the blood.

Routes - Advantages vs Disadvantages		
Route	**Advantages**	**Disadvantages**
Oral	• Safe • Inexpensive • Easy and convenient	• Highly variable absorption • Inactivation by GI tract or first-pass effect • Client must be cooperative and conscious • Contraindications include nausea and vomiting
Intramuscular (Subcutaneous – almost identical)	• Used for poorly soluble medications • Appropriate for preparing medications that are absorbed slowly for an extended period of time (depot preparations)	• Higher cost • Inconvenient • Pain with risk for local tissue damage and nerve damage • Risk for infection
Intravenous	• Onset is rapid • Can control precise amount of medication given • Allows for administration of large volumes of fluid • Irritating medications can be given with free-flowing IV • Absorption of the medication into the blood is immediate providing immediate response.	• Even higher cost • More inconvenient • Absorption of the medication into the blood is immediate. This can be potentially dangerous if the wrong amount of medication is given. • Risk for infection or embolism

- **Distribution** – the transportation of a medication to its site of action by bodily fluids. Distribution may be influenced by:

  ◊ **Circulation** to site of action (e.g., peripheral vascular or cardiac disease may delay medication distribution).

  ◊ **Plasma protein binding**: Medications compete for protein binding sites. One medication can displace another medication from a protein binding site and thus cause the free concentration of that medication to rise. For example, a sulfonamide antibiotic displaces warfarin (Coumadin) from its protein binding sites, which ↑ the concentration of free warfarin and leads to a higher risk for bleeding.

  ◊ **Barriers**: Only medications that have a transport system or are lipid-soluble are able to cross the blood-brain barrier. Neonates should be given reduced dosages of medications that have actions in the brain because their blood-brain barrier is not fully developed.

- **Metabolism** – occurs primarily in the liver. Individuals diagnosed with liver dysfunction have a ↓ ability to metabolize medications and are at risk for undue accumulation of medication and possible toxicity.

  ◊ **Therapeutic consequences of metabolism** can include:

    ° ↑ renal excretion of medication.

    ° Inactivation of medications.

    ° ↑ therapeutic action.

    ° Activation of pro-medications into active forms.

    ° ↓ toxicity when active forms of medications are converted to inactive forms.

    ° ↑ toxicity when inactive forms of medications are converted to active forms.

  ◊ **Factors influencing rate of medication metabolism** can include:

    ° **Age** – infants have limited medication-metabolizing capacity. Take care to avoid injury prior to hepatic maturation of infants. The aging process can also influence medication metabolism, but varies from individual to individual. In general, hepatic medication metabolism tends to decline with age. Observe the client for prolonged medication effects due to ↓ liver function.

    ° Certain medications can cause an ↑ in certain **medication-metabolizing enzymes**. This can cause that particular medication to be metabolized sooner, requiring an ↑ in dosage of that medication to maintain a therapeutic level. It can also cause an ↑ in the metabolism of other medications that are being used concurrently.

    ° **First-pass effect** – some medications are inactivated on their first pass through the liver. It is important to know which medications must be given by a nonenteral route because of their high first-pass effects. Nitroglycerin (Nitrogard) is an example of such a medication. Alternate routes for nitroglycerin administration in order to avoid first-pass effect include intravenous and sublingual routes.

    ° When two medications are metabolized by the same pathway they can interfere with the **metabolism** of one or both of the medications. In this way, the rate of metabolism can be ↓ for one or both of the medications leading to medication accumulation. Observe for an ↑ or ↓ in the levels of the medications when given together.

    ° **Nutritional status** – a malnourished client may be deficient in the factors that are necessary to produce specific medication-metabolizing enzymes. Consequently, medication metabolism may be impaired.

- **Excretion** – the elimination of a medication from the body primarily through the kidneys. Individuals diagnosed with renal dysfunction should be monitored for an ↑ in duration and intensity of medication responses

Δ **Medication responses** – plasma medication levels can be regulated to control medication responses. Medication dosing attempts to maintain plasma levels between the **minimum effective concentration (MEC)** and the toxic concentration. When a medication has achieved plasma levels that are effective and not toxic, the plasma level is within the **therapeutic range.** This can be useful when primary care providers are prescribing certain medications. For example, therapeutic levels are well established for many antiseizure medications. These levels can be used to monitor client response to the medication.

Δ **Therapeutic Index (TI)** – medications with a high TI have a wide safety margin. Therefore, there is no need for routine serum medication level monitoring. Medications with a low TI should have serum medication levels monitored closely. Monitor peak levels based on the route of administration. For example, an oral medication may have a peak of 1 to 3 hr after administration. Whereas, if the medication is given intravenously, the peak time might occur within 10 min. (*Refer to drug reference or pharmacist for specific medication peak times*). For trough levels, blood is drawn immediately before next medication dose regardless of the route of administration.

Δ **Half-life (t1/2)** – may be affected by liver and kidney function. Usually takes four half-lives to achieve steady state of serum concentration (drug intake = drug metabolism and excretion).

Short half-life	Long half-life
Medications leave the body quickly – 4 to 8 hr.	Medications leave the body more slowly – 24+ hr. Greater risk for medication accumulation and toxicity.
Short-dosing interval or minimum effective concentration (MEC) will drop between doses.	Medications are given at longer intervals without loss of therapeutic effects.
	Medications take a longer time to reach steady state.

Δ **Pharmacodynamics** (mechanism of action) describes the interactions between medications and target cells, body systems, and organs to produce effects. Medications interact with cells in one of two ways. Medications can mimic the receptor activity regulated by endogenous compounds or block normal receptor activity regulated by endogenous compounds. For example, morphine is classified as an agonist because it activates the receptors that produce analgesia, sedation, constipation, and other effects. Losartan (Cozaar), an angiotensin II receptor blocker, is classified as an antagonist. Losartan works by blocking angiotensin II receptors on blood vessels, which prevents vasoconstriction.

Medication Category and Classification

Δ   **Prescription medications** are administered under the supervision of primary care providers. These medications may be habit-forming, have potential harmful effects, and require supervision.

- **Uncontrolled substances** – antibiotics are an example of uncontrolled prescription medications. They require monitoring by a primary care provider, but do not pose risk of abuse and/or addiction.

- **Controlled substances** – codeine is an example of a controlled prescription medication. Medications that have a potential for abuse and dependence are categorized into schedules. Heroin is a drug in Schedule I and has no medical use in the United States. Medications categorized in Schedules II through V all have approved applications. Each level has decreasing risk of abuse and dependence. For example, morphine is a Schedule II medication that has a greater risk of abuse and dependence than phenobarbital, which is a Schedule IV medication.

Δ   **FDA pregnancy risk category** (A, B, C, D, X) categorizes medications in terms of their potential harm during pregnancy, with Category A being the safest and Category X the most dangerous. Teratogenesis is most likely to occur during the first trimester. Before giving any medication to a woman who is pregnant (or to one who could be pregnant), determine whether or not it is safe for administration during pregnancy.

Primary Reference:

Lehne, R. A. (2007). *Pharmacology for nursing care* (6th ed.). St. Louis, MO: Saunders.

Additional Resources:

Abrams, A. C., & Goldsmith, T. L. (2003). *Clinical drug therapy: Rationales for nursing practice* (7th ed.). Philadelphia: Lippincott Williams & Wilkins.

Linton, A. D., & Harris, J. A. (2000). *Pharmacology companion for introductory nursing care of adults* (2nd ed.). Philadelphia: Saunders.

Unit 1 Basic Pharmacologic Principles & Safe Administration of Medications
Chapter 1: Basic Pharmacologic Principles

Application Exercises

1. Identify several factors that can influence individual differences in medication response.

2. A client who is pregnant is taking a medication labeled pregnancy risk category B. Is this medication safe for the client? Explain.

3. A client is prescribed phenobarbital for a seizure disorder. Phenobarbital has a long half-life of 4 days. Based on the half-life of phenobarbital, it is most likely that it will be prescribed

   A. once a day.
   B. twice a day.
   C. three times a day.
   D. every other day.

4. An order has been written to "draw peak and trough levels" for a particular medication. When should blood be drawn for each level?

5. After an oral medication has been absorbed, most of the medication is inactivated as the blood initially passes through the liver, producing little therapeutic effect. This is called

   A. tolerance.
   B. first-pass effect.
   C. antagonism.
   D. synergism.

6. A medication has to bind to a _____ in a cell to produce an effect.

7. Medication dosages may need to be decreased for the following reasons. (Select all that apply.)

_____ Increased renal excretion

_____ Increased medication-metabolizing enzymes

_____ Liver failure

_____ Peripheral vascular disease

_____ Concurrent use of medication metabolized by the same pathway

8. The study of medication movement through the body is referred to as _____.

9. When medications act on receptors they can do which of the following? (Select all that apply.)

_____ Mimic the action of the body's own hormones.

_____ Change the enzymes made by the target cell.

_____ Make the receptors respond in new ways.

_____ Change the receptors molecular structure.

_____ Block the action of the body's own compounds.

10. Intravenous administration of a medication eliminates the need for

A. absorption.

B. distribution.

C. metabolism.

D. excretion.

Unit 1 Basic Pharmacologic Principles & Safe Administration of Medications

Chapter 1: Basic Pharmacologic Principles

Application Exercises Answer Key

1. Identify several factors that can influence individual differences in medication response.

    (May include) body weight, age, gender, genetics, biorhythmic cycles, tolerance, accumulation, psychological factors, and medical conditions.

2. A client who is pregnant is taking a medication labeled pregnancy risk category B. Is this medication safe for the client? Explain.

    Medications categorized into the pregnancy safety B category pose more of a risk to a client who is pregnant than those in the A category. Animal studies reveal no fetal risk, but controlled studies have not been done in women. Animal studies show risk of fetal harm, but controlled studies have not demonstrated a risk during the first trimester, and there is no evidence of risk in later trimesters.

3. A client is prescribed phenobarbital for a seizure disorder. Phenobarbital has a long half-life of 4 days. Based on the half-life of phenobarbital, it is most likely that it will be prescribed

    A. once a day.
    B. twice a day.
    C. three times a day.
    D. every other day.

    Medications with long half-lives are able to maintain their therapeutic levels between doses for long periods of time. Therefore, this medication can be administered once a day.

4. An order has been written to "draw peak and trough levels" for a particular medication. When should blood be drawn for each level?

    Peak blood draw depends on the route of administration. Oral medications take longer to peak than medications given by the intravenous route. Trough blood draw should be done immediately before the next medication dose.

5. After an oral medication has been absorbed, most of the medication is inactivated as the blood initially passes through the liver, producing little therapeutic effect. This is called

      A. tolerance.

      B. first-pass effect.

      C. antagonism.

      D. synergism.

Medications that are given orally are taken directly to the liver from the GI tract via the hepatic portal circulation. Some medications will be completely inactivated as they pass through the liver and thus no therapeutic effects will occur. These medications must be administered by a nonenteral route.

6. A medication has to bind to a _____ in a cell to produce an effect.

Receptor. For a medication (which is a chemical) to have an effect on the body, it must interact with other chemicals (the receptors).

7. Medication dosages may need to be decreased for the following reasons. (Select all that apply.)

      _____   Increased renal excretion

      _____   Increased medication-metabolizing enzymes

      __X__   **Liver failure**

      _____   Peripheral vascular disease

      __X__   **Concurrent use of medication metabolized by the same pathway**

Liver failure can decrease metabolism and thus increase the concentration of a medication. When two medications are metabolized in the same way they may compete for metabolism, thereby increasing the concentration of one or both medications. Increased renal excretion may decrease concentration of the medication requiring an increased dosage. Increased medication-metabolizing enzymes can decrease the concentration of the medication. The dose might need to be increased. Peripheral vascular disease may impair distribution, and more of the medication may be needed.

8. The study of medication movement through the body is referred to as _____.

Pharmacokinetics

9. When medications act on receptors they can do which of the following? (Select all that apply.)

    __X__   **Mimic the action of the body's own hormones.**
    _____   Change the enzymes made by the target cell.
    _____   Make the receptors respond in new ways.
    _____   Change the receptors molecular structure.
    __X__   **Block the action of the body's own compounds.**

Medications can only mimic or block the action of endogenous compounds. Medications cannot alter enzymes, cause new responses by receptors, or change molecular structure.

10. Intravenous administration of a medication eliminates the need for

    A. absorption.
    B. distribution.
    C. metabolism.
    D. excretion.

Intravenous administration delivers the medication directly into the bloodstream where it is rapidly distributed throughout the body.

Unit 1   Basic Pharmacologic Principles & Safe Administration of Medications

Chapter 2:   Interactions, Adverse Effects, & Contraindications
Contributor: Judith A. Harris, MSN, RNC

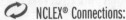 NCLEX® Connections:

Learning Objective: Review and apply knowledge within "**Interactions, Adverse Effects, & Contraindications**" in readiness for performance of the following nursing activities as outlined by the NCLEX® test plans:

Δ   Apply knowledge of the basic mechanisms of drug-drug and drug-food interactions and assess/monitor the client for these interactions.

Δ   Apply knowledge of different types of adverse medication reactions and assess/monitor the client for these effects.

Δ   Demonstrate appropriate nursing care for the client experiencing an adverse medication reaction.

Δ   Assess/monitor the client for contraindications and intervene as appropriate.

Δ   Provide/reinforce teaching to client/family/significant others on how to manage potential adverse effects, interactions, or incompatibilities of all medications taken by the client.

Δ   Demonstrate appropriate documentation of medication administration for clients experiencing medication interactions and adverse effects.

Key Points

Δ   Drug-Drug Interactions

Consequences of Drug-Drug Interactions	
Type of Interaction	Nursing Implications/Interventions
↑ Therapeutic effects	• Some medications may be given together for their ↑ therapeutic effect. For example, clients with asthma are instructed to use albuterol (Proventil), a beta$_2$-adrenergic agonist inhaler, 5 min prior to using triamcinolone acetonide (Azmacort), a glucocorticoid inhaler, in order to ↑ the absorption of Azmacort.
↑ Adverse effects	• Clients may take two medications that have the same side effect. Taking these two medications together ↑ the risk of these side effects. For example, aspirin and warfarin both have anticoagulant effects. When used together, the client has an ↑ risk for bleeding.
↓ Adverse effects	• One medication can be given to counteract the adverse effect of another medication. Antiemetic medications are frequently used for this purpose.
↓ Therapeutic effects	• One medication can ↑ the metabolism of a second medication, thereby decreasing the therapeutic effect of the first medication. For example, clients taking phenytoin (Dilantin), an antiseizure medication, should be advised to avoid alcohol. Alcohol can ↑ the metabolism of phenytoin and thus ↓ its antiseizure effect.

Over-The-Counter (OTC) Medications	
Interactions	**Nursing Implications/Interventions**
Ingredients in OTC medications may interact with other OTC or prescription medications.	• Perform complete medication history.
Inactive ingredients (e.g., dyes, alcohol, preservatives) may cause adverse reactions.	
Potential for overdose exists because of the use of several preparations (including prescription medications) with similar ingredients.	
Interactions of certain prescription and OTC medications can interfere with therapeutic effects.	• Clients are advised to use caution and to check with their primary care provider before using any OTC preparations (e.g., antacids, laxatives, decongestants, cough syrups). For example, antacids can interfere with the absorption of ranitidine (Zantac) and other medications. Advise clients to take antacids 1 hr apart from other medications.

Δ   **Drug-Food Interactions** – food may alter medication absorption and/or may contain substances that react with certain medications.

  • Examples include:

   ◊ Consuming foods with tyramine while taking monoamine oxidase inhibitors (MAOIs) can lead to hypertensive crisis. Clients taking an MAOI should be aware of such foods and avoid them.

   ◊ Vitamin K can ↓ the therapeutic effects of warfarin and place clients at risk for developing blood clots. Clients taking warfarin should avoid eating foods high in vitamin K.

   ◊ Tetracycline can interact with a chelating agent such as milk, and form an insoluble, unabsorbable compound. Instruct clients not to take tetracycline within 2 hr of consuming any dairy products.

   ◊ **Grapefruit juice** seems to act by inhibiting presystemic medication metabolism in the small bowel, thus ↑ absorption of certain oral medications, either ↑ effects or enhancing adverse reactions. Clients should be instructed not to drink grapefruit juice if they are taking such a medication.

Δ   **Adverse Drug Effects** – any unintended or undesired effect that can occur at a normal medication dose. **Side effects** are the secondary medication effects that occur at therapeutic doses. These are usually predictable.

Adverse Medication Effects	Nursing Implications/Nursing Interventions
Central Nervous System (CNS) effects – May result from either CNS stimulation (excitement) or CNS depression.	• If CNS stimulation is expected, clients may be at risk for seizures, and precautions should be taken. • If CNS depression is likely, clients should be advised not to drive or participate in other activities that can be dangerous.
Extrapyramidal symptoms (EPS) (abnormal body movements) – May include involuntary fine motor tremors, rigidity, uncontrollable restlessness, and acute dystonias (spastic movements and/or muscle rigidity affecting the head, neck, eyes, facial area, and limbs).	• Extrapyramidal symptoms are more often associated with medications affecting the CNS, such as those used to treat mental health disorders. • Observe clients for these effects and notify the primary care provider if they occur.
Anticholinergic effects – Many medications have side effects that are a result of muscarinic receptor blockade. The majority of effects are seen in the eye, smooth muscle, exocrine glands, and the heart.	• Clients should be advised of these effects. For example, dry mouth may be relieved by sipping on liquids; photophobia can be managed by use of sunglasses; and urinary retention may be reduced by voiding before taking the medication.
Cardiovascular effects – Cardiovascular effects may result from effects on both blood vessels and the heart.	• For example, orthostatic hypotension can occur with antihypertensives. • Instruct clients about signs of postural hypotension (lightheadedness and dizziness). If these occur, advise the client to sit or lie down. Postural hypotension can be minimized by getting up slowly.
Gastrointestinal effects – Usually result from local irritation of the GI tract, stimulation of the vomiting center in the brain, or ↑ peristalsis. The most serious effects include GI bleeding or ulceration and severe diarrhea.	• For example, advise clients taking opioid analgesics that constipation is a common side effect. Recommend ↑ fluids and dietary fiber.
Hematologic effects – Relatively common and potentially life threatening with some groups of medications. Bone marrow depression/suppression is generally associated with anticancer medications and hemorrhagic disorders with anticoagulants and thrombolytics.	• For example, if clients are taking an anticoagulant, educate them about signs and symptoms of bleeding (e.g., bruising, discolored urine/stool, petechiae, bleeding gums). If the client experiences any of these signs and symptoms, the client should notify the primary care provider.

Adverse Medication Effects	Nursing Implications/Nursing Interventions
Hepatotoxicity – Since most medications are metabolized in the liver, the liver is particularly vulnerable to drug-induced injury. Damage to liver cells can impair metabolism of many medications, causing medication accumulation in the body and producing adverse effects. Many medications can alter normal values of liver function tests with no obvious clinical signs of liver dysfunction.	• When two or more medications that are hepatotoxic are combined, the risk for liver damage is ↑. • Liver function tests should be taken when a client starts a medication known to be hepatotoxic and periodically thereafter.
Nephrotoxicity – May occur with a number of medications, but is primarily the result of certain antimicrobial agents and non-steroidal anti-inflammatory drugs (NSAIDs). Damage to the kidneys may interfere with medication excretion leading to medication accumulation and adverse effects.	• For example, aminoglycosides can cause renal damage. Monitor serum creatinine and BUN levels of clients taking an aminoglycoside.
Toxicity – An adverse medication effect that is considered severe and may be life threatening. It may be caused by an excessive dose, but can also occur at therapeutic dose levels.	• For example, liver damage will occur with an acetaminophen overdose. There is a greater risk of liver damage with chronic alcohol use. The antidote acetylcysteine (Mucomyst) may be used to minimize liver damage.
Allergic reaction – When an individual develops an immune response to a medication. The individual has been previously exposed to the medication and has developed antibodies.	• Allergic reactions range from minor to serious. Mild rash and hives can be treated with diphenhydramine (Benadryl). • Before administering any medications, take a complete medication history.
Anaphylactic reaction – A life-threatening immediate allergic reaction that causes respiratory distress, severe bronchospasm, and cardiovascular collapse.	• Treat with epinephrine, bronchodilators, and antihistamines. Provide respiratory support. Be sure to inform the primary care provider if this response occurs.
Immunosuppression – ↓ or absent immune response.	• For example, glucocorticoids depress the immune response and ↑ the risk for infection. • Clients taking a glucocorticoid should be monitored for signs and symptoms of infection.

Δ   Contraindications and Precautions

- A specific medication may be contraindicated for a client based on the client's condition. For example, penicillin is contraindicated for a client who has an allergy to this medication.

- Precautions should be taken for a client who is more likely to have an adverse reaction than another client. For example, morphine depresses respiratory function, so it should be used with caution for clients who have asthma or impaired respiratory function.

Primary Reference:

Lehne, R. A. (2007). *Pharmacology for nursing care.* (6th ed.). St. Louis, MO: Saunders.

Additional Resources:

Abrams, A. C., & Goldsmith, T. L. (2003). *Clinical drug therapy: Rationales for nursing practice* (7th ed.). Philadelphia: Lippincott Williams & Wilkins.

Linton, A. D., & Harris, J. A. (2000). *Pharmacology companion for introductory nursing care of adults* (2nd ed.). Philadelphia: Saunders.

Unit 1 Basic Pharmacologic Principles & Safe Administration of Medications
Chapter 2: Interactions, Adverse Effects, & Contraindications

Application Exercises

1. Which of the following statements by a client receiving warfarin (Coumadin) indicates a need for further teaching?

        A. "I use a laxative every other day."

        B. "I ate some caramel corn yesterday."

        C. "I use antacids once in a while."

        D. "I always have aspirin with me to use for my headaches."

2. A nurse is ready to administer the first dose of a new oral penicillin prescription to a client. The client states she took penicillin 3 years ago and developed a rash. Based on this information, the nurse should

        A. give the medication as prescribed and observe for a reaction.

        B. administer the medication intravenously to bypass gastric absorption.

        C. withhold the medication and inform the primary care provider of the client's previous reaction.

        D. combine the medication with an antihistamine to decrease the possibility of a reaction.

3. A nursing responsibility for a client receiving an antihypertensive medication is to

        A. increase the dose if the client experiences tachycardia.

        B. teach the client to stand or sit up slowly to avoid dizziness or fainting.

        C. take the client's blood pressure every 4 hr in the same arm in a supine position.

        D. discontinue the client's medication if blood pressure decreases.

4. Do drug-drug interactions produce increased or decreased medication effects? Explain.

5. A nursing student has just been assigned to a new client. When the nurse checks the medication administration record, she observes that the client is on four different medications. When determining if there are any **interactions** between these medications, the nursing student should be concerned if

     A. two of the medications cause drowsiness.

     B. the client is pregnant.

     C. there are no generic forms of the medications available.

     D. the client has difficulty swallowing four pills at one time.

6. When counseling a client who has been prescribed a medication that is highly hepatotoxic, the nurse should instruct the client to

     A. avoid alcohol.

     B. come in for a liver biopsy on a monthly schedule.

     C. avoid strenuous activity and contact sports.

     D. notify her primary care provider immediately if her appetite increases.

7. A client starting on cyclobenzaprine (Flexeril) should be informed that he may experience which of the following anticholinergic side effects?

     A. Dry mouth

     B. Bradycardia

     C. Diarrhea

     D. Urinary frequency

Unit 1 Basic Pharmacologic Principles & Safe Administration of Medications
Chapter 2: Interactions, Adverse Effects, & Contraindications

Application Exercises Answer Key

1. Which of the following statements by a client receiving warfarin (Coumadin) indicates a need for further teaching?

       A. "I use a laxative every other day."

       B. "I ate some caramel corn yesterday."

       C. "I use antacids once in a while."

       D. "I always have aspirin with me to use for my headaches."

    Aspirin decreases platelet aggregation. Warfarin suppresses coagulation. Concurrent use increases the risk for bleeding. If used concurrently, dosage adjustments would need to be made.

2. A nurse is ready to administer the first dose of a new oral penicillin prescription to a client. The client states she took penicillin 3 years ago and developed a rash. Based on this information, the nurse should

       A. give the medication as prescribed and observe for a reaction.

       B. administer the medication intravenously to bypass gastric absorption.

       C. withhold the medication and inform the primary care provider of the client's previous reaction.

       D. combine the medication with an antihistamine to decrease the possibility of a reaction.

    The client was exposed to penicillin 3 years ago and is now sensitized to the medication. Re-exposure to this medication can cause an allergic reaction, ranging from mild to life threatening. Therefore, it is important for the primary care provider to be informed of the client's prior sensitization. The provider may choose to use a different medication.

3. A nursing responsibility for a client receiving an antihypertensive medication is to

> A. increase the dose if the client experiences tachycardia.
>
> **B. teach the client to stand or sit up slowly to avoid dizziness or fainting.**
>
> C. take the client's blood pressure every 4 hr in the same arm in a supine position.
>
> D. discontinue the client's medication if blood pressure decreases.

Orthostatic hypotension is a common side effect of antihypertensives. By changing positions slowly, it allows the body to adjust to the change and prevents dizziness or fainting.

4. Do drug-drug interactions produce increased or decreased medication effects? Explain.

Drug-drug interactions may produce increased or decreased medication effects. These effects can be beneficial or detrimental to the client.

5. A nursing student has just been assigned to a new client. When the nurse checks the medication administration record, she observes that the client is on four different medications. When determining if there are any **interactions** between these medications, the nursing student should be concerned if

> **A. two of the medications cause drowsiness.**
>
> B. the client is pregnant.
>
> C. there are no generic forms of the medications available.
>
> D. the client has difficulty swallowing four pills at one time.

A drug-drug interaction can cause an increased effect. If two of these medications cause drowsiness (CNS depression), they will have a synergistic effect and cause a greater amount of CNS depression. Increasing CNS depression can progress from drowsiness to stupor as well as fatal respiratory depression.

6. When counseling a client who has been prescribed a medication that is highly hepatotoxic, the nurse should instruct the client to

       A. avoid alcohol.

       B. come in for a liver biopsy on a monthly schedule.

       C. avoid strenuous activity and contact sports.

       D. notify her primary care provider immediately if her appetite increases.

Alcohol can damage liver cells, which can then impair metabolism of many medications, leading to medication toxicity.

7. A client starting on cyclobenzaprine (Flexeril) should be informed that he may experience which of the following anticholinergic side effects?

       A. Dry mouth

       B. Bradycardia

       C. Diarrhea

       D. Urinary frequency

Anticholinergic effects include dry mouth. Tachycardia, constipation, and urinary retention are also common anticholinergic side effects.

Unit 1   Basic Pharmacologic Principles & Safe Administration of Medications

Chapter 3:   Basic Dosage Calculation
Contributor: Alison Hewig, MSN, RN

 NCLEX® Connections:

> **Learning Objective:** Review and apply knowledge within **"Basic Dosage Calculation"** in readiness for performance of the following nursing activities as outlined by the NCLEX® test plans:
>
> Δ   Apply knowledge of dosage calculations to determine correct medication dosage for clients.
>
> Δ   Demonstrate use of dimensional analysis and other methods to calculate and monitor client medication dose.

 Key Points

Δ   Basic medication dose conversion and calculation skills are essential to the provision of safe nursing care.

Δ   Regardless of the dosage calculation method used, knowledge of **standard conversions** (e.g., 1 gr = 60 mg) and recognition of **availability data** (e.g., 300 mg/tablet) are used to **solve a clinical problem** (e.g., quantity of tablets to give for a prescribed dose of Tylenol 5 gr).

Δ   **Standard conversion factors** are as follows:
  • 1 mg = 1,000 mcg
  • 1 g = 1,000 mg
  • 1 kg = 1,000 g
  • 1 oz = 30 mL
  • 1 L = 1,000 mL
  • 1 tsp = 5 mL
  • 1 Tbs = 15 mL
  • 1 Tbs = 3 tsp
  • 1 kg = 2.2 lb
  • 1 gr = 60 mg

Δ   General rounding guidelines are to round to the tenths place. For example, 21.81 = 21.8; 21.86 = 21.9.

Methods Used for Dosage Calculations

Δ **Dimensional analysis** – decreases simplicity and efficacy errors in medication administration. Dimensional analysis (or the factor-label method) is a method of dosage calculation that involves **systematically arranging a series of factors into a mathematical equation**.

- For example: $\dfrac{1\,tab}{300\,mg} \bullet \dfrac{60\,mg}{1\,gr} \bullet \dfrac{5\,gr}{1} = \dfrac{300\,mg}{300\,mg} = 1\,tab$

- **Step 1 is to identify your goal** (e.g., to calculate the **quantity** of tablets needed to administer the prescribed Tylenol 5 gr) TIP: Write your goal over 1 to remind yourself that you need to keep gr on top of the equation.

$$\frac{5\,gr}{1}$$

- Identify the conversion and availability factors needed to answer the clinical question. Factors are simply numbers that are related to each other and are written as ratios, which look like fractions. The ratios are not truly fractions because the top number and the bottom number can be switched.

- **Conversion Factors**: For example:

$$\frac{60\,mg}{1\,gr} \quad or \quad \frac{1\,gr}{60\,mg}$$

- **Availability Factors**: For example:

$$\frac{1\,tab}{300\,mg} \quad or \quad \frac{300\,mg}{1\,tab}$$

- Let's apply the dimensional analysis method to the following clinical problem:

  ◊ A primary care provider has prescribed Lasix 40 mg intravenously every day. Available is 10 mg/mL. How many mL should be administered for this dose?

Step	Description	Example
1	Identify your goal. What are you solving for?	**Quantity** of mL required for the prescribed dose: $\dfrac{mL}{1}$
2	Identify what is **available**.	$10\,mg\,/\,mL$
3	Change this to a ratio (or in factor form).	$\dfrac{1\,mL}{10\,mg}$
4	Identify the **desired** dose.	$\dfrac{40\,mg}{1}$
5	Set up your equation. Remember that you are solving for mL. Follow the rules of mathematics which say that to cross out a unit on the top you must do the same to the bottom or vice versa. Therefore, the formula should be set up as:	$\dfrac{mL}{1}=\dfrac{1\,mL}{10\,mg}\cdot\dfrac{40\,mg}{1}$
6	Do the math. Remember to multiply all the way across the top and all the way across the bottom, then divide.	$\dfrac{1\,mL}{10\,mg}\cdot\dfrac{40\,mg}{1}=\dfrac{40\,mL}{10}=4\,mL$

Δ Another dosage calculation method involves the use of **specific formulas**:

$$\frac{Desired}{Available}\cdot Quantity \text{ or } \frac{D}{A}\cdot Q$$

$$\frac{Volume}{Time(min)}\cdot Drop\,Factor\,(gtt/mL) = IV\,Flow\,Rate\,(gtt/min)$$

$$\frac{Volume\,(mL)}{Time\,(min)}\cdot\frac{60\,min}{1\,hr} = IV\,Flow\,Rate\,(mL\,/\,hr)$$

Δ Let's try applying the $\dfrac{D}{A}\cdot Q$ formula to the same clinical problem.

• A primary care provider has prescribed Lasix 40 mg intravenously every day. Available is 10 mg/mL. How many mL should be administered for this dose?

Step	Description	Example
1	What are you solving for?	**What is the quantity** of mL required for the dose?
2	Identify the **desired** dose.	$40\,mg$
3	Identify what is **available.**	$10\,mg$
4	Identify the quantity in which it is available.	$1\,mL$
5	Set up your equation. Remember that you are solving for mL.	$\dfrac{40\,mg}{10\,mg} \bullet 1\,mL$
6	Do the math.	$\dfrac{40\,mg}{10\,mg} \bullet 1\,mL = 4\,mL$

Primary Reference:

Lehne, R. A. (2007). *Pharmacology for nursing care.* (6th ed.). St. Louis, MO: Saunders.

Additional Resources:

Curren, A. M. (2005). *Dimensional analysis for meds.* (3rd ed.) Thomson Delmar Learning. United States.

Mulholland, J. (2006). *The Nurse, the math, the meds: Drug calculations using dimensional analysis.* (1st ed.). Mosby Elsevier.

Unit 1 Basic Pharmacologic Principles & Safe Administration of Medications
Chapter 3: Basic Dosage Calculation

Application Exercises

Directions: For each problem, solve using either the dimensional analysis or formula method. Remember to round to the nearest tenth.

Basic Equations

1. Give 200 mg of metoprolol (Lopressor) now and every morning. The pharmacy sends 100 mg tablets. How many **tablets** should be given?

2. Give methylprednisolone (Solu-Medrol) 5 mg intravenously every 6 hr. Available is 40 mg/2 mL. How many **mL** should be administered for each dose?

3. A client is given acetaminophen (Tylenol) 320 mg orally every 4 to 6 hr when necessary. Available is 160 mg/5 mL. How many **mL** should be given for each dose?

Equations Requiring Conversions

4. Administer aspirin 5 gr every 4 hr when necessary. Available are 325 mg tablets. How many **tablets** should be given for each dose?

5. Give 200 mg of medication every day. Available is 125 mg/tsp. How many **mL** should be given each day?

6. A primary care provider prescribes atropine 0.3 mg intramuscularly on call. The vial is labeled atropine 400 mcg/mL. How many **mL** should be given?

Dosage Calculation from Body Weight

7. A client weighs 27 lb. The primary care provider prescribes Ampicillin 75 mg/kg/day in 4 divided doses. Available is Ampicillin 150 mg/2 mL. How many **mL** per dose should be given?

8. Phenytoin (Dilantin) 5 mg/kg/day is prescribed in 3 divided doses for a child weighing 26 lb. It is available at 50 mg/mL. What is the total daily dosage in **mL** for this child?

9. Kanamycin (Kantrex) 15 mg/kg/day is prescribed in 3 divided doses every 8 hr for an adult weighing 135 lb. It is available at 75 mg/mL. How many **mL** should be given per dose?

IV Flow Rate

10. Give 1 L of normal saline over 8 hr. The tubing drop factor is 20 **gtt/mL**. Calculate how many gtt/min should be delivered per manual control?

11. Keflin 1 g in 50 mL normal saline intravenous piggyback administered over 1 hr. The tubing drop factor is 60 gtt/mL. Calculate how many **gtt/min** should be delivered per manual control?

12. Zantac 50 mg in 100 mL normal saline intravenous piggyback administered over 15 min. The tubing drop factor is 15 gtt/mL. Calculate how many **gtt/min** should be delivered per manual control?

13. A nurse is to administer 500 mL of D_5W over 4 hr. The IV pump should be set to deliver how many mL/hr?

14. An IV medication is to run over 20 min on the pump. The medication is mixed in 50 mL of normal saline. The IV pump should be set to deliver how many **mL/hr**?

15. An IV medication is to run over 45 min on the pump. The medication is mixed in 100 mL of normal saline. The IV pump should be set to deliver how many **mL/hr**?

Unit 1 Basic Pharmacologic Principles & Safe Administration of Medications

Chapter 3: Basic Dosage Calculation

Application Exercises Answer Key

Directions: For each problem, solve using either the dimensional analysis or formula method. Remember to round to the nearest tenth.

Basic Equations

1. Give 200 mg of metoprolol (Lopressor) now and every morning. The pharmacy sends 100 mg tablets. How many **tablets** should be given?

Dimensional Analysis	Formula
$\dfrac{1\,tab}{100\,mg} \bullet \dfrac{200\,mg}{1} = \dfrac{200}{100} = 2\,tabs$	Step 1: Choose formula $\dfrac{D}{A} \bullet Q$ Step 2: Use formula $\dfrac{200\,mg}{100\,mg} \bullet 1\,tab = 2\,tabs$

2. Give methylprednisolone (Solu-Medrol) 5 mg intravenously every 6 hr. Available is 40 mg/2 mL. How many **mL** should be administered for each dose?

Dimensional Analysis	Formula
$\dfrac{2\,mL}{40\,mg} \bullet \dfrac{5\,mg}{1} = \dfrac{10}{40} = 0.25\,mL$ $\dfrac{2\,mL}{40\,mg} \bullet 5$	Step 1: Choose formula $\dfrac{D}{A} \bullet Q$ Step 2: Use formula $\dfrac{5\,mg}{40\,mg} \bullet 2\,mL = \dfrac{10}{40} = 0.25\,mL$

3. A client is given acetaminophen (Tylenol) 320 mg orally every 4 to 6 hr when necessary. Available is 160 mg/5 mL. How many **mL** should be given for each dose?

Dimensional Analysis	Formula
$\dfrac{5\,mL}{160\,mg} \cdot \dfrac{320\,mg}{1} = \dfrac{1{,}600}{160} = 10\,mL$	Step 1: Choose formula $\dfrac{D}{A} \cdot Q$ Step 2: Use formula $\dfrac{320\,mg}{160\,mg} \cdot 5\,mL = \dfrac{1{,}600}{160} = 10\,mL$

Equations Requiring Conversions

4. Administer aspirin 5 gr every 4 hr when necessary. Available are 325 mg tablets. How many **tablets** should be given for each dose?

Dimensional Analysis	Formula
$\dfrac{1\,tab}{325\,mg} \cdot \dfrac{60\,mg}{1\,gr} \cdot \dfrac{5\,gr}{1} = \dfrac{300}{325} = 0.92\ or\ 1\,tab$	Step 1: Choose formula $\dfrac{D}{A} \cdot Q$ Step 2: Conversion $\dfrac{60\,mg}{1\,gr} \cdot \dfrac{5\,gr}{1} = 300\,mg$ Step 3: Use formula $\dfrac{300\,mg}{325\,mg} \cdot 1\,tab = 1\,tab$

5. Give 200 mg of medication every day. Available is 125 mg/tsp. How many **mL** should be given each day?

Dimensional Analysis	Formula
$$\frac{1\,tsp}{125\,mg} \bullet \frac{5\,mL}{1\,tsp} \bullet \frac{200\,mg}{1} = 8\,mL$$	Step 1: Choose formula $$\frac{D}{A} \bullet Q$$ Step 2: Conversion $$1\,tsp = 5\,mL$$ Step 3: Use formula $$\frac{200\,mg}{125\,mg} \bullet 5\,mL = 8\,mL$$

6. A primary care provider prescribes atropine 0.3 mg intramuscularly on call. The vial is labeled atropine 400 mcg/ml. How many **mL** should be given?

Dimensional Analysis	Formula
$$\frac{1\,mL}{400\,mcg} \bullet \frac{1,000\,mcg}{1\,mg} \bullet \frac{0.3\,mg}{1} = 0.75\,mL$$	Step 1: Choose formula $$\frac{D}{A} \bullet Q$$ Step 2: Conversion $$\frac{1,000\,mcg}{1\,mg} \bullet \frac{0.3\,mg}{1} = 300\,mcg$$ Step 3: Use formula $$\frac{300\,mcg}{400\,mcg} \bullet 1\,mL = 0.75\,mL$$

Dosage Calculation from Body Weight

7. A client weighs 27 lb. The primary care provider prescribes Ampicillin 75 mg/kg/day in 4 divided doses. Available is Ampicillin 150 mg/2 mL. How many **mL** per dose should be given?

Dimensional Analysis	Formula
Step 1:	Step 1: Choose formula
$$\frac{1\,kg}{2.2\,lb} \cdot \frac{27\,lb}{1} \cdot \frac{75\,mg}{1\,kg} \cdot \frac{2\,mL}{150\,mg} = \frac{4{,}050}{330}$$ $$= 12.3\,mL\,/\,day$$	$$\frac{D}{A} \cdot Q$$
Step 2: Calculate single dose	Step 2: Conversion
$$\frac{12.3\,mL}{4\,doses} \cdot \frac{1\,dose}{1} = 3.1\,mL$$	$$\frac{1\,kg}{2.2\,lb} \cdot \frac{27\,lb}{1} = 12.3\,kg$$
	Step 3: Calculate dose ordered for client based on weight
	$$\frac{75\,mg}{1\,kg} \cdot \frac{12.3\,kg}{1} = 922.5\,mg\,/\,day$$
	Step 4: Use formula
	$$\frac{922.5\,mg}{150\,mg} \cdot 2\,mL = 12.3\,mL\,/\,day$$
	Step 5: Calculate single dose
	$$\frac{12.3\,mL}{4\,doses} \cdot \frac{1\,dose}{1} = 3.1\,mL$$

8. Phenytoin (Dilantin) 5 mg/kg/day is prescribed in 3 divided doses for a child weighing 26 lb. It is available at 50 mg/mL. What is the total daily dosage in **mL** for this child?

Dimensional Analysis	Formula
Step 1: $$\frac{1\,kg}{2.2\,lb} \bullet \frac{26\,lb}{1} \bullet \frac{5\,mg}{1\,kg} \bullet \frac{1\,mL}{50\,mg} = \frac{130}{110} = 1.2\,mL$$	Step 1: Choose formula $$\frac{D}{A} \bullet Q$$ Step 2: Conversion $$\frac{1\,kg}{2.2\,lb} \bullet \frac{26\,lb}{1} = 11.8\,kg$$ Step 3: Calculate dose ordered for client based on weight $$\frac{5\,mg}{1\,kg} \bullet \frac{11.8\,kg}{1} = 59.1\,mg\,/\,day$$ Step 4: Use formula $$\frac{59.1\,mg}{50\,mg} \bullet 1\,mL = 1.2\,mL\,/\,day$$

9. Kanamycin (Kantrex) 15 mg/kg/day is prescribed in 3 divided doses every 8 hr for an adult weighing 135 lb. It is available at 75 mg/mL. How many **mL** should be given per dose?

Dimensional Analysis	Formula
Step 1:	Step 1: Choose formula
$\dfrac{1\,kg}{2.2\,lb} \cdot \dfrac{135\,lb}{1} \cdot \dfrac{15\,mg}{1\,kg} \cdot \dfrac{1\,mL}{75\,mg} = \dfrac{2,025}{165}$	$\dfrac{D}{A} \cdot Q$
$= 12.3\,mL\,/\,day$	Step 2: Conversion
Step 2: Calculate single dose	$\dfrac{1\,kg}{2.2\,lb} \cdot \dfrac{135\,lb}{1} = 61.4\,kg$
$\dfrac{12.3\,mL}{3\,doses} \cdot \dfrac{1\,dose}{1} = 4.1\,mL$	Step 3: Calculate dose ordered for client based on weight
	$\dfrac{15\,mg}{1\,kg} \cdot \dfrac{61\,kg}{1} = 921\,mg\,/\,day$
	Step 4: Use formula
	$\dfrac{921\,mg}{75\,mg} \cdot 1\,mL = 12.3\,mL/day$
	Step 5: Calculate single dose
	$\dfrac{12.3\,mL}{3\,doses} \cdot \dfrac{1\,dose}{1} = 4.1\,mL$

IV Flow Rate

10. Give 1 L of normal saline over 8 hr. The tubing drop factor is 20 **gtt/mL**. Calculate how many gtt/min should be delivered per manual control?

Dimensional Analysis	Formula
$\dfrac{20\,gtt}{1\,mL} \cdot \dfrac{1,000\,mL}{1\,L} \cdot \dfrac{1\,L}{8\,hr} \cdot \dfrac{1\,hr}{60\,min}$	Step 1: Choose formula
$= 42\,gtt\,/\,min$	$\dfrac{Volume}{Time(min)} \cdot Drop\,Factor\,(gtt\,/\,mL) = IV\,Flow\,Rate\,(gtt\,/\,min)$
	Step 2: Use formula
	$\dfrac{1,000\,mL}{480\,min} \cdot 20\,gtt\,/\,mL = 42\,gtt\,/\,min$

11. Keflin 1 g in 50 mL normal saline intravenous piggyback administered over 1 hr. The tubing drop factor is 60 gtt/mL. Calculate how many **gtt/min** should be delivered per manual control?

Dimensional Analysis	Formula
$$\frac{60\,gtt}{1\,mL} \cdot \frac{50\,mL}{60\,min} = 50\,gtt\,/\,min$$	Step 1: Choose formula $\frac{Volume}{Time(min)} \cdot Drop\ Factor\ (gtt\,/\,mL) = IV\ Flow\ Rate(gtt\,/\,min)$ Step 2: Use formula $$\frac{50\,mL}{60\,min} \cdot 60\,gtt\,/\,mL = 50\,gtt\,/\,min$$

12. Zantac 50 mg in 100 mL normal saline intravenous piggyback administered over 15 min. The tubing drop factor is 15 gtt/mL. Calculate how many **gtt/min** should be delivered per manual control?

Dimensional Analysis	Formula
$$\frac{15\,gtt}{1\,mL} \cdot \frac{100\,mL}{15\,min} = 100\,gtt\,/\,min$$	Step 1: Choose formula $\frac{Volume}{Time(min)} \cdot Drop\ Factor\ (gtt/mL) = IV\ Flow\ Rate(gtt/min)$ Step 2: Use formula $$\frac{100\,mL}{15\,min} \cdot 15\,gtt\,/\,mL = 100\,gtt/min$$

13. A nurse is to administer 500 mL of D_5W over 4 hr. The IV pump should be set to deliver how many mL/hr?

Dimensional Analysis	Formula
$$\frac{500\,mL}{4\,hr} = 125\,mL\,/\,hr$$	Step 1: Choose formula $\frac{Volume(mL)}{Time(min)} \cdot \frac{60min}{1hr} = IVFlowRate(mL\,/\,hr)$ Step 2: Use formula $$\frac{500mL}{240min} \cdot \frac{60min}{1hr} = 125mL\,/\,hr$$

14. An IV medication is to run over 20 min on the pump. The medication is mixed in 50 mL of normal saline. The IV pump should be set to deliver how many **mL/hr**?

Dimensional Analysis	Formula
$$\frac{50\,mL}{20\,min} \cdot \frac{60\,min}{1\,hr} = \frac{3{,}000}{20} = 150\ mL/hr$$	**Step 1: Choose formula** $$\frac{Volume(mL)}{Time(min)} \cdot \frac{60\,min}{1\,hr} = IV\ Flow\ Rate(mL/hr)$$ **Step 2: Use formula** $$\frac{50\,mL}{20\,min} \cdot \frac{60\,min}{1\,hr} = \frac{3{,}000}{20} = 150\ mL/hr$$

15. An IV medication is to run over 45 min on the pump. The medication is mixed in 100 mL of normal saline. The IV pump should be set to deliver how many **mL/hr**?

Dimensional Analysis	Formula
$$\frac{100\,mL}{45\,min} \cdot \frac{60\,min}{1\,hr} = \frac{6{,}000}{45} = 133\ mL/hr$$	**Step 1: Choose formula** $$\frac{Volume(mL)}{Time(min)} \cdot \frac{60\,min}{1\,hr} = IV\ Flow\ Rate(mL/hr)$$ **Step 2: Use formula** $$\frac{100\,mL}{45\,min} \cdot \frac{60\,min}{1\,hr} = \frac{6{,}000}{45} = 133\,mL/hr$$

Unit 1   Basic Pharmacologic Principles & Safe Administration of Medications

Chapter 4:   Medication Administration & Error Reduction
                 Contributor: Judith A. Harris, MSN, RNC

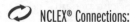 NCLEX® Connections:

> **Learning Objective**: Review and apply knowledge within "**Medication Administration & Error Reduction**" in readiness for performance of the following nursing activities as outlined by the NCLEX® test plans:
>
> Δ   Identify legal issues and nursing responsibilities of medication administration.
>
> Δ   Assess client data (e.g., vital signs, laboratory values, allergies) before medication preparation and administration.
>
> Δ   Prepare and demonstrate safe administration of different routes of medications (e.g., oral, topical, subcutaneous, intramuscular, intradermal, and intravenous).
>
> Δ   Use the nursing process to reduce the risk of medication errors.
>
> Λ   Demonstrate appropriate documentation of all medication administration.
>
> Δ   Evaluate response to medication errors and intervene as indicated.
>
> Δ   Follow legal and facility/agency policies in the administration of controlled substances.
>
> Δ   Identify and use various resources to obtain information regarding medication administration.

 Key Points

Δ   **Preassessment for medication therapy**

   •   The following information should be obtained prior to the institution of medication therapy, and updated as necessary.

      ◊   **Health history**

         °   Age

         °   Diagnosed health problems and current reason for seeking care

         °   All medications currently being taken (prescription and nonprescription): name, dose, route, and frequency of each medication

         °   Any symptoms possibly related to medication therapy

         °   Use of herbal or "natural" products for medicinal purposes

°   Use of caffeine, tobacco, alcohol, and/or street drugs

°   Client's understanding of the purpose of the medications

◊   **Physical examination** – a systemic physical examination permits evaluation of therapeutic effects of medication therapy and detection of possible side and adverse medication effects.

Δ   **Safe medication administration**

- **Six Rights**

  ◊   **Right client** – verify the client's identification each time a medication is given. Check identification band, name, and/or photograph.

  ◊   **Right drug** – correctly interpret medication order (verify completeness and clarity); read label three times: when container is selected, when removing dose from container, and when container is replaced; leave unit-dose medication in its package until administration.

  ◊   **Right dose** – calculate correct medication dose; check drug reference to ensure dose is within usual range.

  ◊   **Right time** – give medication on time to maintain consistent therapeutic blood level. It is generally acceptable to give the medication ½ hr before or after the scheduled time. However, refer to the drug reference or institution policy for exceptions.

  ◊   **Right route** – most common routes of administration are oral, topical, subcutaneous (SC), intramuscular (IM), and intravenous (IV). Select the correct preparation for the ordered route (e.g., otic vs ophthalmic topical ointment or drops). Know how to safely and correctly administer medication.

  ◊   **Right documentation** – immediately record pertinent information, including client's response to the medication.

- **Additional considerations**

  ◊   **Assessment** – appropriate data should be collected before administering medication (e.g., apical heart rate before giving digitalis preparations). Assess the client for physical and psychosocial factors that may affect medication response.

  ◊   **Education** – as part of informed consent, provide accurate information about the medication therapy and its implications (e.g., therapeutic response, side/adverse effects, etc.). To individualize the teaching, determine what the client already knows about the medication, needs to know about the medication, and wants to know about the medication.

  ◊   **Evaluation** – determine the effectiveness of the medication based on the client's response, as well as the occurrence of side/adverse effects.

◊ **Medication refusal** – clients have the right to refuse to take a medication. Determine the reason for refusal, provide information regarding risk of refusal, notify appropriate health care personnel, and document refusal and actions taken.

- **Resources for medication information**

  ◊ Nursing drug handbooks

  ◊ Pharmacology textbooks

  ◊ Professional journals

  ◊ Physicians' Desk Reference (PDR)

  ◊ Professional Web sites

Knowledge required prior to medication administration	
Medication category/class	• Medications may be organized according to pharmacologic action, therapeutic use, body system, chemical makeup, and safe use during pregnancy. For example, lisinopril (Zestril) is classified as an angiotensin-converting enzyme inhibitor (pharmacologic action) and an antihypertensive (therapeutic use).
Mechanism of action	• This is how the medication produces the desired therapeutic effect. For example, glipizide (Glucotrol) is an oral hypoglycemic agent. Glipizide lowers blood glucose levels primarily by stimulating pancreatic islet cells to release insulin.
Therapeutic effect	• This is the primary action for which the medication is administered to a specific client. For example, one client is administered acetaminophen (Tylenol) to lower fever, whereas another client may be administered this medication to relieve pain.
Adverse effects	• These are undesired and sometimes dangerous effects of the medication. Adverse effects are usually identified according to body system.
Toxicity	• Medications can have specific risks and manifestations of toxicity. For example, clients taking digoxin (Lanoxin) should be monitored closely for dysrhythmias, a sign of cardiotoxicity. Hypokalemia places these clients at greater risk for digoxin toxicity.
Medication interactions	• Medications can interact with each other resulting in desired or undesired effects. For example, a desired interaction would be the beta-blocker atenolol (Tenormin) used concurrently with the calcium channel blocker nifedipine (Procardia) to prevent reflex tachycardia. Take complete medication history and be knowledgeable of clinically significant interactions.

Knowledge required prior to medication administration	
Contraindications/ precautions	• Medications may be contraindicated for a client with a specific disease or condition. For example, tetracyclines can stain developing teeth and should not be administered to children under 8 years of age. Some medications should only be used cautiously. For example, vancomycin is excreted unchanged in the kidneys and should be used cautiously in clients with renal impairment.
Preparation, dosage, administration	• It is important to know any special considerations for preparation, recommended dosages, and how to administer the medication. For example, morphine is available in 10 different formulations. Oral doses of morphine are generally higher than parenteral doses due to extensive first-pass effect. Clients with chronic, severe pain, as seen in cancer, are generally given oral doses of morphine.
Nursing implications	• Know how to monitor therapeutic effects, prevent and treat adverse effects, provide for comfort, and instruct clients in the safe use of medications.

Δ Routes of administration

Route	Nursing Implications
Oral or enteral (tablets, capsules, liquids, suspensions, and elixirs)	• Do not give if client is vomiting, has no gag reflex, has difficulty swallowing, or is comatose. • Do not mix with large amounts of food or beverages. • Avoid administration with contraindicated foods or beverages such as grapefruit juice. • Enteric-coated or time-release medications must be swallowed whole. • Administer irritating medications with small amounts of food. • In general, administer oral medications on an empty stomach (1 hr before meals, 2 hr after meals).
Sublingual (under tongue) and **buccal** (between cheek and gum)	• Instruct the client to have medication remain in place until absorbed. Client should not eat or drink while tablet is in place.
Liquids, suspensions, and elixirs	• Determine whether shaking or dilution is required. When administering the medication, the meniscus (lowest fluid line) is at the level of the desired dose.
Transdermal – Medication is stored in a skin patch and absorbed through the skin producing systemic effects.	• In general, to prevent underdosing or overdosing, patches should not be cut. Instruct the client to place the patch on a hairless area of the skin and rotate sites to prevent skin irritation. Wash skin with soap and water, and dry thoroughly before applying a new patch.
Topical	• Apply with a glove, tongue blade, or cotton-tipped applicator. Never apply with bare hand.

Route	Nursing Implications
Instillation (drops, ointments, and sprays) – Generally used for eyes, ears, and nose	• **Eyes** – use surgical aseptic technique when instilling medications in eyes. Rest the dominant hand on the client's forehead, hold dropper above the conjunctival sac approximately 1 to 2 cm, drop medication into the center of sac and have client close eye gently. Apply gentle pressure with the finger and a clean tissue on nasolacrimal duct for 30 to 60 sec to prevent systemic absorption of medication. • **Ears** – medical aseptic technique can be used for medications administered into ears and nose. Ear drops can be administered with the client sitting up or in a side-lying position. The ear canal should be straightened by pulling the auricle upward and outward for adults or down and back for children. Hold the dropper 1 cm above the ear canal, install medication, and then gently apply pressure with finger to tragus of ear. • **Nose** – the client should be supine with his head positioned to allow medication to enter appropriate nasal passage. Use the dominant hand to instill drops supporting the head with the nondominant hand. The client should be instructed to breath through the mouth, stay in a supine position, and cautioned not to blow his nose for 5 min after drop insertion.

Inhalation – Medications usually administered through metered-dose inhalers (MDI) or dry powder inhalers (DPI).	• General principles for inhaled and dry powder medications include:
	  ◊ MDI medications should be shaken vigorously 5 to 6 times prior to use. The client may position her mouth around the device or 2 to 4 cm in front of the mouth.
	  ◊ DPI medications are not to be shaken, and the client should place the mouthpiece between her lips.
	• For both types of devices, the client should exhale, and then inhale the medication deeply through the mouth for 3 to 5 sec, then hold breath for 5 to 10 sec.
	• For MDI, the client will need to depress the canister to deliver the medication. The client should wait a 1 min interval if taking 2 puffs of the same medication. Bronchodilators are taken prior to anti-inflammatory inhalers to ↑ absorption of the anti-inflammatory medication. Advise clients not to exceed recommended dosages. Instruct the client how to take the inhaler on a fixed schedule. A spacer can also be attached to an MDI. The spacer keeps the medication in the device longer and thereby facilitates delivery of the medication to the lungs and ↓ the amount of the medication deposited into the oropharynx. This is beneficial for the delivery of glucocorticoids.

Nasogastric and **gastrostomy** tubes	• Check for proper tube placement. Use a syringe without a plunger or bulb and allow the medication to flow in by gravity. Flush the tube with water between medications and when finished.

Route	Nursing Implications
Suppositories	<ul><li>Keep refrigerated.</li><li>Remove foil wrapper and lubricate suppository if necessary.</li><li>Instruct the client to retain medication and not expel it. Rectal suppositories are inserted beyond internal sphincter. Vaginal suppositories are generally inserted with an applicator.</li></ul>
Parenteral	<ul><li>General considerations for parenteral medications include:<ul><li>◊ The vastus lateralis site is usually the recommended site for infants and children < 2 years of age.</li><li>◊ After age 2, the ventral gluteal site can be used. Both of these sites can accommodate fluid up to 2 mL. The deltoid site has a smaller muscle mass and only can accommodate up to 1 mL of fluid.</li><li>◊ Use a needle size and length appropriate to the type of injection and client size. Syringe size should approximate volume of medication.</li><li>◊ Use a tuberculin syringe for solution volume < 0.5 mL.</li><li>◊ Rotate injection sites to enhance medication absorption, and document each site used.</li><li>◊ Do not use injection sites that are edematous, inflamed, have moles, birthmarks, or scars.</li><li>◊ If medication is given intravenously, immediately monitor the client for therapeutic, side/adverse effects.</li></ul></li></ul>
Intradermal (ID)	<ul><li>Usually used for tuberculin testing or checking for medication/allergy sensitivities.</li><li>May be used for some cancer immunotherapy.</li><li>Use small amounts of solution (0.01 to 0.1 mL) in a tuberculin syringe with a fine gauge needle (26 to 27) in lightly pigmented, thin-skinned, hairless sites (e.g., inner surface mid-forearm or scapular area of back) at a 10 to 15 degree angle.</li></ul>
Subcutaneous	<ul><li>Appropriate for small doses of nonirritating, water-soluble medications. Use a short, fine gauge needle (3/8 to 5/8 in, 25 to 27 gauge) and inject no more than 1.5 mL solution. Use 3/8 in, 25 gauge needle at a 45 degree angle or 1/2 in, 25 gauge needle at a 90 degree angle.</li><li>Sites are selected for adequate fat-pad size (e.g., abdomen, upper hips, lateral upper arms, thighs). Insulin syringes can be 26 to 29 gauge.</li></ul>
Intramuscular	<ul><li>Used for irritating medications, solutions in oils, and aqueous suspensions.</li><li>Most common sites include ventrogluteal, dorsogluteal, deltoid, and vastus lateralis (pediatric).</li><li>Use needle size 18 to 27 (usual 22 to 25 gauge) 1 to 1 ½ in long, and inject at a 90 degree angle. Volume injected is usually 1 to 3 mL. If a greater amount is required, it should be divided into two syringes and two different sites should be used.</li></ul>

Route	Nursing Implications
Z-Track	• Type of IM injection that prevents medication from leaking back into subcutaneous tissue. • It is often used for medications that cause visible and/or permanent skin stains such as certain iron preparations.
Intravenous	• More dangerous route of administration than IM or SC due to rapid onset of medication action. • Preferred sites are peripheral veins in the arm or hand. Ask the client what site he prefers. In neonates, veins of the head, lower legs, and feet may be used. After administration, immediately monitor for therapeutic, side/adverse effects.

Δ   **Medication preparation for administration**

• **Crushing/dissolving tablets or capsules**

◊   Most tablets are scored and can be readily broken in half. Tablets may also be crushed or dissolved according to the manufacturer's instructions.

◊   Capsules are gelatin shells containing powder or time-release beads. Capsules containing powder may be broken apart, and powdered medication dissolved according to manufacturer's instructions. Time-release capsules should not be crushed or diluted as medication will be absorbed at a faster rate than recommended. As a safety measure, try to use a liquid form of the medication instead of crushing the tablets or diluting the powder from capsules. Enteric-coated (hard shell) tablets must not be crushed because of the potential for irritation to gastric mucosa.

• **Mixing injectable medications from two vials**

◊   Draw air into a syringe equal to the amount of solution to be drawn from the first vial. Then, inject air into the first vial, not allowing the needle to touch the solution.

◊   Draw air into the syringe equal to the amount of solution to be drawn from the second vial. Inject air into the second vial and withdraw the desired amount of solution.

◊   Change the needle, unless the entire volume of the first vial will be used.

◊   Withdraw the desired amount of solution from the first vial.

Δ   **Medication errors**

•   **Common medication errors** include:

◊   Wrong medication or IV fluid.

◊   Incorrect dose or IV rate.

◊   Wrong client, route, or time.

◊   Administration of known allergic medication.

◊   Omission of dose.

◊   Incorrect discontinuation of medication or IV fluid.

•   Medication error reduction

Assessment	• Obtain information about the client's medical diagnoses and conditions related to medication administration (e.g., ability to swallow, allergies, heart, liver, and/or kidney disorders).
	• Identify physical and psychosocial risk factors.
	• Learn essential information about each medication to be given.
	• Interpret the medication order accurately. The inappropriate use of abbreviations can lead to errors. For example, ZnSO4, the abbreviation for zinc sulfate, can be mistaken for MS04, morphine sulfate. In both situations, the full name of the medication should be written out. Also, not leaving enough space between the medication name and the dose can lead to error. For example, atenolol 10 mg may be interpreted as atenolol 110 mg. Make sure there is adequate space between the medication name and dose to prevent an inaccurate dose. The Institute for Safe Medication Practices (ISMP) has developed a list of abbreviations, symbols, and dose designations whose use may lead to medication error. For a complete list of error-prone terms go to the ISMP Web site, *www.ismp.org.*
	• Question the primary care provider if the prescription is unclear or seems inappropriate for the client's condition.
	• Check the labels for the medication name and concentration. Read labels correctly and carefully. Different medications may come in similar colors, shapes, and packages. Be aware of look-alike and sound-alike medication names, for example, Keflex and Keflin.
	• To monitor therapeutic responses, dosage changes are usually made gradually. Question the primary care provider if abrupt and excessive changes in dosages are made.
	• Refuse to give a medication if it is believed to be unsafe. Check the prescription with the primary care provider.
Planning	• Calculate doses accurately and verify with a colleague or pharmacist if necessary. Doses are usually 1 to 2 tablets or one single-dose vial. Question multiple tablets or vials for a single dose.
	• Measure doses accurately and double-check high-alert medications (e.g., insulin, heparin) with a colleague.
	• Avoid distractions during medication preparation (e.g., poor lighting, ringing phones). Interruptions may increase the risk of error.

Implementation	<ul><li>Follow Six Rights consistently. Take the medication administration record (MAR) to the bedside.</li><li>Medications should only be administered by the individual who has prepared the medication.</li><li>Follow correct procedures for all routes of administration.</li><li>Communicate clearly both in writing and speaking. Use verbal orders only for emergencies and follow agency protocol for telephone orders.</li><li>Encourage clients to become part of the safety net, teaching them about medications and the importance of proper identification before medications are administered.</li><li>Follow all laws and regulations regarding controlled substances when preparing and administering medications.</li></ul>
Evaluation	<ul><li>Evaluate client response to a medication and document and report appropriately.</li><li>Recognize side/adverse effects, and document and report appropriately.</li><li>Omit or delay doses as indicated by the client's condition, and document and report appropriately.</li><li>Omit or delay a dose if the client says the dose seems too large (e.g., insulin) or oral medications are different (e.g., color, shape) from those usually taken. Verify the prescription order with the primary care provider.</li><li>Report all errors and implement corrective measures immediately. Complete information will facilitate the agency review process and promote solutions to system-based causes. Promptly administer treatment to ↓ injury to the client.</li></ul>

Δ   **Self-administration of medications**

- Self-administration of medications typically takes place in the home and community-based settings. Self-administration may also be used in an institutional setting when clients wish to use their home medications and have the ability to do so safely.

- Careful preassessment is necessary to determine the client's suitability for safe self-medication (e.g., mental status, physical ability).

- Give the client instructions for each medication (written and verbal) regarding dosage, expected responses, side/adverse effects.

- Schedule follow-up visits with the primary care provider to monitor compliance.

Primary Reference:

Lehne, R. A. (2007). *Pharmacology for nursing care*. (6th ed.). St. Louis, MO: Saunders.

Additional Resources:

Abrams, A. C., & Goldsmith, T. L. (2003). *Clinical drug therapy: Rationales for nursing practice* (7th ed.). Philadelphia: Lippincott Williams & Wilkins.

Linton, A. D., & Harris, J. A. (2000). *Pharmacology companion for introductory nursing care of adults* (2nd ed.). Philadelphia: Saunders.

Unit 1 Basic Pharmacologic Principles & Safe Administration of Medications
Chapter 4: Medication Administration & Error Reduction

Application Exercises

1. When administering an oral medication to a client, a nurse should

   A. assess the client's ability to swallow.

   B. administer the medication with grapefruit juice.

   C. not give oral medications to a client with a nasogastric tube in place.

   D. crush enteric coated tablets if the client has trouble swallowing.

2. What is the nurse's responsibility when a client refuses to take a medication?

   the nurse should make a note of it

3. When preparing a medication, a nurse notes that the prescriber has doubled the previous dose of the medication. The nurse should

   A. administer the medication as prescribed.

   B. check the prescription with another nurse before giving the medication.

   C. check with the prescriber regarding the dose prescribed.

   D. record that a doubled dose was prescribed.

4. An aspirin rectal suppository has been prescribed when necessary for fever. The nurse knows that this medication is

   A. expelled within 2 min after insertion to prevent side effects.

   B. administered for local effect.

   C. inserted without any lubrication.

   D. stored in the refrigerator.

5. Nitroglycerin tablets, which are often prescribed for cardiac clients, are given sublingually. This means that the tablets are

   A. dissolved and administered under the skin.

   B. held under the tongue until dissolved.

   C. taken by mouth with a small amount of water.

   D. placed between the cheek and gum.

6. A nurse on a busy medical unit is administering 0600 medications. He enters the client's room, gently shakes the client awake, and calls her name. She awakens slowly and seems groggy. The nurse explains that he has her 0600 medication, which the client quickly takes before falling back to sleep. Outside the room, the nurse looks at the room number and realizes that he just gave the medication to the wrong client. Explain how this medication error could have been prevented.

7. When taking a client's medication history, a nurse knows that

    A. smoking will have no effect on medication action.
    B. over-the-counter medications need to be included.
    C. most medications are not affected by the use of alcohol.
    D. use of herbal products usually has no effect on prescribed medications.

8. Which of the following interventions are included in the nurse's responsibilities when administering medications? (Select all that apply.)

    _/_   Observing for medication side effects
    _/_   Monitoring for therapeutic effects
    _____   Changing the dose if side effects occur
    _/_   Ordering the appropriate dose
    _/_   Maintaining an up-to-date knowledge base

Unit 1 Basic Pharmacologic Principles & Safe Administration of Medications
Chapter 4: Medication Administration & Error Reduction

Application Exercises Answer Key

1. When administering an oral medication to a client, a nurse should

   A. assess the client's ability to swallow.
   B. administer the medication with grapefruit juice.
   C. not give oral medications to a client with a nasogastric tube in place.
   D. crush enteric coated tablets if the client has trouble swallowing.

   Preassessment of clients receiving oral medications includes checking the client's ability to swallow. Many medications interact with grapefruit juice, and water is a better choice of liquid. Oral medications can be given via a nasogastric tube, and crushing enteric coated tablets destroys the protective coating.

2. What is the nurse's responsibility when a client refuses to take a medication?

   Determine the reason for the refusal, provide information regarding risk of refusal, notify the primary care provider, and document the refusal and actions taken.

3. When preparing a medication, a nurse notes that the prescriber has doubled the previous dose of the medication. The nurse should

   A. administer the medication as prescribed.
   B. check the prescription with another nurse before giving the medication.
   C. check with the prescriber regarding the dose prescribed.
   D. record that a doubled dose was prescribed.

   Increases in dosages are usually made gradually. Check with the primary care provider first to determine if the new dosage is correct.

4. An aspirin rectal suppository has been prescribed when necessary for fever. The nurse knows that this medication is

        A. expelled within 2 min after insertion to prevent side effects.

        B. administered for local effect.

        C. inserted without any lubrication.

        D. stored in the refrigerator.

Suppositories should be stored in the refrigerator. A suppository should be retained to produce therapeutic effects. Lubrication is used to facilitate passage of the suppository past the internal anal sphincter.

5. Nitroglycerin tablets, which are often prescribed for cardiac clients, are given sublingually. This means that the tablets are

        A. dissolved and administered under the skin.

        B. held under the tongue until dissolved.

        C. taken by mouth with a small amount of water.

        D. placed between the cheek and gum.

Sublingual medications are correctly administered when placed under the tongue until they are dissolved. They are readily absorbed into the blood stream for systemic effects. Medications placed between the cheek and gums are delivered through the buccal route. The medication should dissolve and is usually used for local effects.

6. A nurse on a busy medical unit is administering 0600 medications. He enters the client's room, gently shakes the client awake, and calls her name. She awakens slowly and seems groggy. The nurse explains that he has her 0600 medication, which the client quickly takes before falling back to sleep. Outside the room, the nurse looks at the room number and realizes that he just gave the medication to the wrong client. Explain how this medication error could have been prevented.

This error occurred because the medication was given to the wrong client. The nurse did not check the client's identification band and relied on the client to respond to her name. Because the client had been asleep she may have simply responded to being awakened.

7. When taking a client's medication history, a nurse knows that

    A. smoking will have no effect on medication action.

    B. over-the-counter medications need to be included.

    C. most medications are not affected by the use of alcohol.

    D. use of herbal products usually has no effect on prescribed medications.

It is important for the nurse to be aware of what over-the-counter medications (OTC) the client is taking. Clients may be self-treating conditions with OTC medications. OTC medications may interact with current or newly prescribed medications.

8. Which of the following interventions are included in the nurse's responsibilities when administering medications? (Select all that apply.)

    __X__   **Observing for medication side effects**

    __X__   **Monitoring for therapeutic effects**

    _____   Changing the dose if side effects occur

    _____   Ordering the appropriate dose

    __X__   **Maintaining an up-to-date knowledge base**

Observing for side effects, monitoring for therapeutic effects, and maintaining an up-to-date knowledge base are all responsibilities of the nurse. The prescriber is responsible for prescribing the appropriate dose and changing the dose if necessary.

Unit 1   Basic Pharmacologic Principles & Safe Administration of Medications

Chapter 5:   Age-Specific and Other Considerations of Medication Administration
Contributor: Judith A. Harris, MSN, RNC

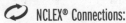 NCLEX® Connections:

> **Learning Objective**: Review and apply knowledge within "**Age-Specific and Other Considerations of Medication Administration**" in readiness for performance of the follow nursing activities as outlined by the NCLEX® test plans:
>
> Δ   Apply knowledge of age-specific and other considerations of medication responses to safely and effectively administer medications.
>
> Δ   Assess/monitor the client for physical and psychosocial factors that impact medication administration.
>
> Δ   Demonstrate appropriate nursing care for the client with an individual variation in medication response.
>
> Δ   Assess/monitor the client for individual medication responses.
>
> Δ   Provide/reinforce teaching to family/significant others/client on how to manage individual variations of medication responses.

 Key Points

Δ   **Factors affecting medication dosages and responses** include:

- **Body weight** – because medications are absorbed and distributed in body tissue, individuals with a greater body mass may require larger doses.

- **Age** – young children with immature liver and kidney function, and older adults, often with reduced liver and kidney function, may require proportionately smaller medication doses.

- **Gender** – females may respond differently to medications than males due to a higher proportion of body fat and the effects of female hormones.

- **Genetics** – genetic factors such as missing enzymes can alter the metabolism of certain medications, thus enhancing or reducing medication action.

- **Biorhythmic cycles** – responses to certain medications vary with the biologic rhythms of the body (e.g., hypnotic medications work better when given at the usual sleep time than at other times).

- **Tolerance** – reduced responsiveness to a medication, either congenital (e.g., genetic factors) or acquired (e.g., stimulation of liver enzymes or other physiologic variations). Cross-tolerance may occur with other chemically similar medications.

- **Accumulation** – ↑ medication concentration in the body due to the inability to metabolize or excrete a medication rapidly enough, resulting in a toxic medication effect. In the older adult, ↓ renal function is the major cause of medication accumulation leading to toxicity.

- **Psychological factors** – emotional state and expectations can influence the effects of a medication. A term used to describe positive medication effects influenced by psychological factors is the **placebo effect.**

- **Medical conditions**

  ◊ Inadequate or inhibited gastric acid inhibits the absorption of medications requiring an acid medium to dissolve.

  ◊ Diarrhea causes oral medications to pass too quickly through the GI tract to be absorbed.

  ◊ Vascular insufficiency prevents distribution of a medication to affected tissue.

  ◊ Liver disease/failure impairs medication metabolism, which may cause toxicity.

  ◊ Kidney disease/failure prevents or delays medication excretion, which may cause toxicity.

Δ **Pharmacology of children**

- While the majority of medications administered to adults are useful for children, the dosages are different. Pediatric dosages are based on **body weight, body surface area (BSA), and maturation of body organs.** **Neonates** (< 1 month old) and **infants** (1 month to 1 year old) have immature liver and kidney function, alkaline gastric juices, and an immature blood-brain barrier. Certain medication dosages are based on **age** due to greater risk for ↓ skeletal bone growth, acute cardiorespiratory failure, or hepatic toxicity.

- Additional **pharmacokinetic factors specific to children** include:

  ◊ ↓ gastric acid production and slower gastric emptying time.

  ◊ ↓ first-pass medication metabolism.

  ◊ ↑ absorption of topical medications (greater body surface area and thinner skin).

  ◊ Lower blood pressure (liver and brain receive greater blood flow and the kidneys receive less).

  ◊ Higher body water content (dilutes water-soluble medications).

  ◊ ↓ serum protein-binding sites (until age 1).

- Be particularly alert when administering medications to children due to high risk for medication error.

  ◊ Dosages are usually based on weight or body surface area.

  ◊ Most medications are not tested on children.

  ◊ Adult medication forms and concentrations may require dilution, calculation, preparation, and administration of very small doses.

  ◊ Limited sites exist for IV medication administration.

Δ **Pharmacology and older adults (65+ years)**

- Physiologic changes associated with aging that impact pharmacokinetics include:

  ◊ ↑ gastric pH (alkaline).

  ◊ ↓ GI motility and gastric emptying time.

  ◊ ↓ blood flow through cardiovascular system, liver, and kidneys.

  ◊ ↓ hepatic enzyme function.

  ◊ ↓ kidney function and glomerular filtration rate.

  ◊ ↓ protein-binding sites.

  ◊ ↓ body water, ↑ body fat, and ↓ lean body mass.

- Other factors affecting medication therapy for older adults include:

  ◊ Impaired memory or altered mental state.

  ◊ Changes in vision and hearing.

  ◊ ↓ mobility and dexterity.

  ◊ Poor client compliance.

  ◊ **Polypharmacy** – the practice of taking several medications simultaneously (prescribed and/or over-the-counter [OTC]) together with diminished bodily functions and certain medical conditions. This can contribute to the potential for medication toxicity.

Δ Nursing interventions for the older adult include:

- ↓ risk of adverse medication effects.

  ◊ Take complete medication history and include all OTC medications.

  ◊ Medications should be started at the lowest possible dose.

  ◊ Monitor/assess the client for therapeutic and adverse effects.

  ◊ Monitor/assess the client for drug-drug and drug-food interactions.

  ◊ Document findings.

  ◊ Notify the primary care provider of adverse effects.

- Promoting compliance.

  ◊ Give clear and concise instructions, verbally and in writing.

  ◊ Ensure dosage form is appropriate. Liquids should be administered to clients who have difficulty swallowing.

  ◊ Provide clearly marked containers that are easy to open.

  ◊ Assist the client to set up a daily calendar with the use of pill containers.

  ◊ Suggest that the client obtain assistance from a friend, neighbor, or relative.

Δ **Pregnancy** – any medication ingested by a woman who is pregnant will be distributed to the fetus as well. Medications are classified according to potential harm to the fetus *(For information, refer to chapter 1, Basic Pharmacologic Principles)*. In general, most medications should be considered potentially harmful to the fetus; therefore, benefits of maternal medication administration must be weighed against possible fetal risk. Medications are most commonly used during pregnancy as nutritional supplements (iron, vitamins, minerals) and for the treatment of nausea, vomiting, gastric acidity, and mild discomforts. Chronic medical conditions such as diabetes or hypertension must be managed with careful maternal-fetal monitoring. **Live virus vaccines** (e.g., measles, mumps, polio, rubella, yellow fever) are contraindicated due to possible teratogenic effects.

Δ **Lactation** – most medications taken by lactating women are secreted in breast milk. However, medication concentration is usually too low to have an effect on the breastfeeding infant. Giving the medication immediately after breastfeeding will minimize medication concentration in the next feeding.

Primary Reference:

Lehne, R. A. (2007). *Pharmacology for nursing care* (6th ed.). St. Louis, MO: Saunders.

Additional Resources:

Abrams, A. C., & Goldsmith, T. L. (2003). *Clinical drug therapy: Rationales for nursing practice* (7th ed.). Philadelphia: Lippincott Williams & Wilkins.

Linton, A. D., & Harris, J. A. (2000). *Pharmacology companion for introductory nursing care of adults* (2nd ed.). Philadelphia: Saunders.

Unit 1 Basic Pharmacologic Principles & Safe Administration of Medications

Chapter 5: Age-Specific and Other Considerations of Medication Administration

Application Exercises

1. Define polypharmacy.   A used of more than one medication at a time

2. Identify physiological factors affecting pharmacokinetics in older adult clients.

3. When giving a medication that is highly protein-bound to an infant, will there be more or less free medication available? Will medication effects be increased or decreased? Explain.

4. A woman who is lactating is to begin taking an antimicrobial medication. She tells the nurse she doesn't want to take the medication because it may harm her baby who is breastfeeding. An appropriate response by the nurse should be,

     A. "You don't have to take the medication if you don't want to."
     B. "Taking the medication immediately after breastfeeding will minimize any effect on your baby."
     C. "You can bottle feed your baby while taking this medication."
     D. "The medication cannot pass through your breast milk to your baby."

5. An older adult client who is hospitalized reports of an inability to sleep at night. The client is given a hypnotic medication at 2200. The next morning the client is drowsy and wants to sleep instead of eating breakfast. The nurse is aware that this effect is most likely due to

     A. reduced cardiac function.
     B. first-pass effect.
     C. reduced hepatic function.
     D. delayed toxic effect.

6. A 65-year-old client's laboratory work indicates hypoalbuminemia. Related to medication therapy, this may result in

     A. reduced therapeutic effect.
     B. decreased medication metabolism.
     C. prolonged half-life of the medication.
     D. excess free medication and possible toxicity.

7. A nurse is providing teaching to an older adult client to promote compliance with medication administration. Which of the following instructions should be included? (Select all that apply.)

_____ Only take medications when not feeling well.

__|__ Place pills in daily pill holders.

____ Contact primary care provider if side effects occur.

____ Ask a relative to check in periodically.

_____ Wait until all medications are finished before refilling prescriptions.

Unit 1 Basic Pharmacologic Principles & Safe Administration of Medications

Chapter 5: Age-Specific and Other Considerations of Medication Administration

Application Exercises Answer Key

1. Define polypharmacy.

   Polypharmacy is the practice of taking several medications simultaneously (prescribed and/or OTC).

2. Identify physiological factors affecting pharmacokinetics in older adult clients.

   Alkaline gastric pH; decreased GI motility and gastric emptying time; decreased CV, hepatic, and renal blood flow; reduced hepatic enzyme function; decreased kidney function and glomerular filtration rate; decreased protein-binding sites; and decreased body water and lean body mass, and increased body fat

3. When giving a medication that is highly protein-bound to an infant, will there be more or less free medication available? Will medication effects be increased or decreased? Explain.

   More free medication will be available due to fewer protein-binding sites. Medication effects will be increased with greater potential for toxicity.

4. A woman who is lactating is to begin taking an antimicrobial medication. She tells the nurse she doesn't want to take the medication because it may harm her baby who is breastfeeding. An appropriate response by the nurse should be,

    A. "You don't have to take the medication if you don't want to."

    B. "Taking the medication immediately after breastfeeding will minimize any effect on your baby."

    C. "You can bottle feed your baby while taking this medication."

    D. "The medication cannot pass through your breast milk to your baby."

Taking any medication right after breastfeeding will decrease the concentration of the medication in the next feeding.

5. An older adult client who is hospitalized reports of an inability to sleep at night. The client is given a hypnotic medication at 2200. The next morning the client is drowsy and wants to sleep instead of eating breakfast. The nurse is aware that this effect is most likely due to

    A. reduced cardiac function.

    B. first-pass effect.

    C. reduced hepatic function.

    D. delayed toxic effect.

Reduced hepatic function may prolong the half-life of a medication and increase the length of response of a medication.

6. A 65-year-old client's laboratory work indicates hypoalbuminemia. Related to medication therapy, this may result in

    A. reduced therapeutic effect.

    B. decreased medication metabolism.

    C. prolonged half-life of the medication.

    D. excess free medication and possible toxicity.

Decreased levels of albumin lead to decreased binding of medications. This can result in increased levels of the free medication.

7. A nurse is providing teaching to an older adult client to promote compliance with medication administration. Which of the following instructions should be included? (Select all that apply.)

_____	Only take medications when not feeling well.
__X__	**Place pills in daily pill holders.**
__X__	**Contact primary care provider if side effects occur.**
__X__	**Ask a relative to check in periodically.**
_____	Wait until all medications are finished before refilling prescriptions.

Placing pills in a daily pill holder reminds the client to take the pills as scheduled; the primary care provider should be notified of side effects to determine if medications need to be adjusted; and assistance from a relative will provide emotional support. The client should take medications on a regular schedule and prescriptions should be filled as each is used up.

Unit 2   Medications Used to Treat Infection
Contributor: Candyce Antley, MSN, PRN

 NCLEX® Connections:

Learning Objective: Review and apply knowledge within **"Medications Used to Treat Infection"** in readiness for performance of the following nursing activities as outlined by the NCLEX® test plans:

Δ   Assess/monitor the client for expected effects of medications.

Δ   Assess/monitor the client for side/adverse effects of medications.

Δ   Assess/monitor the client for actual/potential specific food and medication interactions.

Δ   Identify contraindications, actual/potential incompatibilities, and interactions between medications, and intervene appropriately.

Δ   Identify symptoms/evidence of an allergic reaction, and respond appropriately.

Δ   Evaluate/monitor and document the therapeutic and adverse/side effects of medications.

Δ   Provide/reinforce client teaching on actions, therapeutic effects, potential side/adverse effects, and interactions of medications.

 General Key Points

Δ   Antimicrobial agents **treat bacterial, viral, and fungal infections.**

Δ   Antimicrobials are classified according to the micro-organisms that they treat.

Δ   **Resistance** to micro-organisms is **naturally acquired/inherited or** acquired with **prior exposure** to disease and immunizations.

Δ   **Narrow-spectrum antibiotics** are effective against **a few species** of micro-organisms such as gram-positive cocci, gram-positive bacilli, and gram-negative aerobes.

Δ   **Broad-spectrum antibiotics** are effective against a **wide variety of micro-organisms** including gram-positive cocci and gram-negative bacilli.

Δ   Ideally, **specimens for a culture and sensitivity test** should be collected **prior** to initiation of antimicrobial therapy.

Δ   Prescribed antimicrobial medications should be taken around the clock to maintain therapeutic blood levels.

Δ   Adverse reactions to antimicrobials include:

- **Allergic/hypersensitivity** reactions (e.g., rashes, urticaria), **anaphylaxis** (laryngeal edema, bronchoconstriction, hypotension)

- **Suprainfection** (caused by medication-resistant microbes such as thrush [candidiasis] and results from medication-resistant microbes that emerge during treatment of a primary infection)

- **Organ toxicity** (e.g., **nephrotoxicity, ototoxicity**) ear infection

- Several antimicrobials lower oral contraceptive efficacy. ↑ dosages of oral contraceptives or an alternative form of birth control may be necessary during antimicrobial therapy.

- Misuse/overuse/ineffective use of antimicrobials lead to the development of resistant micro-organisms. Instruct clients to **complete the prescribed course of antibiotic treatment** even though symptoms may improve before the full course of treatment is over.

Key Points

Medication Classification: Penicillins

Select Prototype Medication: **penicillin G (Bicillin LA)**

Other Medications: Broad-spectrum: amoxicillin-clavulanate
(Augmentin)
Antistaphylococcal: nafcillin
(Unipen), methicillin
Antipseudomonas: carbenicillin (Geocillin),
ticarcillin-clavulanate (Timentin), piperacillin-
tazobactam (Zosyn)

Expected Pharmacological Action

Δ   Penicillins destroy bacteria by weakening the bacterial cell wall.

Therapeutic Uses

Δ   Penicillins are the medication of choice for **gram-positive** cocci such as
streptococcus pneumoniae (pneumonia and meningitis), *streptococcus viridans*
(infectious endocarditis), and *streptococcus pyogenes* (pharyngitis).

Δ   Penicillins are the medication of **first choice for meningitis** caused by gram–
negative cocci *Neisseria* meningitides.

Δ   Penicillins are the medication of choice for the treatment of syphilis caused by
spirochete treponema pallidum.

Δ   Extended-spectrum penicillin (e.g., carbenicillin, piperacillin) is effective against
organisms such as *Pseudomonas aeruginosa*, *Enterobacter species*, *Proteus*, *Bacteroides
fragilis*, and *Klebsiella*.

Δ   **Prophylaxis bacterial endocarditis**

Side/Adverse Effects: Nursing Interventions and Client Education

Side/Adverse Effects	Nursing Interventions/Client Education
Allergies/anaphylaxis	• Interview the client for prior allergy. • Wear an allergy identification bracelet. • Observe the client for 30 min following administration of parenteral penicillin.
Renal impairment	• Monitor the client's kidney function. • Monitor the client's intake and output.
Hyperkalemia/dysrhythmias with high doses of penicillin G	• Monitor the client's cardiac status and electrolyte levels.

Contraindications/Precautions

Δ   Penicillins are contraindicated for clients with a severe history of allergies to penicillin, cephalosporin, and/or imipenem.

Δ   Use cautiously in clients with, or at risk for, kidney dysfunction (e.g., acutely ill, older adults, young children).

Δ   Clients who are allergic to one penicillin should be considered cross allergic to other penicillins and at risk for a cross allergy to cephalosporin.

Medication/Food Interactions: Nursing Interventions and Client Education

Aminoglycosides – penicillin inactivates aminoglycosides when mixed in the same IV solution.	• Do not mix penicillin and aminoglycoside in the same intravenous solution.
Oral contraceptives (OC) – ampicillin ↓ OC efficacy.	• Instruct the client to report signs of reduced levels (e.g., breakthrough bleeding). ↑ doses of OC or an alternative form of birth control may be required.

Therapeutic Nursing Interventions and Client Education

Δ   Instruct the client to take oral penicillins with a full glass of water 1 hr before meals or 2 hr after.

Δ   Penicillins such as penicillin V, amoxicillin, amoxicillin-clavulanate, and bacampicillin may be taken with meals.

Δ   Instruct clients to report any signs of an allergic response such as skin rash, itching, and/or hives.

Nursing Evaluation of Medication Effectiveness

Δ   Improvement of infection symptoms (e.g., reduction in fever, pain, inflammation).

Key Points

Medication Classification: Cephalosporins

Select Prototype Medication:	1st generation: **cephalexin (Keflex)**
	2nd generation: **cefaclor (Ceclor)**
	3rd generation: **ceftriaxone (Rocephin)**
	4th generation: **cefepime (Maxipime)**
Other Medications:	1st generation: cephapirin (Cefadyl)
	2nd generation: cefotetan (Cefotan)
	3rd generation: cefotaxime (Claforan)

Expected Pharmacological Action

Δ   Cephalosporins are beta-lactam antibiotics, similar to penicillins that destroy bacterial cell walls causing destruction of micro-organisms.

Δ   Cephalosporins are grouped into four generations. Each generation of cephalosporins is:

- More effective against gram-negative organisms and anaerobes.

- Less likely to be destroyed by beta-lactamase.

- More able to reach cerebrospinal fluid.

Therapeutic Uses

Δ   Cephalosporins are **broad-spectrum** bactericidal medications with a **high therapeutic index** that treat urinary tract infections, postoperative infections, pelvic infections, and meningitis.

Side/Adverse Effects: Nursing Interventions and Client Education

Side/Adverse Effects	Nursing Interventions/Client Education
Allergic/hypersensitivity/anaphylaxis	• If signs of allergy appear (e.g., urticaria, rash, hypotension, and/or dyspnea) stop cephalosporin immediately, and notify the primary care provider.
Bleeding tendencies	• Observe the client for signs of bleeding. • Monitor the client for prothrombin time and bleeding time. • Stop cephalosporin. • Administer parenteral vitamin K.
Thrombophlebitis	• Rotate injection sites. • Administer slowly over 3 to 5 min and in a dilute solution.
Pain with IM injection	• Forewarn the client about pain with injection. • Administer IM injection deep in large muscle mass.
Cross allergy to penicillins	• Assess the client for allergy to penicillin and notify primary care provider. • Instruct the client to observe for and to report signs of allergic reaction (e.g., rash, hives, and/or dyspnea).
Antibiotic associated pseudomembranous colitis	• Observe the client for diarrhea and notify the primary care provider. • Discontinue cephalosporin.

Contraindications/Precautions

Δ   Cephalosporins should not be given to clients who have a history of severe allergic reactions to penicillins.

Δ   Use cautiously in clients with renal impairment.

Δ   Exercise caution if cephalosporins are used in combination with medications that promote bleeding (e.g., anticoagulants, antiplatelets, thrombolytics, nonsteroidal anti-inflammatory agents).

Medication/Food Interactions: Nursing Interventions and Client Education

Medication/Food Interactions	Nursing Interventions/Client Education
Disulfiram reaction (intolerance to alcohol) occurs with combined use of cefmetazole, cefoperazone, or cefotetan and alcohol.	• Instruct the client not to consume alcohol while taking these cephalosporins.
Probenecid delays renal excretion.	• Monitor the client's I&O.

Therapeutic Nursing Interventions and Client Education

Δ   Instruct the client to complete the prescribed course of therapy, even though symptoms may resolve before the full course of antimicrobial treatment is completed.

Δ   Advise clients to take oral cephalosporins with food.

Δ   Instruct clients to store oral cephalosporin suspensions in a refrigerator.

Nursing Evaluation of Medication Effectiveness

Δ   Improvement of infection symptoms (e.g., reduction in fever, pain, and inflammation; clear breath sounds; reduced UTI symptoms, negative urine cultures).

Key Points

Medication Classification: Carbapenems

Select Prototype Medication:	**imipenem (Primaxin)**
Other Medications:	meropenem (Merrem IV)

Expected Pharmacological Action

Δ Carbapenems are beta-lactam antibiotics that destroy bacterial cell walls causing destruction of micro-organisms.

Therapeutic Uses

Δ **Broad antimicrobial spectrum** is **effective for serious infections** such as pneumonia, peritonitis, and urinary tract infections caused by gram-positive cocci, gram-negative cocci, gram-negative bacilli, and mixed aerobic and anaerobic bacteria.

Δ Resistance develops when imipenem is used alone to treat *Pseudomonas aeruginosa*. A combination of antipseudomonal medications should be used to treat this micro-organism.

Side/Adverse Effects: Nursing Interventions and Client Education

Side/Adverse Effects	Nursing Interventions/Client Education
Allergy/hypersensitivity	• Monitor the client for signs of allergic reactions (e.g., rashes, pruritus).
Gastrointestinal symptoms (e.g., nausea, vomiting, diarrhea)	• Observe the client for nausea, vomiting, and diarrhea. • Notify the primary care provider. • Monitor the client's I&O.
Suprainfection	• Monitor the client for signs of colitis, (e.g., diarrhea, oral thrush, vaginal yeast infection) and intervene accordingly.

Contraindications/Precautions

Δ Use cautiously in clients with renal impairment.

Therapeutic Nursing Interventions and Client Education

Δ Instruct the client to complete the prescribed course of antimicrobial therapy, even though symptoms may resolve before the full course is completed.

Nursing Evaluation of Medication Effectiveness

Δ Improvement of infection symptoms (e.g., reduction in fever, pain, and inflammation; clear lung sounds; reduced UTI symptoms, negative urine cultures)

Key Points

Medication Classification: Monobactams

| Select Prototype Medication: | **vancomycin (Vancocin)** |
| Other Medications: | aztreonam (Azactam), fosfomycin (Monurol) |

Expected Pharmacological Action and Therapeutic Uses

Δ   Monobactams are beta-lactam antibiotics that destroy bacterial cell walls causing destruction of micro-organisms.

Therapeutic Uses

Δ   Monobactams are the antimicrobial of choice for **serious infections caused by methicillin resistant *Staph. aureus*** or *Staph. epidermidis*.

Δ   Monobactams are the medication of choice for **antibiotic-associated pseudomembranous colitis** caused by *Clostridium difficile*.

Side/Adverse Effects: Nursing Interventions and Client Education

Side/Adverse Effects	Nursing Interventions/Client Education
Ototoxicity	• Assess the client for signs of hearing loss. • Obtain a baseline hearing test. • Instruct the client to notify the primary care provider if changes in hearing acuity develop. • Monitor vancomycin levels.
Infusion reaction (e.g., rashes, flushing, tachycardia, hypotension)	• Administer vancomycin slowly over 60 min.
Thrombophlebitis	• Rotate injection sites. • Monitor infusion site for redness, swelling, and inflammation.

Contraindications/Precaution

Δ   Use cautiously in clients with renal impairment.

Therapeutic Nursing Interventions and Client Education

Δ   Vancomycin peak blood levels should be collected 1 to 2 hr after completion of IV infusion. Appropriate peak levels are between 30 to 40 µg/mL.

Nursing Evaluation of Medication Effectiveness

Δ   Improvement of infection symptoms (e.g., clear breath sounds; wound healing; improvement of symptoms of antibiotic-associated pseudomembranous colitis symptoms, such as resolution of diarrhea and negative stool cultures for *Clostridium difficile*).

Key Points

Medication Classification: Tetracyclines

Select Prototype Medication:	**tetracycline hydrochloride (Sumycin)**
Other Medications:	doxycycline (Vibramycin)

Expected Pharmacological Action

Δ   Tetracyclines are broad-spectrum antibiotics that inhibit micro-organism growth by preventing protein synthesis (bacteriostatic).

Therapeutic Uses

Δ   Tetracyclines are the medication of choice topically and orally for acne vulgaris.

Δ   First-line medication for rickettsia (e.g., Rocky Mountain spotted fever, typhus fever; infections of the urethra or cervix caused by *Chlamydia trachomatis*; brucellosis; pneumonia caused by *Mycoplasma pneumonia*; Lyme disease; anthrax; **gastrointestinal infections caused by *Helicobacter pylori*; and periodontal disease**).

Side/Adverse Effects: Nursing Interventions and Client Education

Side/Adverse Effects	Nursing Interventions/Client Education
Gastrointestinal discomfort includes cramping, nausea, vomiting, diarrhea, and esophageal ulceration.	• Monitor the client for nausea, vomiting, and diarrhea. • Monitor the client's I&O. • Take oral tetracycline with meals, and avoid giving tetracycline at bedtime to reduce esophageal ulceration.
Yellow/brown tooth discoloration and/or hypoplasia of teeth enamel can occur.	• Avoid administration to children under 8 years of age.
Hepatotoxicity (e.g., lethargy, jaundice) ↑ risk in pregnant and postpartum clients with kidney disease)	• Avoid administration of high doses intravenously.
Photosensitivity such as exaggerated sunburn	• Avoid prolonged exposure to sunlight; wear protective clothing; and use sunscreen.
Suprainfection of the bowel – antibiotic-associated pseudomembranous colitis (e.g., diarrhea, yeast infections of the mouth, pharynx, vagina, bowels)	• Instruct the client to observe for symptoms of diarrhea, and notify the primary care provider.

Contraindications/Precautions

Δ   Tetracyclines should not be administered to clients with renal disease, except for doxycycline and minocycline.

Δ   Use of tetracycline during pregnancy after the fourth month can cause staining of the deciduous teeth, but will not have a permanent effect on permanent teeth.

Medication/Food Interactions: Nursing Interventions and Client Education

Medication/Food Interactions	Nursing Interventions/Client Education
Milk products, calcium supplements, iron supplements, magnesium-containing laxatives, and most antacids – If tetracycline is taken with these medications, nonabsorbable chelates will form, and absorption and effectiveness of oral tetracyclines will result.	• Tetracyclines should be taken on an empty stomach with a full glass of water. • Administer tetracyclines at least 1 hr before and 2 hr after taking food and supplements containing calcium and magnesium.
Oral contraceptives (OC) – tetracycline ↓ the efficacy of OC.	• Instruct the client to report signs of reduced levels, such as breakthrough bleeding. • ↑ doses of OC or an alternative form of birth control may be required.

Therapeutic Nursing Interventions and Client Education

Δ   Tetracyclines should not be given with food, except for doxycycline and minocycline.

Δ   Instruct the client to complete the prescribed course of antimicrobial therapy, even though symptoms may resolve before the full course is completed.

Nursing Evaluation of Medication Effectiveness

Δ   Depending on therapeutic intent, effectiveness may be evidenced by:

•   Improvement of infection symptoms, such as clear breath sounds.

•   Resolution of yeast infections of the mouth, vagina, and bowels.

•   Resolution of acne vulgaris facial lesions.

Key Points

Medication Classification: Bacteriostatic Inhibitors

Select Prototype Medication:	**erythromycin (E-Mycin)**
Other Medications:	clindamycin (Cleocin), azithromycin (Zithromax), clarithromycin (Biaxin)

Expected Pharmacological Action and Therapeutic Uses

Δ Erythromycin slows the growth of micro-organisms by inhibiting protein synthesis (bacteriostatic). At high doses or with susceptible bacteria erythromycin can be bactericidal.

Therapeutic Uses

Δ Bacteriostatic inhibitors are used **to treat infections in clients with a penicillin allergy.**

Δ Bacteriostatic inhibitors are the preferred medication for clients with Legionnaires' disease, whooping cough (pertussis), and acute diphtheria (eliminates the carrier state of diphtheria).

Δ Bacteriostatic inhibitors are the first medication of choice for *Chlamydia* infections (e.g., urethritis and cervicitis; pneumonia caused by *Mycoplasma pneumoniae*; respiratory tract infections caused by ***Streptococcus*** pneumoniae, and group A *Streptococcus pyogenes*).

Δ Bacteriostatic inhibitors are used as an alternative medication to prevent the recurrence of rheumatic fever and bacterial endocarditis for clients who are allergic to penicillin.

Side/Adverse Effects: Nursing Interventions and Client Education

Side/Adverse Effects	Nursing Interventions/Client Education
Gastrointestinal discomfort (e.g., nausea, vomiting, epigastric pain)	• Administer erythromycin with meals. • Observe for GI symptoms and notify the primary care provider.
Thrombophlebitis	• Infusion of intravenous erythromycin should be administered slowly and in a dilute solution.

Contraindications/Precautions

Δ Bacteriostatic inhibitors are contraindicated in clients with pre-existing liver disease.

Medication/Food Interactions: Nursing Interventions and Client Education

Medication/Food Interactions	Nursing Interventions/Client Education
Antihistamines, theophylline (asthma medication), **carbamazepine** (anticonvulsant), and **warfarin** (anticoagulant) – concurrent use with these medications results in toxicity.	• To minimize toxicity, avoid using erythromycin with antihistamines, asthma medication, anticonvulsants, and anticoagulants.

Therapeutic Nursing Interventions and Client Education

Δ   Administer oral preparation on an empty stomach (1 hr before meals and 2 hr after) with a full glass of water.

Δ   Intravenous erythromycin is rarely used. It is only used for very serious infections and is administered by continuous infusion.

Δ   Instruct the client to complete the prescribed course of antimicrobial therapy, even though symptoms may resolve before the full course is completed.

Nursing Evaluation of Medication Effectiveness

Δ   Improvement of infection symptoms (e.g., clear lung sounds; improvement of sore throat, cough, urinary tract symptoms; and resolution of bacterial endocarditis with negative blood cultures).

Key Points

Medication Classification: Aminoglycosides

Select Prototype Medication: **gentamicin (Garamycin)**

Other Medications: amikacin (Amikin), tobramycin sulfate (Nebcin), neomycin, streptomycin, paromomycin (oral)

Expected Pharmacological Action and Therapeutic Uses

Δ   Aminoglycosides are bactericidal antibiotics that destroy micro-organisms by disrupting protein synthesis.

Therapeutic Uses

Δ   Aminoglycosides are the medication of choice against **aerobic gram-negative bacilli** (e.g., *Escherichia coli, Klebsiella pneumoniae, Proteus mirabilis, Pseudomonas aeruginosa*).

Δ   Paromomycin (oral aminoglycoside) is used for intestinal amebiasis and tapeworm infections.

Side/Adverse Effects: Nursing Interventions and Client Education

Side/Adverse Effects	Nursing Interventions/Client Education
Ototoxicity (e.g., cochlear damage [hearing loss] and vestibular damage [loss of balance])	• Monitor the client for symptoms of tinnitus (ringing in the ears), headache, hearing loss, nausea, dizziness, and vertigo. • Instruct the client that if tinnitus, hearing loss, or headaches occur, to notify the primary care provider. • **Stop aminoglycoside if symptoms occur.** Do baseline audiometric studies (hearing test).
Nephrotoxicity related to high total cumulative dose resulting in acute tubular necrosis (e.g., proteinuria, casts in the urine, dilute urine, elevated BUN, creatinine levels)	• Monitor I&O, BUN, and creatinine levels. • Instruct clients to report a significant ↓ in the amount of urine output.
Intensified neuromuscular blockade resulting in respiratory depression	• Closely monitor use in clients with myasthenia gravis, clients on skeletal muscle relaxants, and clients receiving general anesthetics (↑ the risk of excessive neuromuscular blockade and respiratory depression).

Side/Adverse Effects	Nursing Interventions/Client Education
Hypersensitivity (e.g., rash, pruritus, paresthesia of hands and feet, urticaria)	• Monitor clients for allergic symptoms (e.g., rash, pruritus, and tingling of the hands and feet).
Streptomycin	
Neurologic disorder (e.g., peripheral neuritis, optic nerve dysfunction, tingling/numbness of the hands and feet).	• Instruct the client to promptly report any symptoms to the primary care provider.

Contraindications/Precautions

Δ Use cautiously in clients with renal impairment, pre-existing hearing loss, clients with myasthenia gravis, clients on ethacrynic acid (↑ risk for ototoxicity), amphotericin B, cephalosporins, vancomycin (↑ risk for nephrotoxicity), and neuromuscular blocking agents such as tubocurarine.

Δ Clients with renal impairment should receive reduced doses of aminoglycosides.

Medication/Food Interactions: Nursing Interventions and Client Education

Medication/Food Interactions	Nursing Interventions/Client Education
Penicillin – will inactivate aminoglycosides when mixed in the same IV solution.	• Do not mix aminoglycosides and penicillins in the same IV solution.

Therapeutic Nursing Interventions and Client Education

Δ Measure aminoglycoside levels based on dosing schedules. Samples for **peak levels** should be collected **30 min after administration** of aminoglycoside intramuscularly or via an intravenous infusion.

Δ **Trough levels** for clients receiving divided dosing of aminoglycoside, the sample should be collected **prior to the next dose**.

Δ For clients on once-a-day dosing, two samples should be collected (e.g., blood should be drawn 2 and 12 hr after administration). Trough levels are then determined from these values.

Nursing Evaluation of Medication Effectiveness

Δ Improvement of infection symptoms (e.g., clear lung sounds, improvement of urinary tract symptoms, wound healing).

Key Points

Medication Classification: Sulfonamides and Trimethoprim

Select Prototype Medication: **trimethoprim-sulfamethoxazole (TMP-SMZ, Bactrim)**

Other Medications: Cotrim, Septra

Expected Pharmacological Action

Δ Sulfonamides and trimethoprim inhibit bacterial growth by preventing the synthesis of folic acid. Folic acid is essential for the production of DNA, RNA, and proteins.

Therapeutic Uses

Δ TMP-SMZ is the medication of choice for **urinary tract infections** caused by *E. coli* and other infections (e.g., otitis media, bronchitis, shigellosis, pneumonia) caused by *Pneumocystis carinii*.

Side/Adverse Effects: Nursing Interventions and Client Education

Side/Adverse Effects	Nursing Interventions/Client Education
Hypersensitivity including **Stevens-Johnson syndrome**	• Do not administer TMP-SMZ to clients with allergies to sulfonamides (sulfa), thiazide diuretics (hydrochlorothiazide), sulfonylurea-type oral hypoglycemics (tolbutamide), and loop diuretics (furosemide). • Stop TMP-SMZ at the first indication of hypersensitivity, such as rash.
Blood dyscrasias (e.g., hemolytic anemia, agranulocytosis, aplastic anemia)	• Draw the client's baseline and periodic CBC levels to detect any hematologic disorders. • Observe for any bleeding episodes, sore throat, or pallor. • If the above symptoms occur, instruct the client to notify the primary care provider.
Crystalluria	• ↑ oral fluid intake. • Instruct client to drink 8 to 10 glasses of water/day.
Kernicterus (jaundice, ↑ bilirubin levels)	• Avoid administering TMP-SMZ to women who are pregnant near term, breastfeeding mothers, and to infants less than 2 months. • Monitor the client's liver function.

Side/Adverse Effects	Nursing Interventions/Client Education
Photosensitivity	• Avoid prolonged exposure to sunlight, use sunscreen, and wear appropriate protective clothing.

Contraindications/Precautions

Δ TMP-SMZ is contraindicated in clients with folate deficiency (↑ the risk of megaloblastic anemia).

Δ Avoid use in pregnancy and lactation (risk of kernicterus).

Δ Use cautiously in clients with renal dysfunction. Reduce dosage of TMP-SMZ by 50%.

Δ Do not use if creatinine clearance is < 15 mL/min.

Medication/Food Interactions: Nursing Interventions and Client Education

Medication/Food Interactions	Nursing Interventions/Client Education
Warfarin (Coumadin), phenytoin (Dilantin), sulfonylurea oral hypoglycemics-tolbutamide (Orinase) – sulfonamides can ↑ the effects of these medications by inhibiting hepatic metabolism.	• Reduced dosages of these medications may be required during TMP-SMZ therapy.

Therapeutic Nursing Interventions and Client Education

Δ Instruct the client to take TMP-SMZ on an empty stomach with a full glass of water.

Δ Instruct the client to complete the prescribed course of antimicrobial therapy, even though symptoms may resolve before the full course is completed.

Nursing Evaluation of Medication Effectiveness

Δ Depending on therapeutic intent, effectiveness may be evidenced by:

• Improvement of infection symptoms (e.g., clear breath sounds, negative blood cultures, improvement of urinary tract symptoms, [↓ frequency, burning, and pain during urination], negative urine cultures).

• Resolution of diarrhea with negative stool for *Shigella* organism.

• Resolution of otitis media with no ear discharge or earache.

Key Points

Medication Classification: Urinary Tract Antiseptics

Select Prototype Medication: **nitrofurantoin (Macrodantin)**

Expected Pharmacological Action

Δ   This medication is a broad-spectrum urinary antiseptic with bacteriostatic action at low doses and bactericidal action at high doses. Bacterial injury occurs by damaging DNA.

Therapeutic Uses

Δ   Acute urinary tract infections

Δ   Prophylaxis for recurrent lower urinary tract infections

Side/Adverse Effects: Nursing Interventions and Client Education

Side/Adverse Effects	Nursing Interventions/Client Education
Gastrointestinal discomfort (e.g., anorexia, nausea, vomiting, diarrhea)	• Administer nitrofurantoin with milk or meals. • Reduce dosage and use the macrocrystalline tablet to reduce GI discomfort.
Hypersensitivity reactions manifested with pulmonary symptoms (e.g., dyspnea, cough, malaise)	• Stop nitrofurantoin.
Blood dyscrasias (e.g., agranulocytosis, leukopenia, thrombocytopenia)	• Do baseline CBC and perform periodic blood tests, monitor the client for easy bruising, and epistaxis (nose bleeding). • Notify the primary care provider if symptoms occur.
Peripheral neuropathy (e.g., numbness, tingling of the hands and feet, muscle weakness)	• Inform the client about these symptoms and instruct the client to notify the primary care provider if they occur.

Contraindications/Precautions

Δ   Nitrofurantoin is contraindicated in clients with renal dysfunction and creatinine clearance less than 40 mL/min.

    •   With renal impairment, there are low concentrations of nitrofurantoin in the urine. Therefore, levels are not effective enough to eradicate micro-organisms.

    •   Impaired renal function will ↑ the risk of medication toxicity due to inability to excrete nitrofurantoin.

Therapeutic Nursing Interventions and Client Education

Δ   Inform the client that urine will have a brownish discoloration.

Δ   Instruct the client to complete the prescribed course of antimicrobial therapy, even though symptoms may resolve before the full course is completed.

Nursing Evaluation of Medication Effectiveness

Δ   Depending on therapeutic intent, effectiveness may be evidenced by:

- Improvement of infection symptoms (e.g., improvement of urinary tract symptoms [↓ frequency, burning, and pain during urination], negative urine cultures).

- Resolution of diarrhea, nausea, and vomiting.

Key Points

Medication Classification: Antimycobacterial (Antituberculosis)

Select Prototype Medications:	**isoniazid (INH)**
Other Medications:	streptomycin, ethambutol, pyrazinamide

Expected Pharmacological Action and Therapeutic Uses

Δ   This medication is highly specific for mycobacteria. Isoniazid inhibits growth of mycobacteria by preventing synthesis of mycolic acid in the cell wall.

Therapeutic Uses

Δ   Indicated for active and latent tuberculosis

- Latent: INH only – daily for 6 months
- Active: Multiple medication therapy including INH, rifampin, pyrazinamide, and/or pyridoxine daily for 6 months

Side/Adverse Effects: Nursing Interventions and Client Education

Side/Adverse Effects	Nursing Interventions/Client Education
Peripheral neuropathy (e.g., tingling, numbness, burning, and pain resulting from deficiency of pyridoxine, vitamin B_6)	• Instruct the client to observe for symptoms, such as tingling sensations of the hands and feet. • Instruct the client to notify the primary care provider if symptoms occur. • Administer 50 to 200 mg of vitamin B_6 daily.
Hepatotoxicity (e.g., anorexia, malaise, fatigue, nausea, and yellowish discoloration of skin and eyes) with INH and pyrazinamide	• Instruct the client to observe for symptoms and notify the primary care provider if symptoms occur. • Monitor liver function tests and instruct the client to avoid consumption of alcohol. • Stop INH if liver function test results are elevated.

Contraindications/Precautions

Δ   INH is contraindicated for clients with liver disease.

Medication/Food Interactions: Nursing Interventions and Client Education

Medication/Food Interactions	Nursing Interventions/Client Education
Phenytoin – INH interferes with the metabolism of phenytoin with accumulation of phenytoin, resulting in ataxia and incoordination.	• Monitor the client's levels of phenytoin. Dosage of phenytoin may need to be adjusted based on phenytoin levels.
Alcohol, rifampin, and pyrazinamide – use of INH with alcohol, rifampin, and pyrazinamide ↑ the risk for hepatotoxicity.	• Instruct clients to avoid alcohol consumption. • Monitor liver function.

Therapeutic Nursing Interventions and Client Education

Δ   For active tuberculosis, direct observation therapy (DOT) is done to ensure compliance.

Δ   Advise the client to take INH on an empty stomach (1 hr before meals or 2 hr after). Advise clients to take INH with meals if client develops gastric discomfort.

Δ   Instruct the client to complete the prescribed course of antimicrobial therapy, even though symptoms may resolve before the full course is completed.

Nursing Evaluation of Medication Effectiveness

Δ   Improvement of tuberculosis symptoms (e.g., clear breath sounds, no night sweats, ↑ appetite, no afternoon rises of temperature, 3 negative sputum cultures for tuberculosis) usually taking 3 to 6 months to achieve

Key Points

Medication Classification: Anti-Hansen's Disease (Leprosy)

Select Prototype Medications: **dapsone**

Other Medications: clofazimine (Lamprene), rifampin (Rifadin)

Expected Pharmacological Action

Δ   Dapsone is a bactericidal antimicrobial that prevents synthesis of folic acid, which slows the growth of *Mycobacterium leprae*.

Therapeutic Uses

Δ   This medication is indicated for the treatment of Hansen's disease, a chronic disease resulting from infection caused by *M. leprae*. Multi-medication therapy is more effective than monotherapy, so dapsone may be administered in combinations with rifampin, clofazimine, ofloxacin, and minocycline.

Side/Adverse Effects: Nursing Interventions and Client Education

Side/Adverse Effects	Nursing Intervention/Client Education
Discoloration of body fluids caused by ingestion of rifampin	• Inform the client of expected orange color of urine, saliva, sweat, and tears.
Hepatotoxicity (e.g., jaundice, anorexia, fatigue) with the use of rifampin	• Monitor the client's liver function. • Inform the client regarding symptoms of anorexia, fatigue, and malaise, and notify the primary care provider if symptoms occur. • Avoid use in alcoholics.
Mild gastrointestinal discomfort associated with dapsone and rifampin (e.g., anorexia, nausea, abdominal discomfort)	• Abdominal discomfort is mild and does not require any intervention. • Dapsone and rifampin are well-absorbed in the stomach, and effectiveness is reduced by the intake of food.

Contraindications/Precautions

Δ   Use cautiously in clients with liver dysfunction.

Medication/Food Interaction: Nursing Interventions and Client Education

Medication/Food Interaction	Nursing Intervention/Client Education
Warfarin (Coumadin), oral contraceptives, protease inhibitors, and NNRTIs (medications for HIV) – rifampin accelerates metabolism of these medications, resulting in diminished effectiveness.	• ↑ dosages may be necessary.
Oral contraceptives (OC) – rifampin ↓ the efficacy of OC.	• ↑ OC dosages or an alternative form of birth control may be required.

Therapeutic Nursing Interventions and Client Education

Δ   Instruct the client to complete the prescribed course of antimicrobial therapy, even though symptoms may resolve before the full course is completed.

Nursing Evaluation of Medication Effectiveness

Δ   Improvement of Hansen's disease symptoms (e.g., resolution of skin lesions, improvement of mucous membrane lesions, improvement of sensation, negative acid-fast bacilli in smears of skin lesions).

Key Points

Medication Classification: Antiviral

Select Prototype Medication: **acyclovir (Zovirax)**

Other Medications: ganciclovir (Cytovene), interferon alfa, ribavirin (Rebetol), amantadine (Symmetrel), lamivudine (Epivir HBV)

Expected Pharmacological Action

Δ   Acyclovir prevents the reproduction of viral DNA.

Therapeutic Uses

Δ   Antivirals are the medication of choice for herpes simplex virus, varicella–zoster virus, and cytomegalovirus.

Δ   Ganciclovir is the treatment of choice for CMV retinitis in immunocompromised clients with HIV, and transplant clients at risk for CMV infection.

Δ   Ganciclovir is the medication of choice for CMV (cytomegalovirus) retinitis.

Side/Adverse Effects: Nursing Interventions and Client Education

Side/Adverse Effects	Nursing Interventions/Client Education
acyclovir (Zovirax)	
Phlebitis and inflammation at the site of infusion	• Rotate IV injection sites. • Monitor IV sites for swelling and redness.
Nephrotoxicity	• Administer acyclovir infusion slowly over 1 hr. • Ensure adequate hydration during infusion and 2 hr after to minimize nephrotoxicity by increasing oral fluid intake.
Mild discomfort associated with oral therapy (e.g., nausea, headache, diarrhea)	• Observe for symptoms and treat accordingly.

Side/Adverse Effects	Nursing Interventions/Client Education
ganciclovir (Cytovene, Vitrasert)	
Granulocytopenia and thrombocytopenia	• Obtain baseline CBC and platelet count. • Administer granulocyte colony-stimulating factors. • Monitor white blood counts, absolute neutrophil counts, and platelet counts. If absolute neutrophil count is below 500/mm^3, stop treatment. Cell counts improve within 3 to 5 days.
Reproductive toxicity	• Ganciclovir is teratogenic. Advise women to avoid pregnancy during the course of therapy and for 90 days after the end of therapy. • Inform male clients about the risk of sterility.

Contraindications/Precautions

Δ   Ganciclovir is contraindicated during pregnancy (teratogenic) and in clients with a neutrophil count below 500/mm^3.

Δ   Acyclovir should be used cautiously in clients with renal impairment, dehydration, and clients taking nephrotoxic medications.

Δ   Ganciclovir should be used cautiously in clients with pre-existing low white and platelet counts, and clients taking zidovudine and nephrotoxic medications.

Therapeutic Nursing Interventions and Client Education

Δ   For topical administration, advise the client to put on rubber gloves to avoid transfer of virus to other areas of the body.

Δ   Never administer acyclovir by IV bolus.

Δ   Administer IV infusion slowly over 1 hr or longer.

Δ   Inform clients that acyclovir diminishes symptoms but does not cure the virus.

Δ   Instruct clients to wash affected area with soap and water 3 to 4 times/day and to keep the lesions dry after washing.

Δ   Advise clients to refrain from sexual contact while lesions are present.

Δ   Clients with healed herpetic lesions should continue to use condoms to prevent transmission of the virus.

Δ   Surgical intraocular implants for CMV retinitis should be changed every 5 to 8 months.

Δ   Instruct the client to complete the prescribed course of antimicrobial therapy, even though symptoms may resolve before the full course is completed.

Nursing Evaluation of Medication Effectiveness

Δ   Improvement of symptoms (e.g., healed genital lesions, ↓ inflammation and pain, improvement in vision).

Key Points

Medication Classification: Fluoroquinolones

Select Prototype Medication: ciprofloxacin (Cipro)

Expected Pharmacological Action

Δ Fluoroquinolones are bactericidal as a result of inhibition of the enzyme necessary for DNA replication.

Therapeutic Uses

Δ Fluoroquinolones are broad-spectrum antimicrobials used for a wide variety of micro-organisms (e.g., aerobic [requires air for growth] gram-negative bacteria, gram-positive bacteria, *Klebsiella*, and *Escherichia coli*).

Δ Alternative to parenteral antibiotics for clients with severe infections

Δ Respiratory, urinary, and gastrointestinal tract infections; infections of bones, joints, skin, and soft tissues

Δ Medication of choice for prevention of anthrax in clients who have inhaled anthrax spore

Side/Adverse Effects: Nursing Interventions and Client Education

Side/Adverse Effects	Nursing Interventions/Client Education
Gastrointestinal discomfort (e.g., nausea, vomiting, diarrhea)	• Administer medications accordingly.
Achilles tendon rupture	• Instruct the client to observe for signs and symptoms of pain, swelling, redness at Achilles tendon site, and to notify the primary care provider. • Stop ciprofloxacin and refrain from exercise until signs of inflammation subside.
Suprainfection (e.g., thrush, vaginal yeast infection)	• Instruct the client to observe for signs and symptoms of yeast infection (e.g., cottage cheese/curd-like lesions on the mouth and genital area) and to report to the primary care provider if symptoms occur.

Contraindications/Precautions

Δ Ciprofloxacin should not be administered to children < 18 years of age (due to risk of Achilles tendon rupture).

Medication/Food Interactions: Nursing Interventions and Client Education

Medication/Food Interactions	Nursing Interventions/Client Education
Cationic compounds (e.g., aluminum-magnesium antacids, iron salts, sucralfate, milk and dairy products) – ↓ absorption of ciprofloxacin	• Administer cationic compounds 1 hr before or 2 hr after ciprofloxacin.
Theophylline (Theo-Dur) – plasma levels of theophylline can be ↑ with concurrent use of ciprofloxacin	• Monitor levels and adjust dosage accordingly.
Warfarin (Coumadin) – plasma levels of warfarin can be ↑ with concurrent use of ciprofloxacin	• Monitor prothrombin time and INR, and adjust the dosage of warfarin accordingly.

Therapeutic Nursing Interventions and Client Education

Δ   Ciprofloxacin is available in oral and intravenous forms.

Δ   Adjust dosage of ciprofloxacin by decreasing doses in clients with renal dysfunction.

Δ   Intravenous ciprofloxacin should be administered slowly over 60 min.

Δ   For inhalation anthrax infection, ciprofloxacin is administered every 12 hr for 60 days.

Δ   Instruct the client to complete the prescribed course of antimicrobial therapy, even though symptoms may resolve before the full course is completed.

Nursing Evaluation of Medication Effectiveness

Δ   Improvement of symptoms (e.g., clear breath sounds, no signs and symptoms of inflammation, swelling, warmth, and erythema; no evidence of suprainfection [e.g., absence of cottage cheese or curd-like lesions in the mouth and genital areas]).

Key Points

Medication Classification: Antiprotozoals

Select Prototype Medication: **metronidazole (Flagyl)**

Expected Pharmacological Action

Δ   Metronidazole is a broad-spectrum antimicrobial with bactericidal (slows growth of micro-organism) activity against anaerobic (does not require oxygen for growth) micro-organisms.

Therapeutic Uses

Δ   Metronidazole is used to treat protozoal infections (e.g., intestinal *amebiasis, giardiasis, trichomoniasis*). Metronidazole is only effective against obligate anaerobic bacteria (e.g., *Bacteroides fragilis, Clostridium difficile, Gardnerella vaginalis*).

Δ   Medication of choice for infections caused by anaerobic micro-organisms in the CNS, bones and joints, abdominal organs, skin, and soft tissues.

Δ   Used as prophylaxis for clients who will have surgical procedures and are high risk for anaerobic infection (e.g., vaginal, abdominal, colorectal surgery).

Δ   Used to treat *H. pylori* in clients with peptic ulcer disease in combination with use of tetracycline and bismuth salicylate.

Side/Adverse Effects: Nursing Interventions and Client Education

Side/Adverse Effects	Nursing Interventions/Client Education
Gastrointestinal discomfort (e.g., nausea, vomiting, dry mouth, **metallic taste**)	• Advise clients to observe for symptoms and to notify the primary care provider.
Darkening of urine	• Advise clients that this is a harmless effect of metronidazole.
CNS symptoms (e.g., numbness of extremities, ataxia, seizures)	• Advise clients to notify the primary care provider if symptoms occur. • Stop metronidazole.

Contraindications/Precautions

Δ   Use cautiously in clients with renal dysfunction to prevent accumulation of toxic levels with prolonged use.

Δ   Use should be avoided during the first trimester of pregnancy and used with caution during the rest of pregnancy because metronidazole can pass through the placenta.

Medication/Food Interactions: Nursing Interventions and Client Education

Medication/Food Interactions	Nursing Interventions/Client Education
Disulfiram-like reaction with **alcohol** ingestion	• Advise clients to avoid alcohol consumption.
Metronidazole – inhibits inactivation of warfarin	• Monitor prothrombin and INR, and adjust warfarin dosage accordingly.

Therapeutic Nursing Interventions and Client Education

Δ   Instruct the client to complete the prescribed course of antimicrobial therapy, even though symptoms may resolve before the full course is completed.

Nursing Evaluation of Medication Effectiveness

Δ   Improvement of symptoms (e.g., resolution of bloody mucoid diarrhea, formed stools, negative stool results for ameba and *Giardia*, ↓ or absence of watery vaginal/ urethral discharge, negative blood cultures for anaerobic organisms in the CNS, blood, bones and joints, and soft tissues).

Key Points

Medication Classification: Antifungals

Select Prototype Medication: **amphotericin B deoxycholate (Fungizone)**

Other Medications: ketoconazole (Nizoral), nystatin (clotrimazole)

Expected Pharmacological Action

Δ   Amphotericin B deoxycholate is an antifungal agent that acts on fungal cell membranes to ↑ cell permeability, which results in the leakage of intracellular cations leading to cell death. Depending on concentration, these agents can be fungistatic (slow growth on the fungus) or fungicidal (destroys the fungus).

Therapeutic Uses

Δ   Antifungals are the treatment of choice for systemic fungal infection, opportunistic mycoses (e.g., *Candidiasis, Aspergillosis, Cryptococcosis, Mucormycosis*), and nonopportunistic mycoses (e.g., *Blastomycosis, Histoplasmosis, Coccidioidomycosis*).

Δ   Ketoconazole is an antifungal used for the treatment of superficial fungal infections: dermatophytic infections (e.g. *tinea pedis* [ringworm of the foot], *tinea cruris* [ringworm of the groin]).

Side/Adverse Effects: Nursing Interventions and Client Education

Side/Adverse Effects	Nursing Interventions/Client Education
Infusion reactions (e.g., fever, chills, rigors, headache) 1 to 3 hr after initiation	• Pretreat with diphenhydramine (Benadryl) and aspirin. • Meperidine (Demerol) or dantrolene may also be given for rigors. • Hydrocortisone can be used in spite of its immunosuppressant effects if necessary. • Use lipid-based preparation of amphotericin B to minimize reactions.
Thrombophlebitis	• Observe infusion sites for signs of erythema, swelling, and pain. • Rotate injection sites. • Administer in a large vein and administer heparin before infusing amphotericin B.
Nephrotoxicity	• Obtain baseline kidney function (BUN, creatinine) and do weekly kidney function tests. • Monitor I&O. • Notify the primary care provider if there is a ↓ in urine output. • Infuse 1 L of saline on the day of amphotericin B infusion.
Hypokalemia	• Monitor electrolyte levels, especially potassium. • Administer potassium supplements accordingly.
Bone marrow suppression	• Obtain baseline CBC, hematocrit, and monitor weekly.
ketoconazole (Nizoral)	
Hepatotoxicity (e.g., anorexia, nausea, vomiting, jaundice, dark urine, clay-colored stools)	• Obtain baseline liver function studies and monitor liver function monthly. • Notify primary care provider if symptoms occur. • Stop ketoconazole.
Effects on sex hormones in males: **gynecomastia** (enlargement of breast); ↓ sex drive (libido); erectile dysfunction; in females, **irregular menstrual flow**	• Advise the client to observe for these symptoms and to notify the primary care provider.

Contraindications/Precautions

Δ   Antifungals are contraindicated in clients with renal dysfunction due to nephrotoxicity risk.

Medication/Food Interactions: Nursing Interventions and Client Education

Medication/Food Interactions	Nursing Interventions/Client Education
Aminoglycosides (e.g., gentamicin, streptomycin, cyclosporine) – additive nephrotoxic risk when used concurrently with antifungal medications.	• Avoid use of these antimicrobials when clients are taking amphotericin B due to additive nephrotoxicity risk.
Flucytosine – the antifungal effects of flucytosine are potentiated with concurrent use of amphotericin B.	• By potentiating the effects of flucytosine, it allows for a reduction in amphotericin B dosages.

Therapeutic Nursing Interventions and Client Education

Δ   Antifungals are highly toxic and should be reserved for severe life-threatening fungal infections.

Δ   The administration of amphotericin B should be infused slowly over 2 to 4 hr by intravenous route as oral preparation is poorly absorbed in the GI tract.

Δ   Observe solutions for precipitation and discard if precipitates are present.

Δ   Renal damage can be lessened with administration of 1 L saline solution on the day of amphotericin B infusion.

Δ   Instruct the client to complete the prescribed course of antimicrobial therapy, even though symptoms may resolve before the full course is completed.

Nursing Evaluation of Medication Effectiveness

Δ   Improvement of symptoms (e.g., clear breath sounds and negative chest x-rays for fungal lesions).

Primary Reference:

Lehne, R. A. (2007). *Pharmacology for nursing care*. (6th ed.). St. Louis, MO: Saunders.

Additional Resources:

Freeman, J., Queener, S., & Karb, V. (2000). *Pharmacologic basis of nursing practice* (6th ed.). St Louis, MO: Mosby.

Kee, J., Hayes, E., & McCuistion, L. (2005). *Pharmacology: A nursing process approach* (5th ed.). St. Louis, MO: Saunders.

Unit 2 Medications Used to Treat Infection

Application Exercises

Scenario: A client comes to a community clinic complaining of a fever, sore throat, and cough. The client's posterior pharynx is reddened with patches of purulent exudate, and the client states that she experiences pain with swallowing. Her cervical lymph nodes are enlarged and tender to touch. The client's vital signs are: temperature 38.5° C (101.4° F) orally; pulse 96/min; respirations 22/min; and blood pressure 122/84 mm Hg. Based on the symptoms and physical examination, the primary care provider suspects a streptococcal infection, which is confirmed by a quick strep test performed in the clinic. The client is started on amoxicillin-clavulanate (Augmentin) 500 mg orally every 8 hr for 10 days.

1. Before administering the first dose of amoxicillin-clavulanate (Augmentin), what additional assessment data should the nurse collect?

2. When instructing the client on the use of amoxicillin-clavulanate (Augmentin), what should the nurse tell the client is most important?

3. After the first two doses, the client calls and states that she is experiencing an itchy rash. What should the nurse tell the client?

4. The client returns to the clinic and the primary care provider discontinues amoxicillin-clavulanate (Augmentin) and starts the client on cephalexin (Keflex), 250 mg orally every 6 hr for 10 days. The provider provides samples so the client can begin taking the medication immediately. What nursing intervention should the nurse follow? Explain.

Scenario: A client comes to the clinic stating that she has been taking trimethoprim-sulfamethoxazole (Bactrim) for a bladder infection. The client is concerned because she has developed intense perineal itching and a whitish, cheese-like vaginal discharge. She is visiting an out-of-state relative and prefers to see her primary care provider, but cannot wait because the itching is unbearable.

5. How should the nurse respond to the client's concern? What action should the nurse anticipate from the primary care provider?

6. What teaching should the nurse provide to the client to minimize the side effects of Bactrim?

Scenario: A man comes to the clinic complaining of frequency and burning during urination for the past 2 days. A preliminary urinalysis reveals that the urine is cloudy with moderate sediment and ↑ white blood cells. The specimen is sent to the laboratory for a culture and sensitivity test. The primary care provider prescribes nitrofurantoin (Furadantin).

7. Why did the provider choose this particular medication?

8. What client teaching should the nurse provide to the client taking nitrofurantoin?

9. Match the medication of choice for each of the following infections.

Client undergoing colorectal surgery and at risk for anaerobic infection D

Serious systemic fungal infection G

Herpes simplex virus and varicella zoster E

Tuberculosis A

Urinary tract infection B

Serious gram-negative infection F C

Prophylaxis bacterial endocarditis for client allergic to penicillin C F

Acne vulgaris, Lyme disease, and gastrointestinal disease caused by H. pylori H

A. Isoniazid (INH)

B. Trimethoprim-sulfamethoxazole (Bactrim)

C. Gentamicin (Garamycin)

D. Metronidazole (Flagyl)

E. Acyclovir (Zovirax)

F. Erythromycin (E-Mycin)

G. Amphotericin B (Fungizone)

H. Tetracycline hydrochloride (Sumycin)

Unit 2 Medications Used to Treat Infection

Application Exercises Answer Key

Scenario: A client comes to a community clinic complaining of a fever, sore throat, and cough. The client's posterior pharynx is reddened with patches of purulent exudate, and the client states that she experiences pain with swallowing. Her cervical lymph nodes are enlarged and tender to touch. The client's vital signs are: temperature 38.5° C (101.4° F) orally; pulse 96/min; respirations 22/min; and blood pressure 122/84 mm Hg. Based on the symptoms and physical examination, the primary care provider suspects a streptococcal infection, which is confirmed by a quick strep test performed in the clinic. The client is started on amoxicillin-clavulanate (Augmentin) 500 mg orally every 8 hr for 10 days.

1. Before administering the first dose of amoxicillin-clavulanate (Augmentin), what additional assessment data should the nurse collect?

   The nurse should inquire if the client has ever had a reaction to a previous antibiotic, especially if the antibiotic was a penicillin product.

2. When instructing the client on the use of amoxicillin-clavulanate (Augmentin), what should the nurse tell the client is most important?

   Be sure to take the medication with food to avoid gastrointestinal discomfort. Finish taking all of the medication as prescribed, even if the condition improves. Failure to complete a course of antibiotics can result in development of resistant strains of organisms. The client should be advised to never share this medication because some individuals may be allergic to penicillin and may develop a serious reaction. The client should report any signs or symptoms of allergic reaction to the primary care provider.

3. After the first two doses, the client calls and states that she is experiencing an itchy rash. What should the nurse tell the client?

   The nurse should first assess if the client has any other adverse symptoms or is experiencing any difficulty breathing. If so, advise the client to call 9-1-1 immediately. If symptoms are not life-threatening, advise the client to stop taking the medication immediately and come to the clinic for further evaluation.

4. The client returns to the clinic and the primary care provider discontinues amoxicillin-clavulanate (Augmentin) and starts the client on cephalexin (Keflex), 250 mg orally every 6 hr for 10 days. The provider provides samples so the client can begin taking the medication immediately. What nursing intervention should the nurse follow? Explain.

The client should take the first dose and then sit in the waiting room for approximately 30 min. After 30 min, the nurse can assess the client for any possible allergic responses. Cephalosporins have a cross-sensitivity with penicillin medications, so the nurse should ensure that the client is safe. The nurse should carefully document the client's condition prior to sending the client home and consider making a follow-up call to see how the client is doing. Instruct the client to report any further signs or symptoms of allergic reaction immediately to the primary care provider.

Scenario: A client comes to the clinic stating that she has been taking trimethoprim-sulfamethoxazole (Bactrim) for a bladder infection. The client is concerned because she has developed intense perineal itching and a whitish, cheese-like vaginal discharge. She is visiting an out-of-state relative and prefers to see her primary care provider, but cannot wait because the itching is unbearable.

5. How should the nurse respond to the client's concern? What action should the nurse anticipate from the primary care provider?

Inform her that this is a common side effect of antibiotics. The normal bacteria in the body have been altered by the antibiotic, allowing a suprainfection to develop. Most superinfections are fungal in nature. Therefore, the primary care provider will most likely prescribe an antifungal agent, either prescription or over-the-counter.

6. What teaching should the nurse provide to the client to minimize the side effects of Bactrim?

Drink an adequate amount of fluids to maintain a urine output of at least 1,200 to 1,500 mL daily to prevent crystalluria and stone formation. To prevent photosensitivity reactions, avoid direct sunlight and ultraviolet light, and use a sunscreen and protective clothing when going outdoors. If a skin rash, fever, sore throat, mouth sores, unusual bleeding, or bruising develop, notify the primary care provider.

Scenario: A man comes to the clinic complaining of frequency and burning during urination for the past 2 days. A preliminary urinalysis reveals that the urine is cloudy with moderate sediment and ↑ white blood cells. The specimen is sent to the laboratory for a culture and sensitivity test. The primary care provider prescribes nitrofurantoin (Furadantin).

7. Why did the provider choose this particular medication?

Nitrofurantoin (Furadantin) is an antimicrobial agent that achieves good concentration in the urine and is effective against common bacterial pathogens.

8. What client teaching should the nurse provide to the client taking nitrofurantoin?

Warn the client taking nitrofurantoin that the medication may cause urine to appear a rust-brown color. If the client experiences dyspnea, cough, or malaise, he should stop taking the nitrofurantoin, and notify the primary care provider. If the client experiences fever, sore throat, unusual bleeding, numbness and tingling of hands and feet, instruct him to notify the primary care provider.

9. Match the medication of choice for each of the following infections.

Client undergoing colorectal surgery and at risk for anaerobic infection	A. Isoniazid (INH)
Serious systemic fungal infection	B. Trimethoprim-sulfamethoxazole (Bactrim)
Herpes simplex virus and varicella-zoster	C. Gentamicin (Garamycin)
Tuberculosis	D. Metronidazole (Flagyl)
Urinary tract infection	E. Acyclovir (Zovirax)
Serious gram-negative infection	F. Erythromycin (E-Mycin)
Prophylaxis bacterial endocarditis for client allergic to penicillin	G. Amphotericin B (Fungizone)
Acne vulgaris, Lyme disease, and gastrointestinal disease caused by *H. pylori*	H. Tetracycline hydrochloride (Sumycin)

Client undergoing colorectal surgery and at risk for anaerobic infection, D; serious systemic fungal infection, G; herpes simplex virus and varicella-zoster, E; tuberculosis, A; urinary tract infection, B; serious gram-negative infection, C; prophylaxis bacterial endocarditis for client allergic to penicillin, F; acne vulgaris, Lyme disease, and gastrointestinal disease caused by H. pylori, H.

Unit 3   Medications Affecting the Immune System

Contributor: Havovi Patel, MS, MBBS

 NCLEX® Connections:

> **Learning Objective:** Review and apply knowledge within **"Medications Affecting the Immune System"** in readiness for performance of the following nursing activities as outlined by the NCLEX® test plans:
>
> Δ   Assess/monitor the client for expected effects of medications/immunizations.
>
> Δ   Assess/monitor the client for side/adverse effects of medications/immunizations.
>
> Δ   Assess/monitor the client for actual/potential specific food and medication interactions.
>
> Δ   Identify contraindications, actual/potential incompatibilities, and interactions between medications/immunizations, and intervene appropriately.
>
> Δ   Identify symptoms/evidence of an allergic reaction, and respond appropriately.
>
> Δ   Evaluate/monitor and document the therapeutic and adverse/side effects of medications/immunizations.
>
> Δ   Provide/reinforce client teaching on actions, therapeutic effects, potential side/ adverse effects and interactions of medications/immunizations.
>
> Δ   Evaluate a client's immunization status and recognize the need for immunizations based on current immunization guidelines.

 General Key Points

Δ   The immune system protects the body from the invasion of different micro-organisms (e.g., bacteria, viruses, fungi, parasites) by inactivating, removing, or destroying the pathogenic antigens produced by the different micro-organisms, thus protecting the body from disease.

Δ   The body's immune system responds in two ways:

- **Natural immunity or innate-native immunity** is present at birth. Protection is provided by physical barriers against the different micro-organisms. Physical barriers include the skin, mucous membranes, phagocytic cells, and the natural killer cells.

- **Specific acquired immunity** is a response made by the individual's own body producing antibodies to protect itself from the antigens of the invading micro-organisms and/or from immunization.

- **Acquired immunity** can occur in two ways: **active** (having the infection or by the administration of a vaccine or toxoid) and **passive** (administration of preformed antibodies such as immunoglobulins).

- Passive immunity agents such as immunoglobulins have an immediate onset. Active immunity agents such as vaccines may take weeks to months to take effect.

Δ   Major cells of the immune system include:

- **B lymphocytes or B cells** – produce antibodies (e.g., IgA, IgD, IgG, IgE, IgM).

- **Helper T lymphocytes or CD 4 cells** – activate B cells and are responsible for the delayed hypersensitivity reaction.

- **Cytolytic T lymphocytes or CD 8 cells** – destroy target cells directly causing death of the micro-organism.

- **Macrophages and dendritic cells** – phagocytosis.

- **Immunosuppressants** – reduce the proliferation of B cells and cytotoxic T cells.

- **Immunostimulants** – boost the immune system and can assist the body in killing off cancer cells.

Key Points

Medication Classification: Childhood Immunizations

Δ   **Select Prototype Medication and CDC 2006 recommendation for administration** *(See www.cdc.gov for updates.)*:

- **Hepatitis B**: doses at birth, 1 to 2 months, and 6 to 18 months

- **Diphtheria and tetanus toxoids and pertussis vaccine (DTaP)**: doses at 2, 4, 6, 15 to 18 months, and at 4 to 6 years

- **Tetanus and diphtheria toxoids and pertussis vaccine (Tdap)**: 11 to 12 years

- **Tetanus and diphtheria (Td) booster**: every 10 years following DTaP

- **Haemophilus influenza Type B (Hib)**: doses at 2, 4, 6, and at 12 to 15 months

- **Inactivated poliovirus vaccine (IPV)**: doses at 2, 4, 6 to 18 months, and at 4 to 6 years

- **Measles, mumps and rubella vaccine (MMR)**: doses at 12 to 15 months and at 4 to 6 years

- **Varicella vaccine**: single dose at 12 to 18 months or 2 doses administered 4 weeks apart if administered after age 13

- **Pneumococcal conjugate vaccine (PCV)**: doses at 2, 4, 6, and 12 to 15 months

- **Hepatitis A**: 2 doses 6 months apart after age 12 months

- **Influenza vaccine**: annually beginning at age 6 months (October through November ideal time, December is acceptable)

- **Meningococcal vaccine (MCV4)**: a dose at age 11 to 12 years (earlier if specific risk factors)

Expected Pharmacological Action

Δ   Immunizations produce antibodies that provide active immunity. Immunizations may take months to have an effect but confer long-lasting protection against infectious diseases.

Therapeutic Uses

Δ   Eradication of infectious diseases (e.g., polio, smallpox)

Δ   Prevention of childhood infectious diseases and their complications (e.g., measles, diphtheria, mumps, rubella, tetanus, H. influenza)

Side/Adverse Effects: Nursing Interventions and Client Education

Δ   Advise the client to observe for the following side/adverse effects and to report their occurrence to the primary care provider.

Side/Adverse Effects	
MMR	• Local reactions (e.g., rash, fever, swollen glands in cheeks, neck, pain under the jaw) • Anaphylaxis such as difficulty breathing, urticaria, thrombocytopenia, and low platelet count with bruising
DTaP	• Encephalopathy (e.g., fever, irritability, persistent crying that cannot be consoled), seizures, and/or local reaction at the site of injection (e.g., pain, swelling, redness)
IPV	• Vaccine-associated paralytic poliomyelitis and/or local reaction (e.g., pain, redness, swelling)
Hepatitis A&B vaccines	• Local reaction (e.g., anorexia, soreness, fatigue) • Anaphylaxis
Varicella vaccine	• Varicella-like rash, local or generalized (e.g., vesicles on the body)
Pneumococcal vaccine	• Mild local reaction, fever, and no serious adverse effects
Influenza vaccine	• Guillain-Barré syndrome (e.g., ascending paralysis, weakness of lower extremities, difficulty breathing), local reaction, and fever
Meningococcal vaccine	• Mild local reaction and rare risk of allergic response

Contraindications/Precautions

Δ   **MMR** is contraindicated:

•   In pregnant women and children who are allergic to eggs, gelatin, and neomycin.

•   In clients who have a history of thrombocytopenia or thrombocytopenic purpura.

•   In immunocompromised children.

•   In clients with advanced HIV.

•   For clients who recently received blood products or immunoglobulins.

Δ   **DTaP** is contraindicated in children with:

•   Severe febrile illness.

•   A history of prior anaphylactic reaction to the DTaP vaccination.

•   An occurrence of encephalopathy 7 days after the administration of the DTaP immunization.

- An occurrence of seizures within 3 days of the vaccination.

- Uncontrollable crying that cannot be consoled by parents/caregiver. This crying usually lasts more than 3 hr and occurs within 48 hr of the vaccination.

Δ **Hepatitis B** is contraindicated in clients with:

- A prior history of anaphylactic reaction.

- An allergy to Baker's yeast.

Δ **Varicella virus vaccine** is contraindicated:

- For women who are pregnant.

- For clients with cancer.

- For clients with a history of allergy to neomycin and/or gelatin.

- For immunocompromised clients, such as those who have HIV.

- For children with congenital immunodeficiency.

- For clients taking immunosuppressive medications.

Δ **Influenza vaccine is contraindicated** in clients with:

- Acute febrile illness – defer vaccination until symptoms resolve.

- Hypersensitivity to eggs (vaccine is grown in eggs and may contain small amounts of egg proteins) – conduct a skin test prior to administration.

Therapeutic Nursing Interventions and Client Education

Δ Note the date, route, and site of vaccination on the client's immunization record at the time of immunization.

Δ Follow storage and reconstitution directions. If reconstituted, use within 30 min.

Δ In infants and young children, intramuscular vaccinations are given in the vastus lateralis muscle. For older children, adolescents, and adults, vaccinations are given in the deltoid muscle.

Δ Consult the Centers for Disease Control and Prevention for the most current recommended immunization schedule.

Δ Inform the client of possible side/adverse effects, and instruct the client to notify the primary care provider if serious adverse effects occur.

Δ Instruct parents to avoid administration of aspirin to children to treat fever following varicella immunization due to the risk of the development of Reye syndrome.

Δ   There is a small risk of the varicella vaccine virus being transmitted. If a child develops a rash following the vaccination, measures should be taken to protect any pregnant woman and others at risk from exposure, such as those who are immunocompromised.

Δ   Occurrence of vaccine-preventable diseases should be reported to the state or local health department.

Nursing Evaluation of Medication Effectiveness

Δ   Improvement of local reaction to vaccination with absence of pain, fever, and swelling at the site of infection

Key Points

Medication Classification: Adult Immunizations

Δ   **Select Prototype Medication and CDC 2006 recommendation for administration:**

- **Influenza vaccine**: one dose annually after age 50 (earlier if specific risk factors such as chronic disease)

- **Pneumococcal polysaccharide vaccine (PPV)**: one dose at age 65 (earlier if specific risk factors), and revaccinate every 6 to 8 years after initial vaccination

- **Meningococcal vaccine (MCV4)**: students entering college and living in college dormitories if not previously immunized

- **Tetanus diphtheria (Td) booster**: every 10 years

Expected Pharmacological Action

Δ   Adult immunizations prevent infectious diseases through the production of antibodies that provide active immunity.

Therapeutic Uses

Δ   Prevention of infectious diseases and their complications (e.g., pneumonia, tetanus, *H. influenza*)

Side/Adverse Effects: Nursing Interventions and Client Education

Δ   Side/adverse effect include:

- Local reaction (e.g., erythema, swelling, pain) at injection site

- Occurrence of low-grade fever: antipyretic treatment

- Rare risk of systemic allergic reaction (e.g., urticaria, anaphylaxis)

- Influenza vaccine: small risk of Guillain-Barré syndrome

Δ   Contraindications/precautions for the influenza vaccine include:

- Acute febrile illness – defer vaccination until symptoms resolve.

- Hypersensitivity to eggs (vaccine grown in eggs and may contain small amounts of egg proteins) – conduct a skin test prior to administration.

Therapeutic Nursing Interventions and Client Education

Δ   Administer IM vaccines deep in the deltoid muscle.

Δ   Have emergency medications and equipment on standby in case the client experiences an allergic response such as anaphylaxis (rare).

Δ   Note the date, route, and site of vaccination on the client's immunization record at the time of immunization.

Δ   Consult the Centers for Disease Control and Prevention for the most current recommended immunization schedule.

Δ   Inform the client of possible side/adverse effects, and instruct the client to notify the primary care provider if serious adverse effects occur.

Nursing Evaluation of Medication Effectiveness

Δ   No development of infectious disease or serious complications

Key Points

Medication Classification: Immune Globulin

Select Prototype Medication: **Gamma globulin,**
                                         Immunoglobulin G (IgG)

Expected Pharmacological Action

Δ   Immune globulins provide **passive immunity** and provide gamma globulin antibodies.

Therapeutic Uses

Δ   Immunodeficiency syndrome

Δ   Chronic lymphocytic leukemia

Δ   Bone marrow transplantation

Δ   Hepatitis A, hepatitis B exposure

Δ   Measles, rubella, and chickenpox exposure

Side/Adverse Effects: Nursing Interventions and Client Education

Δ   Side/adverse effect include:

•   Local reaction (e.g., erythema, swelling, pain) at injection site

•   Rare risk of systemic allergic reaction (e.g., urticaria, anaphylaxis)

Δ   Contraindications/precautions include:

•   Pregnancy and lactation (Risk category C)

•   Hypersensitivity to medication (previous administration)

Medication/Food Interactions: Nursing Interventions and Client Education

Medication/Food Interactions	Nursing Interventions/Client Education
Live viruses – can lead to disease	• Instruct the client not to have live viruses administered within 3 months of IgG.

Therapeutic Nursing Interventions and Client Education

Δ   Administer IM deep in a large muscle. IV administration is controlled and slow, and rates are based on the client's weight.

Δ   Instruct the client that passive immunity is temporary.

Δ   If the medication is the treatment following disease exposure, identify the date of exposure. IgG should be given within 6 days of measles exposure, 7 days of hepatitis B exposure, and within 14 days of hepatitis A exposure.

Δ   Have emergency medications and equipment on standby in case the client experiences an allergic response such as anaphylaxis (rare).

Nursing Evaluation of Medication Effectiveness

Δ   Medication effectiveness as evidenced by prevention of infection and ↑ platelets

Key Points

Medication Classification: Immunostimulants

Select Prototype Medication: **Interferon Alfa, Aldesleukin (Interleukin-2)**

Expected Pharmacological Action

Δ   Immunostimulants enhance host immune responses and reduce proliferation of cancer cells.

Therapeutic Uses

Δ   Hairy cell leukemia

Δ   Chronic myelogenous leukemia

Δ   Malignant melanoma

Δ   AIDS-related Kaposi's sarcoma

Side/Adverse Effects: Nursing Interventions and Client Education

Side/Adverse Effects	Nursing Interventions/Client Education
Flu-like symptoms (e.g., fever, fatigue, headache, chills, myalgia)	• Administer acetaminophen.
Bone marrow suppression, alopecia, cardiotoxicity, and neurotoxicity (prolonged therapy)	• Monitor CBC, fatigue level, and signs of cardiotoxicity/neurotoxicity. • Monitor the client for signs of infection. • Instruct the client to report dizziness or tingling/numbness of the hands or feet. • Monitor for bruising, bleeding, blood in stools, urine, sputum, or emesis.
Hypotension	• Perform a baseline blood pressure prior to administration. • Monitor blood pressure following administration. • Encourage the client to change positions slowly.

Contraindications/Precautions

- Δ Hypersensitivity to medications (previous administration)

- Δ Pregnancy and lactation (Risk category C)

Medication/Food Interactions: Nursing Interventions and Client Education

Medication/Food Interactions	Nursing Interventions/Client Education
Theophylline (Theo-Dur) – concurrent use can lead to theophylline toxicity.	• Monitor the client for signs of theophylline toxicity. A ↓ in theophylline dosage may be indicated.
Zidovudine (Retrovir) – ↑ the risk of neutropenia	• Monitor the client for ↑ the risk of neutropenia.
Antihypertensives – additive hypotensive effect	• Monitor the client for additive hypotension.

Therapeutic Nursing Interventions and Client Education

- Δ Store the medication in the refrigerator and do not freeze. Administer at room temperature. Do not shake the vial.

- Δ Administer subcutaneously or intramuscularly as prescribed.

Nursing Evaluation of Medication Effectiveness

- Δ Signs of medication effectiveness such as ↓ cell proliferation

Key Points

Medication Classification: Immunosuppressants

Select Prototype Medication: Calcineurin inhibitors: **cyclosporine (Sandimmune, Gengraf, Neoral)**
Glucocorticoids: **prednisone**
Cytotoxics: **azathioprine (Imuran)**

Other Medications: tacrolimus (Prograf), methotrexate (Rheumatrex, Trexall)

Expected Pharmacological Action

Δ   Immunosuppressants act on helper T lymphocytes to suppress production of immune response components, resulting in the suppression of the proliferation of B cells and cytotoxic T cells.

Therapeutic Uses

Δ   Immunosuppressants are used for the treatment of autoimmune disorders (e.g., rheumatoid arthritis, systemic lupus erythematosus, myasthenia gravis, early type 1 diabetes mellitus).

Δ   Immunosuppressants are used to prevent organ rejection in transplant clients (e.g., kidney, liver, and heart transplants). **Lifelong therapy** is necessary to prevent organ rejection.

Side/Adverse Effects: Nursing Interventions and Client Education

Side/Adverse Effects	Nursing Interventions/Client Education
Teratogenesis (Pregnancy Risk Category C)	• Advise the client to avoid use during pregnancy and lactation. • Use contraception measures during medication use.
↑ risk of infection such as fever and/or sore throat	• Advise the client if symptoms occur to notify the primary care provider immediately.
Cyclosporine	
Hepatotoxicity such as jaundice	• Monitor liver function and adjust dosage.
Nephrotoxicity	• Monitor BUN and creatinine. • Measure I&O.
Glucocorticoid	
Osteoporosis	• Monitor bone loss. • Use calcium and vitamin D supplements.
Adrenal insufficiency	• Instruct the client not to stop immunosuppressants abruptly.
Fluid retention	• Monitor for signs of fluid excess (e.g., crackles, weight gain, edema).
Cytotoxic	
Bone marrow depression	• Monitor for neutropenia and thrombocytopenia. • Take precautionary measures.

Contraindications/Precautions

Δ   Cyclosporine is contraindicated in the following situations:

- Pregnancy.

- Recent vaccination with live virus vaccines.

- Recent contact or active infection of chickenpox or herpes zoster.

Δ   Glucocorticoids are contraindicated in the following situations:

- Systemic fungal infections.

- Recurring live virus vaccines (↑ risk of infection).

Medication/Food Interactions: Nursing Interventions and Client Education

Medication/Food Interactions	Nursing Interventions/Client Education
Cyclosporine	
Phenytoin, phenobarbital, rifampin, carbamazepine, and trimethoprim-sulfamethoxazole – cyclosporine level is ↓ with concurrent use of these medications. ↓ can lead to organ rejection.	• Monitor the client's cyclosporine levels and adjust dosage accordingly.
Ketoconazole, erythromycin, and amphotericin B – cyclosporine level is ↑ with concurrent use of these medications, leading to toxicity.	• Monitor cyclosporine dosage and adjust accordingly to prevent toxicity.
Amphotericin B, aminoglycoside, and NSAIDs – all of these medications are nephrotoxic, and concurrent use with cyclosporine ↑ the risk for renal dysfunction.	• Monitor BUN, creatinine, and I&O.
Grapefruit juice – consumption of grapefruit juice ↑ cyclosporine levels by 50%, which poses an ↑ risk of toxicity.	• Advise the client to avoid drinking grapefruit juice.
Glucocorticoids	
Potassium-depleting diuretics – ↑ the risk of hypokalemia.	• Monitor the client's potassium level and administer supplements as needed.
NSAIDs – ↑ the risk of GI ulceration.	• Advise the client to avoid use of NSAIDs. If GI distress occurs, instruct the client to notify the primary care provider.
Glucocorticoids – promote hyperglycemia, thereby counteracting the effects of insulin and oral hypoglycemics	• May need to ↑ dose of hypoglycemic medications.
Azathioprine	
Allopurinol – allopurinol delays the inactivation of azathioprine.	• If taken concurrently, ↓ doses of azathioprine are indicated.

Therapeutic Nursing Interventions and Client Education

Δ   Administer initial dose of cyclosporine over 2 to 6 hr.

Δ   Monitor clients for hypersensitivity reactions. Stay with the client for 30 min after administration of cyclosporine.

Δ   Mix oral cyclosporine with milk or orange juice right before ingestion to ↑ palatability.

Δ   Instruct the client regarding the importance of lifelong therapy to prevent organ rejection.

Δ   Instruct the client to promptly report signs of organ rejection. ↑ doses of immunosuppressants are indicated during periods of organ rejection.

Nursing Evaluation of Medication Effectiveness

Δ   Improvement of symptoms (e.g., absence of signs of organ rejection, ↓ swelling, or absence of joint pain)

Key Points

Medication Classification: Antihistamines

Select Prototype Medication: 1st generation H_1 antagonists: **diphenhydramine (Benadryl), promethazine (Phenergan), and dimenhydrinate (Dramamine)**
2nd generation H_1 antagonists: **loratadine (Claritin), cetirizine (Zyrtec), fexofenadine (Allegra), and desloratadine (Clarinex)**

Expected Pharmacological Action and Therapeutic Uses

Δ   Antihistamine action is on the H_1 receptors, which results in the blocking of histamine release in the small blood vessels, capillaries, and nerves during allergic reactions.

Therapeutic Uses

Δ   1st generation H_1 antagonists are used for:

- Mild allergic reactions (e.g., seasonal allergic rhinitis, urticaria, mild transfusion reaction).

- Anaphylaxis (e.g., hypotension, acute laryngeal edema, bronchospasm).

- Motion sickness.

- Insomnia.

Side/Adverse Effects: Nursing Interventions and Client Education

Side/Adverse Effects	Nursing Interventions/Client Education
1st generation H₁ antagonists	
Sedation	• Advise the client to take the medication at night to minimize daytime sedative effect. • Avoid driving, hazardous activities, consumption of alcohol, and other CNS depressant medications (e.g., barbiturates, benzodiazepines, opioids).
Anticholinergic effects (e.g., dry mouth, constipation)	• Advise the client to take sips of water, suck on sugarless candies, and ↑ fluid intake.
Gastrointestinal discomfort (e.g., nausea, vomiting, constipation)	• Advise clients to take antihistamine with meals.
Acute toxicity (e.g., flushed face, high fever, tachycardia, dry mouth, urinary retention): Children have symptoms of excitation, hallucinations, incoordination and seizures.	• Advise the client to notify the primary care provider if symptoms occur. • Induce vomiting to remove the antihistamine. • Administer activated charcoal and cathartic to ↓ absorption of antihistamine. • Administer acetaminophen for fever. • Apply ice packs or sponge baths.

Contraindications/Precautions

Δ   Antihistamines are contraindicated during the third trimester of pregnancy, for mothers who are breastfeeding, and for newborns. Newborns are sensitive to the adverse effects, such as sedation, of these medications.

Δ   Use cautiously in children and older adults (impact of adverse effects).

Δ   Use cautiously in clients who have asthma, urinary retention, open angle glaucoma, hypertension, and prostate hypertrophy (impact of anticholinergic medications).

Δ   Medication/Food Interactions: Nursing Interventions and Client Education

Medication/Food Interactions	Nursing Interventions/Client Education
CNS depressants/alcohol – additive CNS depression	• Advise clients to avoid alcohol and medications causing CNS depression such as opioids, barbiturates, and benzodiazepines.

Nursing Evaluation of Medication Effectiveness

Δ   Depending on therapeutic intent, effectiveness may be evidenced by:

•   Improvement of allergic reaction (e.g., absence of rhinitis, urticaria).

•   Relief of symptoms of motion sickness (e.g., decreased nausea and vomiting).

Key Points

Medication Classification: Chemotherapy Agents

Select Prototype Medication:

Nitrogen mustards: **cyclophosphamide (Cytoxan, Neosar)**
Platinum compounds: **cisplatin (Platinol AQ)**
Folic acid analog: **methotrexate (Rheumatrex, Trexall)**
Pyrimidine analog: **cytarabine (Cytosar-U)**
Purine analogs: **mercaptopurine (Purinethol)**
Antitumor antibiotics: **doxorubicin (Adriamycin, Rubex)**
Mitotic inhibitors: **vincristine (Oncovin), paclitaxel (Taxol, Onxol)**
Topoisomerase inhibitors: **topotecan (Hycamtin), irinotecan (Camptosar)**
Cytotoxic medications: **asparaginase (Elspar), hydroxyurea (Hydrea), and procarbazine (Matulane)**
Breast cancer: **Antiestrogen: tamoxifen (Nolvadex)**
Prostate cancer: **leuprolide (Lupron)**
Progestins: **megestrol acetate (Megace)**

Expected Pharmacological Action

Δ Anticancer chemotherapeutic agents destroy cancer cells, as well as healthy cells, by preventing the replication of DNA.

Therapeutic Uses

Δ Chemotherapy agents are used in the treatment of a variety of cancers (e.g., leukemias, lymphomas, choriocarcinomas, testicular carcinoma).

Side/Adverse Effects: Nursing Interventions and Client Education

Side/Adverse Effects	Nursing Interventions/Client Education
Bone marrow suppression, such as low white blood cell count or neutropenia, bleeding caused by thrombocytopenia or low platelet count, and anemia or low red blood cells	• Monitor WBC, absolute neutrophil count, platelet count, hemoglobin, and hematocrit. • Assess the client for bruising and bleeding gums. • Instruct the client to avoid crowds and contact with infectious individuals.
Gastrointestinal discomfort, such as nausea and vomiting	• **Administer antiemetic** such as ondansetron (Zofran) in combination with dexamethasone, granisetron (Kytril), or metoclopramide (Reglan) before beginning chemotherapy.
Alopecia	• **Advise clients that hair loss will occur 7 to 10 days after the beginning of treatment and will last for a maximum duration of 2 months after the last administration of the chemotherapeutic agent.** • **Advise clients to select a hairpiece before the occurrence of hair loss.**
Mucositis (GI tract)	• Assess the client's mouth for sores. • Provide frequent oral hygiene using soft toothbrushes and avoiding alcohol mouthwashes.
Reproductive toxicity, such as congenital abnormalities, amenorrhea, menopausal symptoms and atrophy of vaginal epithelium, and sterility in males	• Advise female clients against becoming pregnant while taking these medications. • Advise male clients to consider sperm banking prior to treatment.
Hyperuricemia or elevated levels of uric acid may cause renal damage	• Monitor kidney function, BUN, and creatinine. • ↑ fluid intake and measure I&O. • Administer allopurinol if uric acid level is elevated.
Extravasations of vesicants such as carmustine, dactinomycin, daunorubicin, and vincristine	• Stop chemotherapeutic medications if extravasation occurs. • Only clinically trained personnel should give these medications intravenously.

Therapeutic Nursing Interventions and Client Education

Δ   Dosage for chemotherapeutic agents should be individualized.

Δ   Personnel preparing and administering chemotherapeutic agents should follow safe handling procedures.

Δ   If a chemotherapy spill occurs, follow institutional procedures. Generally, small spills can be handled by following procedures and using supplies contained in a chemo spill kit (e.g., goggles, mask, protective clothing, shoe covers, absorbent pads, detergent cleansers, and chemo waste disposal bags). For large spills, contact the Occupational & Environmental Safety Office (OESO).

Nursing Evaluation of Medication Effectiveness

Δ   Cessation of cancer cell growth and improvement of cancer symptoms

Primary Reference:

Lehne, R. A. (2007). *Pharmacology for nursing care* (6th ed.). St. Louis, MO: Saunders.

Additional Resources:

For information about disease control and prevention, go to the Centers for Disease Control and Prevention Web site: *http://www.cdc.gov/index.htm*.

Ignatavicius, D. D., & Workman, L. M. (2005). *Medical surgical nursing: Critical thinking for collaborative care* (5th ed.). St. Louis, MO: Saunders.

Unit 3 Medications Affecting the Immune System

Application Exercises

1. In which of the following situations is administration of a tetanus diphtheria (Td) booster indicated? (Select all that apply.)

   _____ Finger wound from knife injury while slicing vegetables

   _____ Foot injury from stepping on a nail

   _____ Dog bite injury

   _____ Scald burn injury

   _____ Last tetanus booster 5 years ago

   _____ Compound fracture

   _____ Last tetanus booster 9 years ago

   _____ Last tetanus booster 12 years ago

2. What cautionary measures should be taken when immunizing individuals with an MMR vaccine who have recently received a blood transfusion?

3. Identify which of the following medications has the ability to cause immunosuppression. (Select all that apply.)

   _____ Prednisone

   _____ Azathioprine

   _____ Cyclosporine

   _____ Diphenhydramine (Benadryl)

   _____ Tetanus diphtheria (Td) booster

   _____ loratadine (Claritin)

   _____ Chemotherapy agents

4. In which of the following situations is the administration of a dose of DTaP contraindicated? (Select all that apply.)

   _____ Severe febrile illness

   _____ History of prior anaphylactic reaction to DTaP vaccination

   _____ Occurrence of encephalopathy 7 days after administration of DTaP immunization

   _____ Occurrence of seizures within 3 days of previous vaccination

   _____ Report of low-grade fever occurring within 24 hr of previous DTaP dose

5. Why is it preferable to give the varicella vaccine in childhood rather than in adulthood?

6. What precautions should be taken for a client who has just received a kidney transplant and is taking cyclosporine and phenytoin?

7. What measures need to be taken to reduce development of osteoporosis during steroid therapy?

8. Why is it important that children receiving the varicella vaccine avoid aspirin and salicylates for 6 weeks?

Unit 3 Medications Affecting the Immune System

Application Exercises Answer Key

1. In which of the following situations is administration of a tetanus diphtheria (Td) booster indicated? (Select all that apply.)

_____	Finger wound from knife injury while slicing vegetables
__X__	**Foot injury from stepping on a nail**
__X__	**Dog bite injury**
_____	Scald burn injury
_____	Last tetanus booster 5 years ago
__X__	**Compound fracture**
_____	Last tetanus booster 9 years ago
__X__	**Last tetanus booster 12 years ago**

A foot injury from stepping on a nail, a dog bite injury, a compound fracture, and a tetanus booster received 12 years ago, are all indications for administration of a tetanus booster. Clean, incised, and scald injuries are at low risk for tetanus. Untreated wounds or burns more than 6 hr old, puncture wounds, animal/human bites, compound fractures, wounds that came in contact with soil or manure, and wounds with large amounts of devitalized tissue pose a high risk for tetanus.

2. What cautionary measures should be taken when immunizing individuals with an MMR vaccine who have recently received a blood transfusion?

For individuals who have received immune globulins, such as whole blood, serum, and specific immune globulins, the MMR vaccine should be postponed 3 to 6 months. Immune globulins contain antibodies against viruses in MMR that inhibit the immune response to the vaccine.

3. Identify which of the following medications has the ability to cause immunosuppression? (Select all that apply.)

__X__	**Prednisone**
__X__	**Azathioprine**
__X__	**Cyclosporine**
_____	Diphenhydramine (Benadryl)
_____	Tetanus diphtheria (Td) booster
_____	Loratadine (Claritin)
__X__	**Chemotherapy agents**

Prednisone, azathioprine, cyclosporine, and chemotherapy agents are medications with immunosuppression effects. It is important to monitor for signs of infection and to take precautionary measures during therapy.

4. In which of the following situations is the administration of a dose of DTaP contraindicated? (Select all that apply.)

__X__	**Severe febrile illness**
__X__	**History of prior anaphylactic reaction to DTaP vaccination**
__X__	**Occurrence of encephalopathy 7 days after administration of DTaP immunization**
__X__	**Occurrence of seizures within 3 days of previous vaccination**
_____	Report of low-grade fever occurring within 24 hr of previous DTaP dose

Severe febrile illness, history of prior anaphylactic reaction to DTaP vaccination, occurrence of encephalopathy 7 days after administration of DTaP immunization, and occurrence of seizures within 3 days of previous vaccination are all contraindications for DTaP vaccination. Local reactions and low-grade fever are common side effects following DTAP immunization.

5. Why is it preferable to give the varicella vaccine in childhood rather than in adulthood?

Vaccinating children against chickenpox is vital because it will not only protect them from chickenpox in childhood, but also protect them from serious harm into adulthood. Children who remain unvaccinated may not be diagnosed with chickenpox and may reach adulthood without developing the antibodies to this disease. If adults acquire the disease it is likely to be severe.

6. What precautions should be taken for a client who has just received a kidney transplant and is taking cyclosporine and phenytoin?

Medications that decrease cyclosporine levels are phenytoin, phenobarbital, carbamazepine, rifampin, terbinafine, and trimethoprim-sulfamethoxazole. These can reduce cyclosporine levels and can lead to organ rejection. Increase cyclosporine dosage as needed.

7. What measures need to be taken to reduce development of osteoporosis during steroid therapy?

Bone mineral density of the lumbar spine should be measured before starting therapy with steroids. Glucocorticoids can be administered topically or by inhalation (less bone loss occurs). Several medications can be given to reduce bone loss including calcium and vitamin D supplements, bisphosphonates, calcitonin, and estrogen replacement therapy (in postmenopausal women).

8. Why is it important that children receiving the varicella vaccine avoid aspirin and salicylates for 6 weeks?

Children receiving this vaccine should avoid aspirin and salicylates for 6 weeks due to the risk of developing Reye syndrome. The risk of developing Reye syndrome in this case increases with concurrent use of salicylates.

Unit 4	Medications for Pain and Inflammation
	Contributor: Lora McGuire, RN, MS

 NCLEX® Connections:

Learning Objective: Review and apply knowledge within **"Medications for Pain and Inflammation"** in readiness for performance of the following nursing activities as outlined by the NCLEX® test plans:

Δ   Assess/monitor the client's need for pain medication, and plan and provide care to meet the client's needs for pain intervention.

Δ   Assess/monitor the effectiveness of pain intervention, and advocate for the client's needs as indicated.

Δ   Provide appropriate client education, and reinforce client teaching regarding the purposes and possible effects of pain medications.

Δ   Assess/monitor the client for expected effects of medications.

Δ   Assess/monitor the client for side/adverse effects of medications.

Δ   Assess/monitor the client for actual/potential specific food and medication interactions.

Δ   Identify contraindications, actual/potential incompatibilities, and interactions between medications, and intervene appropriately.

Δ   Identify symptoms/evidence of an allergic reaction, and respond appropriately.

Δ   Evaluate/monitor and document the therapeutic and adverse/side effects of medications.

 General Key Points

Δ   **Analgesics** are medications that **relieve pain**

   •   Narcotics

   •   Nonsteroidal anti-inflammatory drugs (NSAIDs)

   •   Antimigraine agents

Δ   **Anti-inflammatory agents** are medications that **reduce inflammation**

   •   Salicylates

   •   Glucocorticoids

- Antigout medications

- Disease-modifying antirheumatic drugs (DMARDs)

Δ Certain anti-inflammatory medications have properties that **reduce fever** (antipyretic), such as salicylates and ibuprofen.

Δ Salicylates and NSAIDs **reduce platelet aggregation** and can be used therapeutically to reduce a client's risk of thrombosis. This antiplatelet effect can also pose a greater risk for bleeding and requires careful monitoring of clients.

Δ Salicylates, NSAIDs, and glucocorticoids **pose the risk for gastric ulceration**.

Δ Acetaminophen (Tylenol) has analgesic and antipyretic effects, does not have anti-inflammatory effects, and does not reduce platelet aggregation.

Δ Acetaminophen overdose poses a risk for severe injury to the liver.

Δ Prolonged use of narcotic analgesics, such as morphine and/or meperidine (Demerol), may result in:

- Tolerance.

- Physical dependence.

- Addiction.

Δ Nurses have a **priority responsibility** for the **continuous assessment of clients' pain levels** and to provide effective interventions.

Key Points

Medication Classification: Nonsteroidal Anti-Inflammatory Drugs

Select Prototype Medication: 1st generation **NSAIDs** (COX-1 and COX-2 Inhibitor): **aspirin**
2nd generation **NSAIDs** (selective COX-2 Inhibitor): **celecoxib (Celebrex)**

Other Medications: 1st generation: ibuprofen (Motrin, Advil), naproxen (Naprosyn), ketorolac (Toradol)
2nd generation: valdecoxib (Bextra)

Expected Pharmacological Action

Δ   Inhibition of cyclooxygenase: Inhibition of COX-2 results in ↓ inflammation, pain, and fever. Inhibition of COX-1 results in the ↓ of platelet aggregation.

Therapeutic Uses

Δ   Inflammation suppression

Δ   Analgesia for mild to moderate pain

Δ   Fever reduction

Δ   Dysmenorrhea

Δ   Low level suppression of platelet aggregation

Side/Adverse Effects: Nursing Interventions and Client Education

Side/Adverse Effects	Nursing Interventions/Client Education
Gastrointestinal discomfort (e.g., dyspepsia, abdominal pain, heartburn, nausea): **Aspirin-induced gastric ulcer, perforation, and bleeding**	• Advise the client to take aspirin with food or with a full glass of water. • Advise the client about prolonged use. • Observe for signs of bleeding (e.g., passage of black or dark-colored stools, severe abdominal pain, nausea, vomiting). • Administer a proton pump inhibitor, such as omeprazole (Prilosec), and an H_2 receptor antagonist, such as ranitidine (Zantac) to ↓ the risk of ulcer formation. • Use prophylaxis agents such as misoprostol (Cytotec).
Renal dysfunction (e.g., ↓ urine output, weight gain, ↑ BUN and creatinine levels)	• Monitor I&O and kidney function (e.g., BUN, creatinine).
Salicylism (e.g., tinnitus, sweating, headache and dizziness, respiratory alkalosis)	• Advise the client if symptoms occur, to notify the primary care provider, and to stop taking aspirin.
Reye syndrome is rare, but serious in childhood; occurs when aspirin is used for fever reduction in children who have a viral illness, such as chickenpox or influenza	• Advise the client to avoid giving aspirin when a child has a viral illness (e.g., chickenpox, influenza).

Contraindications/Precautions

Δ   **Aspirin contraindications** include:

- Peptic ulcer disease.

- Bleeding disorders (e.g., hemophilia, vitamin K deficiency)

- Hypersensitivity to aspirin and other NSAIDs.

- Pregnancy (Pregnancy Risk Category D).

- Children with chickenpox or influenza.

Δ   **Use NSAIDs cautiously** in older adults, clients who smoke cigarettes, and in clients with *H. pylori* infection, hypovolemia, hay fever, chronic urticaria, and/or a history of alcoholism.

Medication/Food Interactions: Nursing Interventions and Client Education

Medication/Food Interactions	Nursing Interventions/Client Education
Warfarin – ↑ risk of bleeding	• Monitor the client's prothrombin time, and INR, and advise the client about the potential risk of bleeding when an NSAID is combined with warfarin.
Glucocorticoids – ↑ risk of gastric bleeding	• Advise the client to take antiulcer prophylaxis, such as misoprostol (Cytotec), to ↓ the risk for gastric ulcer.
Alcohol – ↑ risk of bleeding	• Advise the client to avoid consuming alcoholic beverages to ↓ the risk of GI bleeding.
Ibuprofen – ↓ antiplatelet effects of low-dose aspirin used to prevent MI	• Advise the client not to take ibuprofen.

Therapeutic Nursing Interventions and Client Education

Δ   Advise the client to stop aspirin 1 week before an elective surgery or expected date of childbirth.

Δ   Advise the client to take aspirin **with food, milk, or a full glass of water to reduce gastric discomfort**.

Δ   Instruct the client not to chew or crush enteric-coated or sustained-release aspirin tablets.

Δ   Advise the client to notify the primary care provider if signs and symptoms of gastric discomfort or ulceration occur.

Δ   Clients unable to tolerate aspirin due to GI ulceration, risk of bleeding, or renal impairment should be prescribed a 2nd generation **NSAID,** such as celecoxib (Celebrex).

Δ   One 1st generation NSAID, **ketorolac (Toradol), is used for short-term treatment of moderate to severe pain** such as that associated with postoperative recovery.

  •   Ketorolac provides analgesia without anti-inflammatory effect.

  •   When ketorolac is used concurrently with opioids, the analgesic effect of opioids is enhanced without the occurrence of adverse effects associated with opioids (e.g., respiratory depression, constipation).

  •   When ketorolac is used with other NSAIDs serious adverse effects can occur; therefore, ketorolac should be used no more than 5 days. Usually started as parenteral administration and then progresses to oral doses.

Nursing Evaluation of Medication Effectiveness

Δ   Depending on therapeutic intent, effectiveness may be evidenced by:

- Reduction in inflammation.

- Reduction of fever.

- Relief from mild to moderate pain or dysmenorrhea.

- Platelet aggregation suppression.

Key Points

Medication Classification: Acetaminophen

Select Prototype Medication: **acetaminophen (Tylenol)**

Expected Pharmacological Action

    Δ   Acetaminophen slows the production of prostaglandins in the central nervous system.

Therapeutic Uses

    Δ   Analgesic (relief of pain) effect

    Δ   Antipyretic (reduction of fever) effects

Side/Adverse Effects: Nursing Interventions and Client Education

Side/Adverse Effects	Nursing Interventions/Client Education
Acute toxicity that results in liver damage with early symptoms of nausea, vomiting, diarrhea, sweating, and abdominal discomfort progressing to hepatic failure, coma, and death	• Advise the client to take acetaminophen as prescribed and not to exceed 4 g per day. • Administer the antidote, acetylcysteine (Mucomyst).

Contraindications/Precautions

    Δ   Use cautiously in clients who consume three or more alcoholic drinks/day and those taking warfarin (interferes with metabolism).

Medication/Food Interactions: Nursing Interventions and Client Education

Medication/Food Interactions	Nursing Interventions/Client Education
• **Alcohol** – ↑ the risk of liver damage	• Advise the client about the potential risk of liver damage with consumption of alcohol.
• **Warfarin (Coumadin)** – acetaminophen slows the metabolism of warfarin leading to ↑ levels of warfarin. This places the client at risk for bleeding.	• Instruct the client to observe for signs of bleeding (e.g., bruising, petechiae, hematuria). • Monitor prothrombin time and INR levels and adjust dosages of warfarin accordingly.

Therapeutic Nursing Interventions and Client Education

Δ   Acetaminophen is a component of multiple prescribed and over-the-counter medications. Keep a running total of daily acetaminophen intake and follow recommended dosages as prescribed by the primary care provider to prevent toxicity, not to exceed 4 g per day.

Δ   In the event of an acetaminophen overdose, liver damage can be reduced by administering a weight-based dosage of the antidote acetylcysteine (Mucomyst) in a diluted form via an oroduodenal tube (has an unpleasant odor that ↑ risk of emesis).

Nursing Evaluation of Medication Effectiveness

Δ   Depending on therapeutic intent, effectiveness may be evidenced by:

•   Relief of pain.

•   Reduction of fever.

Key Points

Medication Classification: Opioid Agonists

Select Prototype Medication:	**Morphine sulfate**
Other Medications:	fentanyl (Sublimaze, Duragesic), meperidine (Demerol), methadone (Dolophine), codeine, oxycodone (OxyContin)

Expected Pharmacological Action

Δ   Opioid agonists, such as morphine, codeine, meperidine, and other morphine-like medications (fentanyl), act on the mu receptors, and to a lesser degree on kappa receptors. Activation of mu receptors produces analgesia, respiratory depression, euphoria, and sedation, whereas kappa receptor activation produces analgesia, sedation, and ↓ GI motility.

Therapeutic Uses

Δ   Relief of moderate to severe pain (e.g., postoperative pain, myocardial infarction pain, cancer pain)

Δ   Sedation

Δ   Reduction of bowel motility

Δ   Codeine: cough suppression

Side/Adverse Effects: Nursing Interventions and Client Education

Side/Adverse Effects	Nursing Interventions/Client Education
Respiratory depression	• Monitor the client's vital signs. • Stop opioids if the client's respiratory rate is less than 12/min, and then notify the primary care provider. • Avoid the use of opioids with CNS depressant medications (e.g., barbiturates, benzodiazepines, and consumption of alcohol).
Constipation	• ↑ fluid intake and physical activity. • Administer a stimulant laxative, such as bisacodyl (Dulcolax), to counteract ↓ bowel motility, or a stool softener, such as docusate sodium (Colace), to prevent constipation.
Orthostatic hypotension	• Advise the client to sit or lie down if symptoms of lightheadedness or dizziness occur. • Avoid sudden changes in position by slowly moving the client from a lying to a sitting or standing position. • Provide assistance with ambulation as needed.
Urinary retention	• Advise the client to void every 4 hr. • Monitor I&O. • Assess the client's bladder for distention by palpating the lower abdomen area every 4 to 6 hr.
Cough suppression	• Advise the client to cough at regular intervals to prevent accumulation of secretions in the airway. • Auscultate the client's lungs for crackles, and instruct the client to ↑ intake of fluid to liquefy secretions.
Sedation	• Advise the client to avoid hazardous activities such as driving or operating heavy machinery.
Biliary colic	• Avoid giving morphine to clients who have a history of biliary colic. Use meperidine as an alternative.
Emesis	• Administer an antiemetic such as promethazine (Phenergan).
Opioid overdose triad of coma, respiratory depression, and pinpoint pupils	• Monitor the client's vital signs. • Place the client on a ventilator. • Administer opioid antagonists, such as naloxone (Narcan) or nalmefene (Revex).

Contraindications/Precautions

Δ   Morphine is contraindicated after biliary tract surgery.

Δ   **Morphine is contraindicated** for premature infants (during and after delivery due to respiratory depressant effects).

Δ   **Use cautiously with:**

- Clients who have asthma, emphysema, and/or head injuries due to the risk of respiratory depression.

- Infants and older adult clients due the risk of respiratory depression.

- Pregnant clients due to the risk of physical dependence of the fetus.

- Clients in labor due to the risk of respiratory depression in the newborn and inhibition of labor by decreasing uterine contractions.

- Clients who are extremely obese. Obese clients are at a greater risk for prolonged side effects due to the accumulation of medication that is metabolized at a slower rate.

- Clients with inflammatory bowel disease due to the risk of megacolon or paralytic ileus.

- Clients with an enlarged prostate due to the risk of acute urinary retention.

Δ   **Repeated use of meperidine** can result in the accumulation of normeperidine, which can result in **seizures and neurotoxicity.** Do not administer more than 600 mg/24 hr, and **limit its use to less than 48 hr.**

Medication/Food Interactions: Nursing Interventions and Client Education

Medication/Food Interactions	Nursing Interventions/Client Education
CNS depressants (e.g., barbiturates, phenobarbital, benzodiazepines, alcohol) – additive CNS depression action	• Warn the client about the use of these medications in conjunction with opioid agonists. • Advise the client to avoid consumption of alcohol when taking opioid agonists.
Anticholinergic agents, such as antihistamines (diphenhydramine [Benadryl]), and tricyclic depressants (amitriptyline [Elavil]) – additive anticholinergic effects (e.g., constipation, urinary retention)	• Advise the client about the potential risk of morphine-induced constipation and urinary retention. • Advise the client to ↑ fluids and dietary fiber to prevent constipation.
Monoamine oxidase inhibitors (MAOIs) – may cause hyperpyrexic coma, characterized by excitation, seizures, and respiratory depression	• Avoid the use of meperidine with MAOIs to prevent occurrence of this syndrome.
Antihypertensives – additive hypotensive effects	• Warn the client to refrain from using opioids with antihypertensive agents because it can further lower blood pressure.

Therapeutic Nursing Interventions and Client Education

Δ   Assess the client's pain level on a regular basis. Document the client's response.

Δ   Take the client's baseline vital signs. If the client's respiratory rate is less than **12/min**, notify the primary care provider, and **withhold** the medication.

Δ   Follow controlled substance procedures.

Δ   Double check opioid doses with another nurse prior to administration.

Δ   Administer opioids **intravenously slowly over a period of 4 to 5 min**; have naloxone (Narcan) and resuscitation equipment available.

Δ   Warn the client not to ↑ dosage without consulting the primary care provider.

Δ   Administer opioids to clients with cancer on a fixed schedule around the clock, not when necessary. Also, administer supplemental doses as needed.

Δ   Advise the client with physical dependence not to discontinue opioids abruptly. Opioids should be withdrawn slowly, and the dosage should be tapered slowly over a period of 3 days.

Δ   Closely monitor patient-controlled analgesia pump (PCA) settings (dose, lockout interval, and 4-hr limit). Reassure the client regarding safety measures that safeguard against self-administration of excessive doses. Encourage the client to use PCA prophylactically prior to activities likely to augment pain levels.

Δ   When switching clients from PCA to oral doses of opioids, make sure the client receives adequate PCA dosing until the onset of oral medication takes place.

Δ   Parenteral fentanyl is used primarily in surgery to induce anesthesia. It is approximately 100 times more potent (milligram potency) than morphine.

Δ   With the first administration of a transdermal fentanyl patch, it will take numerous hours to achieve the desired therapeutic effect. Administer short-acting opioids prior to onset of therapeutic effects and for breakthrough pain.

Nursing Evaluation of Medication Effectiveness

Δ   Depending on the therapeutic intent, effectiveness may be evidenced by:

•   Relief of moderate to severe pain (e.g., postoperative pain, cancer pain, myocardial pain).

•   Cough suppression.

•   Resolution of diarrhea.

Key Points

Medication Classification: Agonists-Antagonists Opioids

Select Prototype Medication: **pentazocine (Talwin)**

Other Medications: butorphanol (Stadol)

Expected Pharmacological Action

Δ   These medications act as **antagonists** to mu receptors; therefore, activation of these receptors that usually cause analgesia, euphoria, respiratory depression, sedation, physical dependence, and ↓ GI motility does not occur.

Δ   These medications act as **agonists** to kappa receptors; therefore, activation of these receptors can cause analgesia, sedation, and ↓ GI motility.

Δ   Compared to pure opioid agonists, agonist-antagonists have:

•   A low potential for abuse causing little euphoria. In fact, high doses can cause adverse effects (e.g., anxiety, restlessness, mental confusion).

•   Less respiratory depression. Kappa receptors will cause a certain degree of respiratory depression and then no more (have a "ceiling").

Therapeutic Uses

Δ   Agonists-antagonists opioids relieve mild to moderate pain; not used for treatment of severe pain.

Side/Adverse Effects: Nursing Interventions and Client Education

Side/Adverse Effects	Nursing Interventions/Client Education
Abstinence syndrome (cramping, hypertension, vomiting)	• May be precipitated when given to clients who are physically dependent on opioid agonists. • Advise clients to stop opioid agonists, such as morphine sulfate before using agonist-antagonist medications, such as pentazocine (Talwin). • Avoid giving to clients if undisclosed opioid use is suspected.

Contraindications/Precautions

△ Use cautiously in clients with a history of myocardial infarction (↑ cardiac workload) and clients who are physically dependent on opioids.

Therapeutic Nursing Interventions and Client Education

△ Take the client's baseline vital signs. If the client's respiratory rate is less than 12/min, withhold the medication and notify the primary care provider.

△ Warn the client not to ↑ dosage without consulting the primary care provider.

Nursing Evaluation of Medication Effectiveness

△ Monitor for improvement of symptoms, such as relief of pain.

Key Points

Medication Classification: Opioid Antagonists

Select Prototype Medication:	**naloxone (Narcan)**
Other Medications:	naltrexone (Re Via, Depade), nalmefene (Revex)

Expected Pharmacological Action

Δ   Opioid antagonists interfere with the action of opioids by competing for opioid receptors. Opioid antagonists have no effect in the absence of opioids.

Therapeutic Uses

Δ   Treatment of opioid overdose

Δ   Reversal of effects of opioids, such as respiratory depression

Δ   Reversal of respiratory depression in an infant

Side/Adverse Effects: Nursing Interventions and Client Education

Side/Adverse Effects	Nursing Interventions/Client Education
Tachycardia and tachypnea	• Monitor the client's heart rhythm (risk of ventricular tachycardia) and respiratory function. • Have resuscitative equipment, including oxygen, on standby during administration.
Abstinence syndrome (cramping, hypertension, vomiting)	• These symptoms may occur when given to clients physically dependent on opioid agonists.

Contraindications/Precautions

Δ   Hypersensitivity

Δ   Opioid dependency

Δ   Pregnancy Risk Category B

Therapeutic Nursing Interventions and Client Education

Δ   Naloxone has rapid first-pass inactivation and should be administered IV, IM, or SC. Do not administer orally.

Δ   Observe the client for withdrawal symptoms and/or abrupt onset of pain. Be prepared to address the client's need for analgesia (e.g., if given for postoperative opioid-related respiratory depression).

Nursing Evaluation of Medication Effectiveness

Δ   Reversal of respiratory depression (e.g., respirations are regular, client is without shortness of breath, respiratory rate is 16 to 20/min in adults and 40 to 60/min in newborns)

Key Points

Medication Classification: Adjuvant Medications for Pain

Select Prototype Medication:

Tricyclic antidepressants: amitriptyline (Elavil)
Anticonvulsants: carbamazepine (Tegretol), gabapentin (Neurontin), phenytoin (Dilantin
CNS stimulants: methylphenidate (Ritalin), dextroamphetamine (Dexedrine)
Antihistamines: hydroxyzine (Vistaril)
Glucocorticoids: dexamethasone (Decadron), prednisone (Deltasone)
Bisphosphonates: etidronate (Didronel), pamidronate (Aredia)

Expected Pharmacological Action

Δ   Adjuvant medications for pain enhance the effects of opioids.

Therapeutic Uses

Δ   Used in combination with opioids – cannot be used as a substitute for opioids

•   Treating pain with an adjuvant medication allows for lower dosages of opioids, and thereby ↓ the adverse effects experienced with opioids (e.g., sedation and constipation).

Δ   Help alleviate other symptoms that aggravate pain (e.g., depression, seizures, dysrhythmias)

Δ   Used in the treatment of neuropathic pain (e.g., cramping, aching, burning, darting and lancinating pain).

Δ   Used in cancer-related conditions (e.g., ↑ intracranial pressure, spinal cord compression, bone pain).

Side/Adverse Effects: Nursing Interventions and Client Education

Side/Adverse Effects	Nursing Interventions/Client Education
Tricyclic antidepressants (TADs): amitriptyline (Elavil) (Used to relieve neuropathic pain)	
Orthostatic hypotension	• Advise the client to sit or lie down if symptoms of lightheadedness or dizziness occur. • Avoid sudden changes in positions by slowly moving the client from a lying to a sitting or standing position. • Provide assistance with ambulation as needed. • Monitor the client's blood pressure while the client is lying down, sitting, and standing.
Sedation	• Advise the client to avoid hazardous activities, such as driving or operating heavy machinery.
Anticholinergic effects (e.g., dry mouth, urinary retention, constipation)	• ↑ the client's fluid intake. • Instruct the client to ↑ physical activity by engaging in a regular exercise routine. • Administer a stimulant laxative, such as bisacodyl (Dulcolax) to counteract ↓ bowel motility, and a stool softener, such as docusate sodium (Colace) to prevent constipation. • Advise the client to void every 4 hr. • Monitor the client's I&O, and assess the client's bladder by palpating the lower abdomen area for bladder distention every 4 to 6 hr.
Anticonvulsants: carbamazepine (Tegretol), gabapentin (Neurontin) (Used to relieve neuropathic pain)	
Bone marrow suppression	• Periodically monitor the client's complete blood count and platelets. • Advise the client to observe for signs of easy bruising and bleeding, and to notify the primary care provider if they occur.
CNS stimulants: dextroamphetamine (Dexedrine), methylphenidate(Ritalin)	
Weight loss	• Monitor the client's weight.
Insomnia	• Avoid dosing late in the day.

Side/Adverse Effects	Nursing Interventions/Client Education
Antihistamines: hydroxyzines (Vistaril)	
Sedation	• Advise the client to avoid hazardous activities, such as driving or operating heavy machinery.
Glucocorticoids: dexamethasone (Decadron) **(Used in cancer-related conditions, such as increased intracranial pressure and epidural spinal cord compression).**	
Adrenal insufficiency (e.g., hypotension, dehydration, weakness, lethargy, vomiting, diarrhea) associated with prolonged use	• Advise the client to observe for symptoms, and to notify the primary care provider if symptoms occur. • Administer fluids such as normal saline, salt, and hydrocortisone IV.
Osteoporosis	• Advise the client to take calcium supplements, vitamin D, and/or bisphosphonate (e.g., alendronate [Fosamax]) as prescribed.
Hypokalemia	• Monitor the client's potassium levels and administer potassium supplements as needed to maintain a level between 3.0 to 5.0 mEq/L.
Glucose intolerance	• Monitor the client's blood glucose levels.
Peptic ulcer disease	• Advise the client to take the medication with meals. • Prophylactic use of H_2 antagonist such as ranitidine (Zantac).
Bisphosphonate: etidronate (Didronel), pamidronate (Aredia) **(Used for relief of cancer-induced bone pain)**	
Transient flu-like symptoms	• Advise the client to notify the primary care provider if symptoms occur.
Venous irritation at injection site	• Monitor the injection site and infuse with sufficient IV fluids.

Therapeutic Nursing Interventions and Client Education

△   Clients should receive a pain management plan.

△   Encourage the client to voice fears and concerns about cancer, cancer pain, and pain treatment.

△   Advise the client that dosing of pain medications should be given on a fixed schedule around the clock, and not as needed.

△   Advise the client that physical dependence is not considered addiction.

Nursing Evaluation of Medication Effectiveness

△   Depending on the therapeutic intent, effectiveness may be evidenced by:

•   Relief of depression, seizures, dysrhythmias, and other symptoms that aggravate the client's pain level.

•   ↓ opioid side effects.

•   Relief of neuropathic pain.

•   ↓ cancer bone pain.

Key Points

Medication Classification: Antigout Medication

Select Prototype Medication: **colchicine**

Other Medications: indomethacin (Indocin), allopurinol
                                      (Zyloprim), probenecid

Expected Pharmacological Action

Δ   Colchicine and indomethacin ↓ inflammation in clients with gout by possibly
     preventing infiltration of leukocytes. These medications do not effect uric acid
     production or excretion.

Δ   Allopurinol inhibits uric acid production.

Δ   Probenecid inhibits uric acid reabsorption by the renal tubules.

Therapeutic Uses

Λ   Colchicine and indomethacin:

•   Treatment of acute gout attacks.

•   If given in response to precursor symptoms of an acute gout attack, can abort
     the attack.

•   ↓ in the incidence of acute attacks for clients with chronic gout.

Δ   Allopurinol and probenecid:

•   Hyperuricemia (chronic gout secondary to cancer chemotherapy).

Δ   Probenecid:

•   Prolongs the effects of penicillins and cephalosporins by delaying their
     elimination.

Side/Adverse Effects: Nursing Interventions and Client Education

Side/Adverse Effects	Nursing Interventions/Client Education
Colchicine – GI toxicity (e.g., abdominal pain, diarrhea, nausea, vomiting) Others – mild GI distress	• Take oral medications with food. • Provide antidiarrheal agents as prescribed. • If severe symptoms occur, stop colchicine.
Probenecid – Renal injury	• Alkalinize the urine and encourage intake of 2 to 3 L of fluids/day.

Contraindications/Precautions

Δ Avoid use of colchicine during pregnancy (FDA Pregnancy Risk Category C, if used orally; Category D, if used intravenously).

Δ Use colchicine cautiously in older adults, debilitated clients, and clients with renal, cardiac, and gastrointestinal dysfunction.

Medication/Food Interactions: Nursing Interventions and Client Education

Medication/Food Interactions	Nursing Interventions/Client Education
allopurinol (Zyloprim)	
Warfarin (Coumadin) – slows the metabolism of warfarin within the liver, which places the client at risk for bleeding.	• Instruct the client to observe for signs of bleeding (e.g., bruising, petechiae, hematuria). • Monitor the client's prothrombin time and INR levels and adjust dosages of warfarin accordingly.
Probenecid	
Salicylates – lessens the effectiveness of probenecid.	• Advise the client not to use salicylates during probenecid therapy.

Therapeutic Nursing Interventions and Client Education

Δ Instruct the client to concurrently take preventive measures such as avoiding alcohol and foods high in purine (e.g., red meat, scallops, cream sauces). The client should ensure an adequate intake of water, exercise regularly, and maintain an appropriate body weight.

Nursing Evaluation of Medication Effectiveness

Δ Depending on the therapeutic intent, effectiveness may be evidenced by:

• Improvement of pain caused by a gout attack (e.g., ↓ in joint swelling, redness, and uric acid levels).

• ↓ in number of gout attacks.

• ↓ in uric acid levels.

Key Points

Medication Classification: Migraine Medications

Select Prototype Medication:

Ergot alkaloids: ergotamine (Ergostat)
Serotonin receptor agonists (Triptans): sumatriptan (Imitrex)
Beta-blockers: propanolol (Inderal)
Anticonvulsants: divalproex (Depakote ER)
Tricyclic antidepressants (TADs): amitriptyline (Elavil)
Calcium channel blockers: verapamil (Calan)
Estrogens: estrogen gel and estrogen patches (Alora, Climara, and Estraderm)

Other Medications:

Ergot alkaloids: ergotamine and caffeine (Cafergot)
Triptans: almotriptan (Axert), frovatriptan (Frova), naratriptan (Amerge), zolmitriptan (Zomig)

Expected Pharmacological Action

Δ   Migraine medications prevent the inflammation and dilation of the intracranial blood vessels, thereby relieving migraine pain.

Therapeutic Uses

Δ   To abort acute migraine attack

Δ   Prevention of migraine attack

Side/Adverse Effects: Nursing Interventions and Client Education

Side/Adverse Effects	Nursing Interventions/Client Education
Ergot alkaloids: ergotamine	
Gastrointestinal discomfort such as nausea and vomiting	• Administer metoclopramide (Reglan).
Ergotism (e.g., muscle pain, paresthesias in fingers and toes, cold pale extremities)	• Stop medication, and immediately notify the primary care provider if symptoms occur.
Physical dependence	• Advise the client not to exceed the prescribed medication dose. • Inform the client regarding symptoms of withdrawal (e.g., headache, nausea, vomiting, restlessness). • Instruct the client to notify the primary care provider if symptoms occur.
Abortion	• Avoid using medication during pregnancy. • Use adequate contraception during therapy.
Serotonin receptor antagonists (Triptans): sumatriptan (Imitrex)	
Chest symptoms, such as heavy arms or chest pressure	• Warn the client about symptoms, and reassure the client that symptoms are not dangerous; symptoms are self-limiting.
Coronary vasospasm/angina	• Do not administer to a client with, or at risk for, coronary artery disease (CAD).
Teratogenic	• Avoid use during pregnancy. • Use adequate contraception during therapy.
Beta-blockers: propanolol (Inderal)	
Extreme tiredness, fatigue, depression, and asthma exacerbation	• Advise the client to observe for symptoms, and if symptoms occur, to notify the primary care provider.
Anticonvulsants: divalproex (Depakote)	
Neural tube defects	• Avoid use during pregnancy. • Use adequate contraception during therapy.

Side/Adverse Effects	Nursing Interventions/Client Education
Tricyclic antidepressants (TADs): amitriptyline (Elavil)	
Anticholinergic effects (e.g., dry mouth, constipation, urinary retention, blurred vision, and tachycardia)	• ↑ fluid intake. • ↑ physical activity by engaging in regular exercise. • Administer stimulant laxatives, such as bisacodyl (Dulcolax) to counteract ↓ bowel motility, or stool softeners, such as docusate sodium (Colace) to prevent constipation. • Advise the client to void every 4 hr. • Monitor the client's I&O. • Assess the client's bladder by palpating the lower abdomen area for bladder distention every 4 to 6 hr. • Monitor the client's visual acuity and vital signs. • Notify the primary care provider if symptoms occur.
Calcium channel blockers: verapamil (Calan)	
Orthostatic hypotension	• Advise the client to sit or lie down if symptoms of lightheadedness or dizziness occur. • Avoid sudden changes in position by slowly moving the client from a lying to a sitting or standing position. • Provide assistance with ambulation as needed. • Monitor the client's blood pressure while the client is lying down, sitting, and standing.
Constipation	• ↑ fluid intake. • ↑ physical activity by engaging in regular exercise. • Administer stimulant laxatives, such as bisacodyl (Dulcolax) to counteract ↓ bowel motility, or stool softeners, such as docusate sodium (Colace) to prevent constipation.
Estrogens: estrogen gel and estrogen patches (Alora, Climara, and Estraderm) are used for menstrual headaches. *(For information, refer to unit 12, Medications Affecting Reproduction).*	

Contraindications/Precautions

Δ **Ergotamine** is contraindicated in clients with renal and/or liver dysfunction, sepsis, CAD, and during pregnancy.

Δ **Triptans** are contraindicated in clients with ischemic heart disease, a history of myocardial infarction, uncontrolled hypertension, and other heart diseases.

Medication/Food Interactions: Nursing Interventions and Client Education

Medication/Food Interactions	Nursing Interventions/Client Education
Ergotamine (Ergostat), Triptan: sumatriptan (Imitrex) – can lead to spastic reaction of the blood vessels.	• Avoid concurrent use of these medications to prevent spastic reaction of the blood vessels.
Triptans with monoamine oxidase inhibitors (MAOIs) – concurrent use can lead to MAO toxicity.	• Do not give triptans within 2 weeks of stopping MAOIs.

Therapeutic Nursing Interventions and Client Education

Δ   Advise clients with migraines to avoid trigger factors that cause stress such as consumption of alcohol, fatigue, and tyramine-containing foods (wine and aged cheese).

Nursing Evaluation of Medication Effectiveness

Δ   Depending on the therapeutic intent, effectiveness may be evidenced by:

- Reduction in intensity and frequency of migraine attacks.

- Prophylaxis against migraine attacks.

- Termination of migraine headaches.

Key Points

Medication Classification: Medications for Rheumatoid Arthritis

Select Prototype Medication:

Disease Modifying Antirheumatic Medications (DMARDs):

Cytotoxic medications: methotrexate Rheumatrex)
Gold salts: aurothioglucose (Solganal)
Antimalarial agents: hydroxychloroquine (Plaquenil)
Sulfasalazine: (Azulfidine)
Biologic response modifiers: etanercept (Enbrel) and infliximab (Remicade)
Penicillamine: (Cuprimine, Depen)

Glucocorticoids: prednisone (Deltasone)
Immunosuppressants: cyclosporine (Sandimmune, Neoral)
NSAIDs: naproxen (Naprosyn) and celecoxib (Celebrex)

Expected Pharmacological Action

Δ   DMARDs slow joint degeneration and progression the of rheumatoid arthritis.

Δ   Glucocorticoids provide symptomatic relief of inflammation and pain.

Δ   NSAIDs provide rapid, symptomatic relief of inflammation and pain.

Therapeutic Uses

Δ   Analgesia for pain, swelling, and joint stiffness

Δ   Maintenance of joint function

Δ   Slows/delays the worsening of the disease (DMARDs, glucocorticoids)

Δ   Short-term therapy until long-acting DMARDs take effect (NSAIDs, glucocorticoids)

Side/Adverse Effects: Nursing Interventions and Client Education

Side/Adverse Effects	Nursing Interventions/Client Education
Cytotoxic agents: methotrexate (Rheumatex) (First choice of DMARDs for RA)	
Hepatic fibrosis	• Monitor liver function test. • Advise the client to observe for symptoms of anorexia, abdominal fullness, and jaundice. The client should notify the primary care provider if symptoms occur.
Bone marrow suppression	• Obtain the client's baseline CBC and platelet counts. Repeat every 3 to 6 months.
GI ulceration	• Advise the client to take the medication with food or a full glass of water. • Stop the medication if symptoms occur. • Prophylactic use of H_2 antagonists, such as ranitidine (Zantac).
Fetal death/congenital abnormalities	• Avoid use during pregnancy. • Use adequate contraception during therapy.
Gold salts: aurothioglucose (Solganal) (Use in clients who do not respond to other DMARDS)	
Toxicity (e.g., intense pruritus, rashes, stomatitis)	• Stop medication. • Notify the primary care provider if symptoms occur.
Renal toxicity such as proteinuria	• Stop medication. • Monitor I&O, BUN, creatinine, and UA.
Blood dyscrasias (e.g., thrombocytopenia, leukopenia, agranulocytosis, aplastic anemia)	• Monitor CBC, WBC, and platelet counts periodically. • Advise the client to observe for signs of bruising and gum bleeding. • Instruct the client to notify the primary care provider if symptoms occur.
Hepatitis	• Monitor liver function tests.
GI discomfort (e.g., nausea, vomiting, abdominal pain)	• Observe for symptoms, and notify the primary care provider.

Side/Adverse Effects	Nursing Interventions/Client Education
Antimalarial agents: hydroxychloroquine (Plaquenil) (Delayed onset of action; improves long-term outcomes of RA)	
Retinal damage such as blindness	• Advise the client to have baseline eye examination and follow-up eye exams every 6 months with an ophthalmologist. • Stop medication if symptoms of blurred vision occur, and notify the primary care provider.
Sulfasalazine (Azulfidine)	
Gastrointestinal discomfort (e.g., nausea, vomiting, diarrhea, and abdominal pain)	• Use enteric-coated preparation and divide dosage daily.
Hepatic dysfunction	• Monitor liver function tests.
Bone marrow suppression	• Monitor CBC and platelet counts.
Biologic response modifiers (tumor necrosis blockers): ctanercept (Enbrel), infliximab (Remicade)	
Injection-site irritation (e.g., redness, swelling, pain, itching)	• Monitor the client's injection site, and stop the medication if signs of irritation occur.
Penicillamine (Cuprimine, Depen)	
Bone marrow suppression	• Obtain the client's baseline CBC, platelet counts, and repeat every 3 to 6 months.
Glucocorticoids: prednisone (Deltasone)	
Osteoporosis	• Advise the client to take calcium supplements, vitamin D, and/or bisphosphonate (etidronate).
Adrenal suppression	• Advise the client to observe for symptoms, and to notify the primary care provider if symptoms occur. • Administer fluids such as normal saline, salt, and hydrocortisone IV.
GI discomfort	• Advise the client to observe for symptoms, and to notify the primary care provider if symptoms occur. • Prophylactic use of H_2 antagonists.

Therapeutic Nursing Interventions and Client Education

Δ   Anticipate the use of DMARDs within 3 months of RA diagnosis to delay joint degeneration.

Δ   Anticipate the use of glucocorticoids.

•   Short-term management of RA

•   Supplement to other medications when there is RA flare up

•   Control of symptoms when response to DMARDs is still developing

Nursing Evaluation of Medication Effectiveness

Δ   Depending on the therapeutic intent, effectiveness may be evidenced by:

- Improvement of symptoms of rheumatoid arthritis (e.g., ↓ swelling of joints, absence of joint stiffness, ability to maintain joint function, and absence of pain).

- ↓ in systemic complications (e.g., weight loss and fatigue).

Primary Reference:

Lehne, R. A. (2007). *Pharmacology for nursing care* (6th ed.). St. Louis, MO: Saunders.

Additional Resources:

McCaffery, M. & Pasero, C. (1999). *Pain: Clinical manual* (2nd ed.). St. Louis, MO: Mosby.

American Pain Society (2003). *Principles of analgesic use in the treatment of acute pain and cancer pain* (5th ed.). Glenview, IL: Author.

For information about headache education, go to the American Council for Headache Education's Web site, *www.achenet.org.*

For information about headaches, go to the National Headache Foundation's Web site, *www.headaches.org.*

Unit 4 Medications for Pain and Inflammation

Application Exercises

1. Match the following medications with their appropriate therapeutic use.

Morphine sulfate	A. 80 to 100 times more potent than morphine
Fentanyl	B. Opioid antagonist/reversal agent
Codeine	C. Cough suppression
Amitriptyline (Elavil)	D. Gold standard opioid used for moderate to severe acute/chronic pain
Naloxone (Narcan)	E. Neuropathic pain

2. Which of the following methods provides the most effective pain control?

   A. Administering opioid analgesics when necessary
   B. Responding promptly to a client's request for pain relief
   C. Administering analgesics on a fixed schedule around the clock
   D. Encouraging clients to wait until pain becomes severe before asking for analgesics

3. A client taking colchicine to prevent acute gout attacks calls his primary care provider reporting diarrhea, nausea, and vomiting. Which of the following instructions should the client be given?

   A. Take an antacid, and call back in the morning
   B. Get plenty of rest to prevent dehydration
   C. Stop taking the medication, and come in to see his primary care provider now
   D. Take the medication every other day until the symptoms subside

4. Which of the following are potential adverse effects of aspirin? (Select all that apply.)

   _____ Tinnitus
   _____ GI upset/ulceration
   _____ Hepatoxicity
   _____ Platelet interference
   _____ Reye's syndrome

5. Which of the following opioids cause CNS toxicities with repetitive dosing and should not be used for more than 48 hr?

        A. Dolophine (Methadone)

        B. Hydromorphone (Dilaudid)

        C. Meperidine (Demerol)

        D. Morphine sulfate

6. Which of the following opioids is available as a transdermal patch?

        A. Fentanyl

        B. Meperidine (Demerol)

        C. Morphine sulfate

        D. Oxycodone

7. Sumatriptan (Imitrex) is contraindicated for clients with

        A. peptic ulcer disease.

        B. coronary artery disease.

        C. asthma.

        D. diabetes.

Unit 4 Medications for Pain and Inflammation

Application Exercises Answer Key

1. Match the following medications with their appropriate therapeutic use.

Morphine sulfate	A. 80 to 100 times more potent than morphine
Fentanyl	B. Opioid antagonist/reversal agent
Codeine	C. Cough suppression
Amitriptyline (Elavil)	D. Gold standard opioid used for moderate to severe acute/ chronic pain
Naloxone (Narcan)	E. Neuropathic pain

Morphine sulfate (D); Fentanyl (A); Codeine (C); Amitriptyline (Elavil) (E); and Naloxone (Narcan) (B).

2. Which of the following methods provides the most effective pain control?

 A. Administering opioid analgesics when necessary

 B. Responding promptly to a client's request for pain relief

 C. Administering analgesics on a fixed schedule around the clock

 D. Encouraging clients to wait until pain becomes severe before asking for analgesics

A fixed schedule provides for continuous pain relief. Administering opioid analgesics only when necessary delays relief of pain and promotes periods of uncontrolled unnecessary discomfort.

3. A client taking colchicine to prevent acute gout attacks calls his primary care provider reporting diarrhea, nausea, and vomiting. Which of the following instructions should the client be given?

 A. Take an antacid, and call back in the morning

 B. Get plenty of rest to prevent dehydration

 C. Stop taking the medication, and come in to see his primary care provider now

 D. Take the medication every other day until the symptoms subside

Diarrhea, nausea, and vomiting are signs of GI toxicity. The medication should be discontinued and the client should be seen by the primary care provider as soon as possible.

4. Which of the following are potential adverse effects of aspirin? (Select all that apply.)

    __X__   **Tinnitus**

    __X__   **GI upset/ulceration**

    _____   Hepatoxicity

    __X__   **Platelet interference**

    __X__   **Reye's syndrome**

Hepatotoxicity is a potential adverse effect of acetaminophen overdoses.

5. Which of the following opioids cause CNS toxicities with repetitive dosing and should not be used for more than 48 hr?

    A. Dolophine (Methadone)

    B. Hydromorphone (Dilaudid)

    C. Meperidine (Demerol)

    D. Morphine sulfate

Repeated use of meperidine can result in accumulation of normeperidine, which can result in seizures and neurotoxicity. Do not administer more than 600 mg/24 hr, and limit use to less than 48 hr.

6. Which of the following opioids is available as a transdermal patch?

    A. Fentanyl

    B. Meperidine (Demerol)

    C. Morphine sulfate

    D. Oxycodone

With the first administration of a transdermal fentanyl patch, it will take numerous hours to achieve therapeutic effect. Administer short-acting opioids prior to onset of therapeutic effects and for breakthrough pain.

7. Sumatriptan (Imitrex) is contraindicated for clients with

   A. peptic ulcer disease.
   B. coronary artery disease.
   C. asthma.
   D. diabetes.

A client with coronary artery disease has impaired coronary blood flow. Sumatriptan can cause coronary vasospasms, which could further compromise coronary blood flow. There are no contraindications in peptic ulcer disease, asthma, and/or diabetes.

Unit 5	Medications Affecting the Nervous System

Contributor: Judith A. Harris, MSN, RNC

 NCLEX® Connections:

Learning Objective: Review and apply knowledge within **"Medications Affecting the Nervous System"** in readiness for performance of the following nursing activities as outlined by the NCLEX® test plans:

Δ   Assess/monitor the client for expected effects of medications.

Δ   Assess/monitor the client for side/adverse effects of medications.

Δ   Assess/monitor the client for actual/potential specific food and medication interactions.

Δ   Identify contraindications, actual/potential incompatibilities, and interactions between medications, and intervene appropriately.

Δ   Identify symptoms/evidence of an allergic reaction, and respond appropriately.

Δ   Evaluate/monitor and document the therapeutic and adverse/side effects of medications.

Δ   Provide/reinforce client teaching on actions, therapeutic effects, potential side/adverse effects, and interactions of medications.

 General Key Points

Δ   Medications affecting the peripheral and central nervous systems exert their action on:

Peripheral nervous system (PNS)	Central nervous system (CNS)
• Somatic nervous system – voluntary muscles	• Brain
• Autonomic nervous system – involuntary processes of the: ◊ Heart. ◊ Secretory glands (e.g., salivary, sweat, gastric, bronchial glands). ◊ Smooth muscle of bronchi, blood vessels, and GI and GU tracts.	• Spinal cord

Δ   Autonomic nervous system is divided into:

Parasympathetic nervous system (PNS)		Sympathetic nervous system (SNS)	
<ul><li>↓ HR (conservation of energy by ↓ cardiac workload)</li><li>↑ secretion of GI tract</li><li>Assists with emptying bladder and bowel</li><li>Assists with vision by focusing eye for near vision and constriction of pupil</li><li>Bronchial smooth muscle contraction</li></ul>		<ul><li>Regulation of the heart and blood vessels</li><li>Control of body temperature</li><li>Initiation of "fight or flight" response</li></ul>	
Classifications	**Example**	**Classifications**	**Example**
Muscarinic agonists or parasympathomimetic medications mimic or imitate the activity of the PNS.	• Bethanechol	Adrenergic agonists or sympathomimetic medications mimic or imitate the activity of the SNS.	• Epinephrine
Muscarinic antagonists or anticholinergic (ACh) medications block ACh at muscarinic receptors.	• Atropine	Adrenergic antagonists or sympatholytic medications block alpha$_1$, alpha$_2$, beta$_1$, and beta$_2$ receptors.	• Prazosin (Minipress) is an alpha-adrenergic antagonist. Propranolol (Inderal) is a beta-adrenergic antagonist.
Ganglionic-stimulating agents selectively mimic the effects of ACh at nicotinic$_N$ receptors	• Nicotine		
Cholinesterase inhibitors prevent the enzyme cholinesterase (ChE) from inactivating acetylcholine (ACh) leading to ↑ ACh available at receptor sites.	• Physostigmine (Neostigmine)		
Neuromuscular-blocking agents selectively block the effects of ACh at nicotinic$_M$ receptors at the neuromuscular junction.	• Tubocurarine		

Δ   Acetylcholine (ACh), epinephrine, and norepinephrine are the three major transmitters of the ANS.

Δ   Activation of receptors has important significance in medication action/effects as illustrated in the following table.

Receptor Activation	Response
Nicotinic $_N$ receptors	• Release of epinephrine from adrenal medulla
Nicotinic $_M$ receptors	• Skeletal muscle contraction
Muscarinic receptors	• ↓ in the secretion from the lungs, stomach, intestines, and sweat glands • ↓ in HR • Smooth muscle contraction in bronchi and GI tract • In the eye, miosis (↓ in the diameter of the pupil) results from contraction of the sphincter muscle of the iris • In the eye, focusing for near vision results from ciliary muscle contraction. • In the bladder, voiding results from contraction of the detrusor muscle and relaxation of the trigone and sphincter muscles.
Alpha$_1$ receptors	• In the eye(s), radial muscle contraction leads to mydriasis (↑ in the diameter of the pupil). • Veins and arterioles are activated to constrict. • Male sex organs are activated to promote ejaculation. • Activation of alpha$_1$ receptors cause the prostatic capsule, and trigone, and sphincter muscles to contract.
Beta$_1$ receptors	• ↑ HR, ↑ the force of contraction, ↑ conduction through the AV node • Release of renin by the kidney
Beta$_2$ receptors	• Dilates bronchi • Relaxes uterine smooth muscle • Vasodilation of arterioles in heart, lungs, and skeletal muscles • ↑ glycogenolysis in the liver • Skeletal muscle contraction
Dopamine receptors	• Dilates blood vessels in the kidneys

Δ   Numerous compounds work as transmitters in the CNS.

Δ   CNS medications are used for a wide variety of purposes including treatment of Parkinson's disease, seizure disorders, mental health disorders, and to provide analgesia and anesthesia.

Δ   The blood-brain barrier protects the brain from potential harm, but it also prevents entry of medications, limiting their therapeutic effects.

Δ   Limited knowledge of CNS disorders and how the brain functions prevents absolute certainty of how these medications produce their therapeutic effects.

Δ   Adaptive changes occur in the brain with prolonged exposure to medications.

↑ therapeutic effects	• Full therapeutic effects are delayed for several weeks. The desired effect may not be a result of the medication action on synaptic function, but rather from an adaptive change in the brain. Antipsychotic and antidepressant medications may take several weeks before full therapeutic effect is attained.
↓ side effects	• Initial use of medication may result in side effects that diminish over time without a decrease in the therapeutic effect. For example, the conventional antipsychotic medication chlorpromazine (Thorazine) causes sedation during the early stage of treatment. Sedation will subside with continued use, but the therapeutic effects of chlorpromazine continue.
Tolerance and physical dependence	• Tolerance produces ↓ response to the medication requiring a larger dose to elicit the same response. Physical dependence results in adaptive changes in the brain that require continued use of the medication for the brain to continue to function as it had before. A withdrawal or abstinence syndrome will occur if the medication is stopped abruptly. Most CNS medications must be withdrawn slowly.

Δ   CNS disorders are responsive to a variety of medications from different classifications. Medication selection may be based on individual client factors (e.g., age, gender, comorbid disorders, concurrent medication use, presence of risk factors).

Δ   Medications used for CNS disorders usually have more than one therapeutic indication.

Δ   Most medications used for CNS disorders have a delayed onset of therapeutic effect and usually require several weeks to reach their peak.

Δ   Most medications used for CNS disorders should not be withdrawn suddenly, but slowly by tapering dose.

Δ   Treatment of **Parkinson's disease** involves the use of two main classes of medications:

   • Medications that activate dopamine receptors directly or indirectly.

   • Medications that block acetylcholine receptors.

Δ   Treatment goals for **seizure disorders** include achieving adequate seizure control with minimal side effects.

- Different types of seizures are responsive to different types of medications. Therefore, a client must have a complete evaluation to determine the appropriate medication.

- Clients usually require life-long management with medications, so compliance is extremely important.

- Clients taking medications with established safe and effective plasma levels should have periodic blood tests to evaluate the effectiveness of the medication.

- Discontinuation of antiepileptic medications must be done slowly, taking 6 weeks to several months to complete withdrawal.

Δ   The clinical course of **schizophrenia** usually involves acute exacerbations with intervals of semi-remission.

- Medications will be used to treat positive symptoms (e.g., agitation, delusions); negative symptoms (e.g., social withdrawal, poor self-care); and cognitive symptoms (e.g., difficulties with memory and learning).

- A conventional antipsychotic, such as chlorpromazine (Thorazine) is more effective for treating positive symptoms, whereas an atypical antipsychotic, such as clozapine (Clozaril), is effective for both positive and negative symptoms.

- Initial therapy usually requires high doses that should be divided throughout the day. Maintenance doses should be kept at the lowest effective dose and can be given once a day at bedtime.

Δ   Clients starting antidepressant medication therapy for **depression** need to be advised that symptom relief can take 1 to 3 weeks and possibly 2 to 3 months for full benefits to be achieved. Encourage continued compliance.

- Antidepressant medications are classified into three main groups:

◊   Tricyclic antidepressants

◊   Selective serotonin reuptake inhibitors (SSRIs)

◊   Monamine oxidase inhibitors (MAOIs)

Δ   **Bipolar disorders** are primarily managed with mood stabilizers. Antipsychotic and antidepressant medications may be used during acute episodes of mania and/ or depression.

- The three main mood stabilizer medications used for **bipolar disorder** are lithium, valproic acid (Depakote), and carbamazepine (Tegretol).

Key Points

Medication Classification: Cholinesterase Inhibitors

Select Prototype Medication: **neostigmine (Prostigmin)**

Other Medications: physostigmine

Expected Pharmacological Action

Δ   Cholinesterase inhibitors prevent the enzyme cholinesterase (ChE) from inactivating acetylcholine (ACh), thereby increasing the amount of ACh available at receptor sites. Transmission of nerve impulses is increased at all sites responding to ACh as a transmitter.

Therapeutic Uses

Δ   Neostigmine (Prostigmin) ↑ muscle strength by ↑ ACh effects at motor neurons in myasthenia gravis.

Δ   Neostigmine causes reversal of nondepolarizing neuromuscular blocking agents (tubocurarine) following surgery

Side/Adverse Effects: Nursing Interventions and Client Education

Side/Adverse Effects	Nursing Interventions/Client Education
Excessive muscarine stimulation as evidenced by ↑ GI motility, ↑ GI secretions, bradycardia, and urinary urgency	• Advise the client of potential side effects. If effects become intolerable, instruct the client to notify the primary care provider. • Side effects may be treated with atropine.
Cholinergic crisis – excessive muscarinic stimulation and respiratory depression from neuromuscular blockade	• Muscarinic effects can be treated with atropine. • Provide respiratory support through mechanical ventilation and oxygen.

Contraindications/Precautions

Δ   Pregnancy Risk Category C

Δ   Contraindicated in clients with obstruction of GI and GU system

Δ   Use cautiously in clients with seizure disorders, hyperthyroidism, peptic ulcer disease, asthma, bradycardia, and hypotension.

Medication/Food Interactions: Nursing Interventions and Client Education

Medication/Food Interactions	Nursing Interventions/Client Education
Atropine – counteracts the effects of neostigmine	• Atropine is used to treat neostigmine toxicity. • Monitor the client closely and provide mechanical ventilation until the client has regained full muscle function.
Tubocurarine	• Neostigmine reverses neuromuscular blockade after surgical procedures and overdose. • Monitor the client for return of respiratory function. Support respiratory function as necessary. If used to treat overdose, provide mechanical ventilation until the client has regained full muscle function.
Succinylcholine – ↑ neuromuscular blockade.	• Avoid concurrent use.

Therapeutic Nursing Interventions and Client Education

Δ   Instruct the client to take medications as prescribed.

Δ   Advise the client that dosage is very individualized and starts at very low doses and is titrated until desired muscle function is achieved.

Δ   Encourage the client to participate in self-dosage adjustments. This can be accomplished by having the client:

•   Keep records of medication administration and effects.

•   Recognize signs of inadequate dosing, such as difficulty swallowing and signs of overmedication, such as urinary urgency.

•   Modify dosage based on response.

Δ   Advise the client to wear a medical alert bracelet.

Nursing Evaluation of Medication Effectiveness

Δ   Decreased episodes of extreme fatigue

Δ   Improved muscle strength as demonstrated by chewing, swallowing, and performing personal hygiene and other desired tasks

Key Points

Medication Classification: Neuromuscular Blocking Agents

Select Prototype Medication: Nondepolarizing neuromuscular blocker: tubocurarine (Tubarine)
Depolarizing neuromuscular blocker: succinylcholine (Anectine)

Other Medications: Nondepolarizing neuromuscular blockers: pancuronium (Pavulon)

Expected Pharmacological Action

Δ   Neuromuscular blocking agents block ACh at the neuromuscular junction resulting in muscle relaxation and hypotension. They do not cross the blood-brain barrier, so complete paralysis can be achieved without loss of consciousness or decreased pain sensation.

Therapeutic Uses

Δ   Neuromuscular blocking agents are used as adjuncts to general anesthesia to promote muscle relaxation.

Δ   Neuromuscular blocking agents are used to control spontaneous respiratory movements in clients receiving mechanical ventilation.

Δ   These medications are used to diagnose myasthenia gravis.

Δ   Succinylcholine is the preferred agent for:

- Seizure control during electroconvulsive therapy.
- Endotracheal intubation.
- Endoscopy.

Side/Adverse Effects: Nursing Interventions and Client Education

Side/Adverse Effects	Nursing Interventions/Client Education
Respiratory arrest from paralyzed respiratory muscles	• Continuously monitor the client's respiratory function and vital signs. • Have equipment ready for resuscitation and mechanical ventilation. • Monitor the client for return of respiratory function when medication is discontinued.
Hypotension resulting from histamine release and ganglionic blockade. Other cardiac effects include bradycardia and dysrhythmias.	• The client must be on continuous monitoring during therapy with life support equipment accessible. • Treat with antihistamine or per agency protocol.
succinylcholine (Anectine)	
Low pseudocholinesterase activity can lead to prolonged apnea in clients.	• Test the client's blood, or administer a small test dose for clients suspected of having low levels of pseudocholinesterase. • Do not administer medication if pseudocholinesterase activity is low.
Malignant hyperthermia – signs include muscle rigidity accompanied by ↑ temperature, reaching a level as high as 43° C (109.4° F).	• Monitor the client's vital signs. • Stop succinylcholine and other anesthetics. • Ice or infusion of iced saline can be used to cool the client. • Administer dantrolene to ↓ metabolic activity of skeletal muscle.
After 12 to 24 hr postoperative, clients may experience muscle pain in upper body and back.	• Advise clients that response is not unusual and eventually will subside. • Notify the primary care provider to consider short-term use of muscle relaxant.
Hyperkalemia	• Monitor potassium levels.

Contraindications/Precautions

Δ Pregnancy Risk Category C

Δ Succinylcholine (Anectine) is contraindicated in clients with risk of hyperkalemia (e.g., major trauma, severe burns).

Δ Use cautiously in clients with myasthenia gravis, respiratory dysfunction, and fluid and electrolyte imbalances.

Medication/Food Interactions: Nursing Interventions and Client Education

Medication/Food Interactions	Nursing Interventions/Client Education
General anesthetics – often used concurrently in surgery.	• Dosage of tubocurarine should be reduced to prevent extreme neuromuscular blockade.
Aminoglycosides, tetracyclines can ↑ the effects of neuromuscular blockade.	• Take complete medication history of clients who are to receive neuromuscular blockade.
Neostigmine (Prostigmin) and other cholinesterase inhibitors – ↓ the effects of nondepolarizing neuromuscular blockers, such as tubocurarine; ↑ the effects of depolarizing neuromuscular blockers, such as succinylcholine.	• Monitor the client during neuromuscular blockade reversal after surgery.

Therapeutic Nursing Interventions and Client Education

Δ   Clients must be on continuous cardiac monitoring during therapy.

Δ   Monitor the client for respiratory depression and have life support equipment available.

Δ   Carefully monitor the client for return of respiratory function.

Nursing Evaluation of Medication Effectiveness

Δ   Depending on therapeutic intent, effectiveness may be evidenced by:

• Muscle relaxation during surgery.

• No spontaneous respiratory movements in clients on mechanical ventilation.

• Absence of seizures in clients receiving electroconvulsive therapy.

• Successful endotracheal intubation.

Key Points

Medication Classification: Anti-Parkinson's Medications

Select Prototype Medication:

Dopaminergics: levodopa (Dopar, Larodopa)
Dopamine agonists: pramipexole (Mirapex)
Centrally acting anticholinergics: benztropine (Cogentin)
Dopamine releaser (Antiviral): amantadine (Symmetrel)

Other Medications:

Dopaminergics: levodopa plus carbidopa (Sinemet)
Dopamine agonists: ropinirole (Requip), bromocriptine (Parlodel)
Centrally acting anticholinergics: trihexyphenidyl (Artane)

Classifications	Medications	Expected Pharmacological Action
Dopaminergics	Levodopa (Dopar, Larodopa), levodopa plus carbidopa (Sinemet)	• Levodopa crosses the blood-brain barrier and is taken up by dopaminergic nerve terminals and converted to dopamine (DA). This newly synthesized DA is released into the synaptic space and causes stimulation of DA receptors. • Carbidopa does not possess any therapeutic effects, but is used to augment levodopa. Carbidopa inhibits conversion of levodopa to DA in the intestine and periphery, and thereby allows for ↑ amounts of levodopa to reach the CNS.
Dopamine agonists	Pramipexole (Mirapex), ropinirole (Requip), bromocriptine (Parlodel)	• Act directly on DA receptors.

Classifications	Medications	Expected Pharmacological Action
Centrally acting Anticholinergics	Benztropine (Cogentin), Trihexyphenidyl (Artane)	• These medications block acetylcholine at muscarinic receptors, which assists in maintaining the balance between dopamine and acetylcholine in the brain.
Antiviral	Amantadine (Symmetrel)	• Antivirals stimulate DA release, prevent dopamine reuptake, and may block cholinergic and glutamate receptors.

Therapeutic Uses

Δ   These medications do not halt the progression of Parkinson's disease (PD); however, they do offer symptomatic relief from dyskinesias (e.g., bradykinesia, resting tremors, muscle rigidity).

Δ   Levodopa may be used as a first-line medication for PD treatment.

Δ   Pramipexole (Mirapex) is used as monotherapy in early-stage PD, and used in conjunction with levodopa in late-stage PD. It is used more often in younger clients who are more able to tolerate daytime drowsiness and postural hypotension.

Side/Adverse Effects: Nursing Interventions and Client Education

Side/Adverse Effects	Nursing Interventions/Client Education
Dopaminergics: levodopa (Dopar, Larodopa) - Usually dose dependent	
Nausea and vomiting, drowsiness	• Administer in small doses at the start of treatment and with food.
Dyskinesias (e.g., head bobbing, tics, grimacing, tremors)	• Decrease dosage of medication, but the decrease may result in resumption of PD symptoms.
Orthostatic hypotension	• Monitor the client's blood pressure. • Instruct the client about signs of postural hypotension (lightheadedness, dizziness). If these occur, advise the client to sit or lie down. Postural hypotension can be minimized by getting up slowly. Advise the client to avoid sudden changes of position.

Side/Adverse Effects	Nursing Interventions/Client Education
Cardiovascular effects from beta$_1$ stimulation (e.g., tachycardia, palpitations, irregular heartbeat)	• Monitor the client's vital signs. • Monitor ECG. • Notify the primary care provider if symptoms occur. • Use cautiously in clients with cardiovascular disorders.
Psychosis (e.g., visual hallucinations, nightmares)	• Administer antipsychotic medications such as clozapine (Clozaril) if symptoms occur.
Discoloration of sweat and urine	• Advise the client that this is a harmless side effect.
Activation of malignant melanoma	• Avoid use of medication in clients with skin lesions that have not been diagnosed.
Dopamine Agonists: pramipexole (Mirapex)	
Sleep attacks	• Advise the client to notify the primary care provider immediately if these occur.
Daytime sleepiness	• Advise the client of the potential for drowsiness and to avoid hazardous activities. • Advise the client to avoid the use of other CNS depressants such as alcohol.
Orthostatic hypotension	• Instruct the client about the signs of postural hypotension (lightheadedness, dizziness). If these occur, advise the client to sit or lie down. Postural hypotension can be minimized by getting up slowly. Advise the client to avoid sudden changes of position.
Psychosis (e.g., visual hallucinations, nightmares)	• Administer antipsychotic medications, such as Clozaril if symptoms occur.
Dyskinesias (e.g., head bobbing, tics, grimacing, tremors)	• Decrease dosage of medication.
Nausea	• Advise the client to take medication with food.
Centrally acting anticholinergics: benztropine (Cogentin)	
Nausea, vomiting	• Administer in small doses at the start of treatment and with food.
Atropine-like effects (e.g., dry mouth, blurred vision, mydriasis, urinary retention, constipation)	• Advise the client to observe for symptoms, and notify the primary care provider. • Monitor I&O and assess the client for urinary retention. • Advise the client to chew sugarless gum, eat foods high in fiber, and increase water intake to at least 8 to 10 glasses of water/day.

Side/Adverse Effects	Nursing Interventions/Client Education
Antihistamine effects (e.g., sedation, drowsiness)	• Advise the client to avoid hazardous activities while taking the medication.
Antiviral: amandatine (Symmetrel)	
CNS effects (e.g., confusion, dizziness, restlessness)	• Advise the client to avoid hazardous activities while taking the medication.
Atropine-like effects (e.g., dry mouth, blurred vision, mydriasis, urinary retention, constipation)	• Advise client to observe symptoms and notify the primary care provider. • Monitor I&O, and assess the client for urinary retention. • Advise the client to chew sugarless gum, eat high-fiber foods, and increase water intake to at least 8 to 10 glasses of water/day.
Discoloration of skin, also called livido reticularis	• Advise the client that discoloration of the skin will subside when the medication is discontinued.
levodopa plus carbidopa (Sinemet)	
Abnormal movements, psychiatric disorders	• Advise the client of potential side effects, and to notify the primary care provider if they occur.

Contraindications/Precautions

Δ   Levodopa

• Pregnancy Risk Category C

• Contraindicated in clients with malignant melanoma

• Do not use within 2 weeks of MAOI use.

• Use cautiously in clients with heart disease and psychiatric disorders.

Δ   Pramipexole (Mirapex)

• Pregnancy Risk Category C

• Use cautiously in clients with liver and kidney impairment.

Δ   Anticholinergic agents

• Contraindicated in clients with narrow-angle glaucoma

• Use cautiously in older adults, the very young, clients with enlarged prostate glands, and a history of urinary retention.

Medication/Food Interactions: Nursing Interventions and Client Education

Medication/Food Interactions	Nursing Interventions/Client Education
Dopaminergics: levodopa (Dopar, Larodopa)	
Proteins interfere with levodopa absorption and transport across the blood-brain barrier. High protein meals ↓ therapeutic effects.	• Proteins trigger an "off episode." • Advise the client to eat protein in several portions during the day.
Conventional-antipsychotic agents (e.g., chlorpromazine [**Compazine**], haloperidol [**Haldol**]) ↓ therapeutic effects.	• Avoid use with levodopa. • To treat levodopa-induced psychosis, use the atypical antipsychotic clozapine (Clozaril).
Pyridoxine ↓ therapeutic effects.	• Advise the client to avoid vitamin preparations that contain pyridoxine.
MAOIs cause hypertension.	• Avoid concurrent use.
Carbidopa, dopamine agonists, anticholinergics, COMT inhibitors, and dopamine releasers ↑ therapeutic effects.	• These medications can be used concurrently to increase the beneficial effects of levodopa.
Dopamine agonists: pramipexole (Mirapex)	
Levodopa – concurrent use has beneficial and harmful interactions. Use with levodopa can ↓ motor control fluctuations and allow for lower dosage of levodopa. Concurrent use can also ↑ the risk of orthostatic hypotension and dyskinesias.	• Monitor the client for these interactions.
Levodopa plus carbidopa (Sinemet)	
Beneficial interactions include – allowing for lower dosage of levodopa, ↓ cardiovascular responses to dopamine in the periphery, and ↓ nausea.	• Monitor the client for therapeutic effects.

Therapeutic Nursing Interventions and Client Education

Δ   Instruct family members to assist the client with the medication at home.

Δ   Instruct the client about the possible sudden loss of the effects of medication and to notify the primary care provider if symptoms occur.

Δ   Inform the client that effects of the medication may not be noticeable for several weeks to several months.

Δ   Medication "holidays" may be indicated, but must be monitored in hospital setting.

Nursing Evaluation of Medication Effectiveness

Δ   Improvement of symptoms (e.g., ability to perform activities of daily living [ADLs] such as bathing, walking, eating, dressing), absence of tremors, and reduction of irritability and stiffness

Key Points

Medication Classification: Antiepileptics (AEDs)

Select Prototype Medication:	**Barbiturates: phenobarbital (Luminal)** **Hydantoins: phenytoin (Dilantin)** **Benzodiazepines: diazepam (Valium)** **lorazepam (Ativan)** **carbamazepine (Tegretol)** **ethosuximide (Zarontin)** **valproic acid (Depakote)** **gabapentin (Neurontin)**
Other Medications:	lamotrigine (Lamictal), oxcarbazepine (Trileptal), clonazepam (Klonopin)

Expected Pharmacological Action

Δ   AEDs control seizure disorders by various mechanisms, which include:

- Slowing the entrance of sodium and calcium back into the neuron and, thus extending the time it takes for the nerve to return to its active state.

- Suppressing neuronal firing, which decreases seizure activity and prevents propagation of seizure activity into other areas of the brain.

- Potentiating the inhibitory effects of gamma butyric acid (GABA) and thereby suppressing seizure activity.

Therapeutic Uses

Δ   Treatment of generalized seizures

- Tonic clonic (Grand mal)
- Absence seizures (Petit mal)
- Atonic seizures
- Myoclonic seizures
- Status epilepticus
- Febrile seizures

Δ   Treatment of partial seizures

- Simple partial
- Complex partial

Δ   Complete eradication of seizure activity

Medications	Therapeutic Uses
Phenobarbital (Luminal)	• Phenobarbital is used for partial seizures and generalized tonic–clonic seizures. • This medication is not effective against **absence seizures**.
Phenytoin (Dilantin)	• Phenytoin is effective against all major forms of epilepsy except absence seizures. • Use IV route for status epilepticus. • Antidysrhythmic
Carbamazepine (Tegretol)	• Carbamazepine is used for the treatment of partial (simple and complex) seizures, tonic-clonic seizures, bipolar disorder and trigeminal and glossopharyngeal neuralgias.
Ethosuximide (Zarontin)	• Ethosuximide is only indicated for **absence seizures.**
Valproic acid (Depakote)	• Valproic acid is used for partial, generalized and absence seizures, bipolar disorder, and migraine headaches.
Gabapentin (Neurontin)	• Gabapentin is used as a single agent for control of partial seizures. This medication is also used for neuropathic pain and the prevention of migraine headaches.
Diazepam (Valium)	• Diazepam is used in status epilepticus.

Side/Adverse Effects: Nursing Interventions and Client Education

Side/Adverse Effects	Nursing Interventions/Client Education
Barbiturates: phenobarbital (Luminal)	
CNS effects in adults manifest as drowsiness, sedation, confusion, and anxiety; In children, CNS effects manifest as irritability and hyperactivity	• Advise clients to observe for symptoms. If symptoms occur, the client should be instructed to notify the primary care provider. • Advise clients to avoid hazardous activities, such as driving.
Toxicity (e.g., nystagmus, ataxia, respiratory depression, coma, pinpoint pupils, hypotension, death)	• Stop medication. Administer oxygen and maintain respiratory function with ventilatory support. • Monitor the client's vital signs.
Hydantoins-phenytoin (Dilantin)	
CNS effects (e g., nystagmus, sedation, ataxia, double vision)	• Monitor for symptoms and notify the primary care provider if symptoms occur.
Gingival hyperplasia – softening and overgrowth of gum tissue resulting in tenderness and bleeding gums.	• Advise the client to maintain good oral hygiene (e.g., dental flossing, massaging gums).
Skin rash	• Stop medication if rash develops.
Teratogenic (e.g., cleft palate, heart defects)	• Avoid use in pregnancy.
Cardiovascular effects (e.g., dysrhythmias, hypotension)	• Administer at slow IV rate and in dilute solution to prevent adverse CV effects.
Endocrine and other effects (e.g., coarsening of facial features, hirsutism, and interference with vitamin D metabolism)	• Instruct the client to report changes. • Encourage the client to consume adequate amounts of calcium and vitamin D.
carbamazepine (Tegretol)	
Cognitive function is minimally affected, but CNS effects (e.g., nystagmus, double vision, vertigo, staggering gait, headache) can occur.	• Administer in low doses initially and then gradually increase dosage. • Administer dose at bedtime.
Blood dyscrasias (e.g., leukopenia, anemia, thrombocytopenia)	• Obtain the client's baseline CBC and platelets. Perform ongoing monitoring of CBC and platelets. • Observe the client for signs of bruising and bleeding of gums.
Teratogenesis	• Advise the client to avoid use in pregnancy.
Hypo-osmolarity – promotes secretion of ADH which inhibits water excretion by the kidneys, and places the client with heart failure at risk for fluid overload.	• Monitor serum sodium periodically. • Monitor the client for edema, ↓ in urine output, and hypertension.

Side/Adverse Effects	Nursing Interventions/Client Education
Skin disorders (e.g., dermatitis, rash, Stevens-Johnson syndrome)	• Treat mild reactions with anti-inflammatory or antihistamine medications. • Medication should be discontinued if there is a severe reaction.
ethosuximide (Zarontin)	
Gastrointestinal effects (e.g., nausea, vomiting)	• Administer with food.
CNS effects (e.g., sleepiness, lightheadedness, fatigue)	• Administer low initial dosage. • Advise the client to avoid hazardous activities, such as driving.
valproic acid (Depakote)	
Gastrointestinal effects (e.g., nausea vomiting, indigestion)	• Advise the client to take medication with food. Enteric-coated formulation can ↓ symptoms.
Hepatotoxicity (e.g., anorexia, abdominal pain, jaundice)	• Assess baseline liver function and monitor liver function periodically. • Advise the client to observe for signs (e.g., anorexia, nausea, vomiting, abdominal pain, jaundice), and notify the primary care provider if symptoms occur. • Avoid using in children younger than 3 years old. • Medication should be prescribed in lowest effective dose.
Pancreatitis as evidenced by nausea, vomiting, and abdominal pain	• Advise the client to observe for symptoms and to notify the primary care provider immediately if these symptoms occur. • Monitor amylase levels. • Medication should be discontinued if pancreatitis develops.
Thrombocytopenia	• Advise the client to observe for symptoms such as bruising, and to notify the primary care provider if these occur. • Monitor the client's platelet counts.
gabapentin (Neurontin)	
CNS effects (e.g., drowsiness, nystagmus)	• Administer low initial dosage. • Advise the client to avoid hazardous activities, such as driving.
Benzodiazepines: diazepam (Valium)	
Respiratory depression	• Monitor the client's vital signs. • Have resuscitation equipment ready. • Administer oxygen.

Side/Adverse Effects	Nursing Interventions/Client Education
Anterograde amnesia	• Monitor the client for memory loss. • Notify the primary care provider if symptoms occur.
Teratogenic (e.g., cleft palate, heart defects)	• Advise the client to avoid use in pregnancy.

Contraindications/Precautions

Δ   The following medications are in Pregnancy Risk Category D.

- **Barbiturates** – contraindicated in clients with intermittent porphyria

- **Phenytoin** – contraindicated in clients with sinus bradycardia, sinoatrial blocks, second-and third-degree AV block, or Stokes-Adams syndrome

- **Carbamazepine** – contraindicated in clients with bone marrow suppression or with bleeding disorders

- **Valproic Acid** – contraindicated in clients with liver disorders

Medication/Food Interactions: Nursing Interventions and Client Education

Medication/Food Interactions	Nursing Interventions/Client Education
phenytoin (Dilantin)	
Oral contraceptives, warfarin (Coumadin), and glucocorticoids – phenytoin causes a ↓ in the effects of these medications due to the stimulation of hepatic drug-metabolizing enzymes.	• Advise the client to increase dose of oral contraceptives. • Monitor for therapeutic effects of warfarin and glucocorticoids. Dosages may need to be adjusted.
Alcohol, diazepam (Valium), cimetidine (Tagamet), and valproic acid ↑ phenytoin levels.	• Advise the client to avoid concomitant use. • Monitor serum levels.
Carbamazepine (Tegretol), phenobarbital, and chronic alcohol use ↓ phenytoin levels.	• Encourage the client to avoid use of alcohol.
CNS depressants (e.g., **barbiturates, alcohol**) – additive CNS depressant effects can occur with concurrent use.	• Advise clients to avoid concurrent use of alcohol and other CNS depressants.
carbamazepine (Tegretol)	
Oral contraceptives and warfarin (Coumadin) – carbamazepine causes ↓ in the effects of these medications due to stimulation of hepatic drug-metabolizing enzymes.	• Advise the client to increase dose of oral contraceptives. • Monitor for therapeutic effects of warfarin. • Dosages may need to be adjusted.
Grapefruit juice – Inhibits metabolism, and thus ↑ carbamazepine levels.	• Advise clients to avoid intake of grapefruit juice.
Phenytoin and phenobarbital – ↓ the effects of carbamazepine.	• Advise the client to avoid concomitant use.
valproic acid (Depakote)	
Phenytoin and phenobarbital – concurrent use with valproic acid ↑ the levels of these medications.	• Monitor phenytoin and phenobarbital levels. • Adjust dosage of medications as needed.

Therapeutic Nursing Interventions and Client Education

Δ   Advise clients taking antiepileptic medications that treatment provides for control of seizures, not cure of disorder.

Δ   Encourage the client to keep a seizure frequency diary to monitor effectiveness of therapy.

Δ   Advise clients to take medications as prescribed and not to stop medications without consulting the primary care provider.

Δ   Advise clients to avoid hazardous activities (e.g., driving, operating heavy machinery) until seizures are fully controlled.

Δ   Advise clients who are traveling to carry extra medication to avoid interruption of medications in case stranded in locations where their medication is not available.

Δ   Advise clients of childbearing age to avoid pregnancy, as medications may cause birth defects and congenital abnormalities.

Δ   Advise the client that phenytoin (Dilantin) doses must be individualized. Dosing usually starts twice a day and can be switched to once a day dosing with an extended-release form when maintenance dose has been established.

Δ   Advise client that phenytoin (Dilantin) has a narrow therapeutic range, and strict adherence to the medication regimen is imperative to prevent toxicity or therapeutic failure.

Nursing Evaluation of Medication Effectiveness

Δ   Absence or decreased occurrence of seizures

Δ   Ability to perform all ADLs and function normally

Key Points

Medication Classification: Muscle Relaxants and Antispasmodics

Select Prototype Medication: Centrally acting muscle relaxants: diazepam (Valium)
Peripherally acting muscle relaxants: dantrolene (Dantrium)

Other Medications: Centrally acting muscle relaxants: baclofen (Lioresal), cyclobenzaprine (Flexeril), metaxalone (Skelaxin)

Expected Pharmacological Action

Medications	Expected Pharmacologic Action	Therapeutic Uses
Diazepam (Valium)	• Acts in the CNS to enhance GABA and produce sedative effects.	• Relief of **muscle spasm** related to muscle injury • Anxiety and panic disorders • Insomnia • Status epilepticus • Alcohol withdrawal • Anesthesia induction
Baclofen (Lioresal), cyclobenzaprine (Flexeril), metaxalone (Skelaxin)		• Relief of muscle spasm related to muscle injury
Diazepam (Valium), baclofen (Lioresal)	• Acts in the CNS to depress spasticity of muscles. • May be a result of enhancement of GABA in the spinal cord and brain.	• Relief of spasticity related to cerebral palsy and multiple sclerosis
Dantrolene (Dantrium)	• The only peripherally acting muscle relaxant, this medication acts **directly** on spastic muscles and inhibits muscle contraction by preventing release of calcium in skeletal muscles.	• Relief of spasticity related to cerebral palsy and multiple sclerosis • Treatment of malignant hyperthermia

Side/Adverse Effects: Nursing Interventions and Client Education

Side/Adverse Effects	Nursing Interventions/Client Education
CNS depression (e.g., sleepiness, lightheadedness, fatigue)	• Start at low doses. • Warn the client of potential side effects. • Advise clients to avoid hazardous activities, such as driving, and concurrent use of other CNS depressants, such as alcohol.
Metaxalone (Skelaxin) and dantrolene (Dantrium) – hepatic toxicity (e.g., anorexia, nausea, vomiting, abdominal pain, jaundice)	• Obtain the client's baseline liver function studies and perform periodic follow-up liver function tests. • Observe the client for signs of toxicity, and notify the primary care provider if symptoms occur. • Start at low dose.
Physical dependence from chronic long-term use	• Advise the client not to discontinue medication abruptly.
Baclofen (Lioresal) – nausea, constipation, and urinary retention	• Advise the client of side effects and notify the primary care provider if symptoms occur. • Monitor the client's I&O. • Advise the client to increase intake of high fiber foods.

Contraindications/Precautions

Δ   Baclofen (Lioresal) and dantrolene (Dantrium)

  • Pregnancy Risk Category C

Δ   Diazepam (Valium)

  • Pregnancy Risk Category D

Δ   Use both of these medications cautiously in clients with impaired liver and renal function.

Medication/Food Interactions: Nursing Interventions and Client Education

Medication/Food Interactions	Nursing Interventions/Client Education
CNS depressants **(e.g., alcohol, opioids, antihistamines)** – additive CNS depressant effects with concurrent use	• Start at low doses. • Warn the client of potential side effects. • Advise clients to avoid hazardous activities, such as driving, and concurrent use of other CNS depressants, such as alcohol.

Therapeutic Nursing Interventions and Client Education

Δ   Instruct clients to take medications as prescribed.

Δ   Advise client not to stop taking medication abruptly to avoid withdrawal reaction.

Δ   Advise client to avoid CNS depressants while using these medications.

Δ   Provide assistance as needed in performance of ADLs and self-medication.

Nursing Evaluation of Medication Effectiveness

Δ   Absence of muscle rigidity and spasms, good range of motion

Δ   Absence of pain

Δ   Increased ability to perform ADLs

Key Points

Medication Classification: Local Anesthetics

Select Prototype Medication:

Other Medications:

Amide type: lidocaine (Xylocaine)

Ester type: tetracaine (Pontocaine), Ester type: procaine (Novocain)

Expected Pharmacological Action

Δ   These medications decrease pain by blocking conduction of pain impulses in a circumscribed area. Loss of consciousness does not occur.

Therapeutic Uses

Δ   Parenteral administration includes:

- Dental procedures.

- Minor surgical procedures.

- Labor and delivery.

- Diagnostic procedures.

Δ   Topical administration includes:

- Skin and mucous membrane disorders.

Side/Adverse Effects: Nursing Interventions and Client Education

Side/Adverse Effects	Nursing Interventions/Client Education
CNS excitation (e.g., seizures, followed by respiratory depression, leading to unconsciousness)	• Monitor the client's vital signs and respiratory status. • Monitor for signs of seizure activity, sedation, change in mental status (e.g., decrease in level of consciousness). • Have equipment ready for resuscitation. • Administer benzodiazepines (e.g., midazolam [Versed] or diazepam [Valium]) to treat seizures.
Hypotension, cardio suppression as evidenced by bradycardia, heart block, and cardiac arrest	• Monitor the client's vital signs and ECG. • If symptoms occur, administer treatment accordingly as prescribed.
Allergic reactions – more likely with ester-type agents, such as procaine	• Amide-type agents are less likely to cause allergic reactions, therefore are used for injection. • Observe for symptoms of allergy to anesthetics such as allergic dermatitis or anaphylaxis. • Treat with antihistamines or agency protocol.
Labor and delivery – labor can be prolonged due to a ↓ in uterine contractility. Local anesthetics can cross the placenta and result in fetal bradycardia and CNS depression.	• Use cautiously in women who are in labor. • Monitor uterine activity for effectiveness. • Monitor fetal heart rate (FHR) for bradycardia and decreased variability.
Spinal headache	• Monitor clients for signs of severe headache. • Advise client to remain flat in bed for 12 hr postprocedure.
Urinary retention	• Monitor the client's urinary output. • Notify the primary care provider if the client has not voided within 8 hr.

Contraindications/Precautions

Δ   Pregnancy Risk Category B

Δ   Contraindicated in clients with allergy to ester-type local anesthetics (e.g., procaine [Novocain])

Δ   Contraindicated in clients with supraventricular dysrhythmias and/or heart block

Δ   Use cautiously in clients with liver and kidney disfunction, heart failure, and myasthenias gravis.

Therapeutic Nursing Interventions and Client Education

Δ   Advise the client to avoid hazardous activities when recovering from anesthesia.

Δ   Maintain the client in a comfortable position during recovery.

Δ   Prepare injection site of local anesthetic.

Δ   Maintain IV access for administration of emergency medications if necessary.

Δ   Have equipment ready for resuscitation.

Nursing Evaluation of Medication Effectiveness

Δ   Client undergoes procedure without experiencing pain.

Key Points

Medication Classification: General Inhalation Anesthetics

Select Prototype Medication: **halothane (Fluothane)**

Other Medications: isoflurane (Forane), nitrous oxide (laughing gas)

Expected Pharmacological Action

Δ   Inhalation anesthesia produces loss of consciousness, loss of all sensation (pain, touch, temperature), relaxation of muscles, and memory loss (amnesia).

Therapeutic Uses

Δ   Anesthesia for surgery

Δ   Diagnostic procedures

Δ   Cardiological procedures

Δ   Relief of pain (analgesia)

Δ   Muscle relaxation

Side/Adverse Effects: Nursing Interventions and Client Education

Side/Adverse Effects	Nursing Interventions/Client Education
Hypotension	• Continuously monitor the client's vital signs: blood pressure, pulse rate, and respiratory rate.
Respiratory and cardiovascular depression	• Provide continuous monitoring of vital signs and ECG. • Provide mechanical ventilation during procedure. • Have equipment ready for resuscitation.
Malignant hyperthermia: signs include muscle rigidity accompanied by ↑ temperature, reaching a level as high as 43° C (109.4° F).	• Monitor the client's vital signs. • Stop succinylcholine and other anesthetics. • Ice or infusion of ice saline can be used to cool client. • Administer dantrolene to ↓ metabolic activity of skeletal muscle.

Side/Adverse Effects	Nursing Interventions/Client Education
Hepatotoxicity especially in adults	• Assess baseline liver function and monitor liver function periodically. • Observe for signs of anorexia, nausea, vomiting, abdominal pain, and jaundice.
Gastric contents aspiration due to depressed gag reflex	• Endotracheal tube placement • Monitor client following removal of tube.
Risk for toxicity in operating room personnel.	• Operating rooms must have adequate ventilation to prevent toxicity.

Contraindications/Precautions

Δ   Use cautiously in clients with hypersensitivity reaction with previous use of anesthetics.

Δ   Use cautiously in clients with chronic respiratory disease (e.g., asthma, COPD, emphysema) and chronic liver disorders.

Medication/Food Interactions: Nursing Interventions and Client Education

Medication/Food Interactions	Nursing Interventions/Client Education
CNS depressants (e.g., **barbiturates, benzodiazepines, alcohol**) – additive CNS depression	• Dose of anesthetic can be reduced. • Have equipment ready for resuscitation. • Monitor the client's vital signs.
CNS stimulants (e.g., **amphetamines, cocaine**) – additive CNS stimulant effect	• Obtain history of drug use. • Monitor the client's vital signs. • The client will need a greater dose of anesthetic.
Opioid analgesics such as **morphine sulfate** – provide analgesia and cough suppression: Constipation and urinary retention may occur.	• Dose of anesthetic can be reduced due to analgesia provided by opioid. • Monitor the client's bowel and bladder function. • Encourage early ambulation and assist the client to void.
Succinylcholine – provides muscle relaxation	• Administer ventilatory support. • Monitor the client's vital signs, especially respirations.

Therapeutic Nursing Interventions and Client Education

Δ   Obtain the client's complete medical history, especially side effects of anesthetic used.

Δ   Advise the client not to consume any food or drink for 6 to 8 hr prior to the surgical procedure.

Δ   Allow clients to express their fears, and reassure them that anesthetics will provide sleep and pain relief during surgical procedures.

Δ   Monitor the client for nausea and vomiting. Treat per agency protocol.

Δ   Provide postoperative care to assist lung expansion and elimination of anesthetic agents. Encourage/assist the client to turn or change position every 2 hr, cough and deep breathe, and use incentive spirometer.

Δ   Encourage early ambulation.

Nursing Evaluation of Medication Effectiveness

Δ   The client will undergo a surgical procedure with loss of consciousness and elimination of pain.

Δ   Postoperative recovery as evidenced by:

•   Vital signs return to baseline.

•   Client is responsive and oriented to time, place, and person.

•   Return of bowel sounds.

•   Voiding within 8 hr of surgery.

•   Absence of or control of nausea and vomiting.

Key Points

Medication Classification: Intravenous Anesthetics

Select Prototype Medication: Barbiturates: thiopental (Pentothal)
                                     Benzodiazepines: diazepam (Valium)
                                     Ketamine (Ketalar)
                                     Propofol (Diprivan)

Other Medications: Benzodiazepines: midazolam (Versed)

Expected Pharmacological Action

Δ   These medications produce loss of consciousness and elimination of response to painful stimuli.

Therapeutic Uses

Δ   Adjunct to inhalation anesthetics

Δ   Induction and maintenance of anesthesia

Δ   Amnesia

Δ   Midazolam (Versed) and an opioid analgesic such as fentanyl result in conscious sedation (e.g., client is sedated, does not experience pain or anxiety, but responds to verbal commands).

Δ   Ketamine (Ketalar) can be used safely with children.

Side/Adverse Effects: Nursing Interventions and Client Education

Side/Adverse Effects	Nursing Interventions/Client Education
Respiratory and cardiovascular depression including hypotension	• Provide continuous monitoring of the client's vital signs and ECG. • Provide mechanical ventilation during procedure. • Have equipment ready for resuscitation.
Bacterial infection – propofol (Diprivan)	• Use opened vial within 6 hr. • Monitor for signs of infection (e.g., fever, malaise after surgery).
Ketamine – psychologic reaction (e.g., hallucinations, unsettling dreams, and mental confusion): Occurs less in children under 15 years and adults over 65.	• Premedicate with diazepam to ↓ the risk of reaction. • Avoid using in clients with a history of mental illness.

Contraindications/Precautions

Δ   Ketamine should be avoided in clients with psychiatric disorders.

Medication/Food Interactions: Nursing Interventions and Client Education

Medication/Food Interactions	Nursing Interventions/Client Education
CNS depressants (e.g., **barbiturates, benzodiazepines, alcohol)** – additive CNS depression	• Dose of anesthetic can be reduced. • Have equipment ready for resuscitation. • Monitor the client's vital signs.
CNS stimulants (e.g., **amphetamines, cocaine)** – additive CNS stimulation	• Obtain history of drug use. • Monitor the client's vital signs. • The client will need a greater dose of anesthetic.
Opioid analgesics, such as morphine sulfate – provide analgesia and cough suppression: Constipation and urinary retention may occur.	• Dose of anesthetic can be reduced due to analgesia provided by opioid. • Monitor the client's bowel and bladder function. • Encourage early ambulation and assist client to void.

Therapeutic Nursing Interventions and Client Education

Δ   Midazolam (Versed) should be injected slowly over 2 or more min to decrease side effects. Wait another 2 min or more before administering additional doses.

Δ   Propofol (Diprivan) should be injected in a large vein to decrease pain at injection site. IV lidocaine should be used as a local anesthetic before injecting propofol.

Δ   If receiving sedation in outpatient setting, advise the client of the need to be driven home following the procedure.

Nursing Evaluation of Medication Effectiveness

Δ Client undergoes surgical procedure with loss of consciousness and elimination of pain.

Δ Postoperative recovery as evidenced by:

- Vital signs return to baseline.
- Client is responsive and oriented to time, place, and person.
- Return of bowel sounds.
- Voiding within 8 hr of surgery.
- Control of nausea and vomiting.

Key Points

Medication Classification: Antipsychotics-Conventional

Select Prototype Medication: **Low potency: chlorpromazine (Thorazine)**
                                          High potency: haloperidol (Haldol)

Other Medications: fluphenazine (Prolixin), molindone (Moban), perphenazine (Trilafon), thiothixene (Navane)

Expected Pharmacological Action

Δ   Dopamine, acetylcholine, histamine, and norepinephrine receptors in the brain and periphery are blocked. Inhibition of psychotic symptoms is believed to be a result of dopamine$_2$ blockade in the brain.

Therapeutic Uses

Δ   Treatment of acute and chronic psychosis includes:

  • Schizophrenia.

  • Bipolar disorders.

  • Tourette's syndrome.

  • Delusional disorders.

  • Schizoaffective disorders.

  • Dementia and other organic mental syndromes.

  • Huntington's chorea.

Side/Adverse Effects: Nursing Interventions and Client Education

Side/Adverse Effects	Nursing Interventions/Client Education
Early extrapyramidal symptoms (EPS) – Acute dystonia (e.g., client experiences severe spasms of tongue, neck, face, and back) Parkinsonism (e.g., bradykinesia, rigidity, shuffling gait, drooling) tremors Akathisia (e.g., inability to stand still or sit, pacing)	• EPS may develop very soon (within hours) of first dose. • Severe cases should be treated with IM or IV dose of an anticholinergic medication (e.g., benztropine [Cogentin] or diphenhydramine [Benadryl]). Otherwise, can manage with oral doses of anticholinergic medications. • Symptoms usually appear within 1 month of initiation of therapy. Manage symptoms with anticholinergic medications (e.g., benztropine [Cogentin] or diphenhydramine [Benadryl]). Symptoms usually resolve within a few months. • Medication can be discontinued to determine if symptoms return. If symptoms persist, the client can be switched to an atypical antipsychotic agent, such as risperidone (Risperdal). • Effects usually develop within 2 months of the initiation of treatment. • Manage symptoms with beta-blocker, benzodiazepine, or anticholinergic medication.
Late extrapyramidal symptoms (EPS) – tardive dyskinesia (TD) (e.g., twisting or worm-like movement of the tongue and face, lip-smacking)	• Clients should be on lowest dosage possible to control symptoms. • Evaluate the client after 12 months of therapy and then every 3 months. If signs of TD appear, the client should be switched to an atypical agent.
Neuroleptic malignant syndrome (e.g., sudden high-grade fever, blood pressure fluctuations, dysrhythmias, muscle rigidity, change in level of consciousness developing into coma)	• Stop antipsychotic medication. • Monitor the client's vital signs. • Apply cooling blankets. • Administer antipyretics (e.g., aspirin, acetaminophen). • Increase the client's fluid intake. • Administer benzodiazepines to control anxiety. • Administer dantrolene (Dantrium) to induce muscle relaxation. • Wait 2 weeks before resuming therapy. Consider switching to an atypical agent.

Side/Adverse Effects	Nursing Interventions/Client Education
Anticholinergic effects (e.g., dry mouth, visual disturbances, acute urinary retention, constipation, tachycardia)	• Assess the client for urinary retention. • Monitor the client's I&O. • Advise the client to chew sugarless gum, eat foods high in fiber, and increase water intake to at least 8 to 10 glasses of water a day. • Teach the client to monitor HR and report noteworthy increases. These effects are more likely with low-potency agents.
Orthostatic hypotension	• The client should develop tolerance in 2 to 3 months. • Instruct the client about signs of postural hypotension (e.g., lightheadedness, dizziness). If these occur, advise the client to sit or lie down. Orthostatic hypotension can be minimized by getting up slowly.
Sedation	• Administer dose at bedtime. • Effect should diminish within a week. • Advise the client not to drive until sedation has subsided.
Neuroendocrine effects (e.g., gynecomastia [breast enlargement], galactorrhea, menstrual irregularities)	• Advise the client to observe for symptoms and to notify the primary care provider if these occur.
Seizures – greatest risk in clients with existing seizure disorder	• Advise the client to report seizure activity and report to the primary care provider. • An increase in antipsychotic medication may be necessary.
Sexual dysfunction – common in both males and females	• Advise the client of possible side effects. • Encourage that the client report side effects to the primary care provider. • The client may need dosage lowered or be switched to a high-potency agent.
Skin effects – photosensitivity resulting in severe sunburn, contact dermatitis from handling medications	• Advise clients to avoid excessive exposure to sunlight, to use sunscreen, and to wear protective clothing. • Advise the client to avoid direct contact with medication.
Agranulocytosis	• Advise the client to observe for signs of infection (e.g., fever, sore throat), and to notify the primary care provider if these occur. If signs of infection appear, obtain the client's baseline WBC and discontinue medication if laboratory test indicates the presence of infection.

Side/Adverse Effects	Nursing Interventions/Client Education
Severe dysrhythmias	• Obtain the client's baseline ECG and potassium level prior to treatment and periodically throughout the treatment period. • Avoid concurrent use with other medications that prolong QT interval.

Contraindications/Precautions

Δ   Contraindicated in clients in a coma, clients with severe depression, Parkinson's disease, prolactin-dependent cancer of the breast, and severe hypotension

Δ   Use cautiously in clients with glaucoma, paralytic ileus, prostate enlargement, heart disorders, liver or kidney disease, and seizure disorders.

Medication/Food Interactions: Nursing Interventions and Client Education

Medication/Food Interactions	Nursing Interventions/Client Education
Anticholinergics agents – concurrent use with other anticholinergic medications will ↑ effects.	• Advise the client to avoid OTC medications that contain anticholinergic agents (e.g., sleep medications, antihistamines).
CNS depressants (e.g., **alcohol, opioids, antihistamines)** – additive CNS depressant effects with concurrent use	• Advise the client to avoid alcohol and other medications that cause CNS depression. • Advise clients to avoid hazardous activities, such as driving.
Levodopa – by activating dopamine receptors, levodopa counteracts effects of antipsychotic agents.	• Clients receiving antipsychotic medications for treatment of psychiatric disorders should not use levodopa and other direct dopamine receptor agonists concurrently.

Therapeutic Nursing Interventions and Client Education

Δ   Client's should be carefully assessed to distinguish between EPS and worsening of psychotic disorder.

Δ   Early EPS symptoms can be controlled with the use of anticholinergics, beta-blockers, and benzodiazepines. If symptoms are intolerable, a client can be switched to a low-potency or an atypical antipsychotic agent.

Δ   Advise clients that antipsychotic medications do not cause addiction.

Δ   Advise clients to take medication as prescribed and to take it on a regular schedule.

Δ   Instruct the client in ways to minimize anticholinergic side effects, which include:

- Sipping fluids and sucking on hard candy to ↓ dry mouth.

- Avoiding hazardous activities if visual disturbances occur.

- Wearing sunglasses outside to prevent photophobia.

- Voiding just before taking medication to minimize urinary retention.

- ↑ intake of dietary fiber and fluids to prevent constipation.

- Not participating in strenuous exercising in warm weather due to suppression of sweating.

Δ   Advise clients that effective treatment occurs in 4 to 6 weeks.

Δ   Advise clients that liquid preparation should be protected from sunlight.

Δ   Advise clients to avoid skin contact of liquid preparation to avoid developing dermatitis.

Δ   Administer medication in equally divided doses until effective dose is attained. When effective dose is determined, advise the client to take the total dose at bedtime to decrease sedative side effects.

Δ   Consider depot preparations for clients with difficulty maintaining medication regimen. Inform the client that lower doses can be used with depot preparations, which will decrease the risk of developing tardive dyskinesia.

Nursing Evaluation of Medication Effectiveness

Δ   Improvement of symptoms (e.g., prevention of acute psychotic symptoms, absence of hallucinations, delusions, anxiety, hostility)

Δ   Improvement in ability to perform ADLs

Δ   Improvement in ability to interact socially with peers

Δ   Improvement of sleeping and eating habits

Key Points

Medication Classification: Antipsychotics-Atypical

Select Prototype Medication:	**clozapine (Clozaril)**
Other Medications:	risperidone (Risperdal), olanzapine (Zyprexa), quetiapine (Seroquel), aripiprazole (Abilify)

Expected Pharmacological Action

Δ   The primary actions of these antipsychotic medications result from blocking **serotonin,** and to a lesser degree, **dopamine** receptors. These medications also block receptors for norepinephrine, histamine, and acetylcholine. In comparison to conventional antipsychotics, these medications cause a similar reduction of positive symptoms, a greater reduction of negative symptoms, and less likelihood of EPS and development of tardive dyskinesia.

Therapeutic Uses

Δ   Severe schizophrenia

Δ   Psychosis induced by levodopa therapy

Side/Adverse Effects: Nursing Interventions and Client Education

Side/Adverse Effects	Nursing Interventions/Client Education
Agranulocytosis	• Obtain the client's baseline WBC and then monitor weekly. • Medication is discontinued with WBC count < 3,000/mm³ or granulocyte count < 1,500/mm³. • Monitor the client for signs of infection (e.g., fever, sore throat, lesions in mouth), and notify the primary care provider if symptoms occur.
Seizures	• Avoid use in clients with seizure disorders. • Advise the client to report seizure activity.
New onset of diabetes or loss of glucose control in clients with diabetes, (e.g., polyuria [↑ urination], polyphagia [↑ appetite], polydipsia [↑ thirst])	• Obtain the client's baseline fasting blood glucose FBG and monitor periodically throughout treatment. • Instruct the client to report signs such as ↑ thirst, urination, and appetite. • If the client has achieved good control of psychotic symptoms, consider managing diabetes with insulin or oral hypoglycemic.
Weight gain	• Advise the client to follow a healthy, low-caloric diet, engage in regular exercise, and monitor weight gain. • Cholesterol, triglycerides, and blood glucose should be monitored if weight gain is > 14 kg (30 lb).
Inflammation of heart muscle as evidenced by dyspnea, ↑ RR, lethargy, chest pain, palpitations	• Advise the client to observe for symptoms, and to notify the primary care provider if symptoms occur. • Stop medication.

Contraindications/Precautions

Δ   Pregnancy Risk Category B

Δ   Contraindicated in clients with a history of agranulocytosis and bone marrow depression

Δ   Contraindicated in clients on anticancer medications

Δ   Use cautiously in clients with seizure disorders and diabetes.

Medication/Food Interactions: Nursing Interventions and Client Education

Medication/Food Interactions	Nursing Interventions/Client Education
Immunosuppressive medications, such as anticancer medications	• Avoid use in clients.

Therapeutic Nursing Interventions and Client Education

Δ   Advise clients that low doses of medication are given initially and are then gradually increased.

Δ   Advise the client that clozapine (Clozaril) has less likelihood of causing EPS symptoms, including tardive dyskinesia.

Δ   Advise the client to observe for signs of diabetes (e.g., increased thirst, urination), infection (e.g., fatigue, fever), and weight gain. Advise the client to report these signs to the primary care provider.

Nursing Evaluation of Medication Effectiveness

Δ   Improvement of symptoms (e.g., prevention of acute psychotic symptoms, absence of hallucinations, delusions, anxiety, hostility)

Δ   Improvement in ability to perform ADLs

Δ   Improvement in ability to interact socially with peers

Δ   Improvement of sleeping and eating habits

Key Points

Medication Classification: Antidepressants-Tricyclic (TCA)

Select Prototype Medication: **amitriptyline (Elavil)**

Other Medications: imipramine (Tofranil), doxepin (Sinequan)

Expected Pharmacological Action

Δ   These medications block reuptake of the monoamine neurotransmitters norepinephrine and serotonin in the synaptic space, thereby intensifying the effects that they produce.

Therapeutic Uses

Δ   Depression

Δ   Bipolar disorders

Side/Adverse Effects: Nursing Interventions and Client Education

Side/Adverse Effects	Nursing Interventions/Client Education
Orthostatic hypotension	• Instruct clients about the signs of postural hypotension (lightheadedness, dizziness). If these occur, advise the client to sit or lie down. Orthostatic hypotension can be minimized by getting up slowly. • Monitor the client's blood pressure and heart rate for the hospitalized client. Take orthostatic blood pressures, waiting at least 1 min between lying down and sitting or standing. If a significant change in blood pressure and HR is noted, do not administer the medication, and notify the primary care provider.
Anticholinergic effects (e.g., dry mouth, blurred vision, photophobia, acute urinary retention, constipation, tachycardia)	• Instruct the client on ways to minimize anticholinergic effects. • Advise the client to chew sugarless gum, eat foods high in fiber, and increase water intake to at least 8 to 10 glasses of water/day. • Teach the client to monitor HR and report noteworthy increases. • Advise the client to notify the primary care provider if symptoms are intolerable.

Side/Adverse Effects	Nursing Interventions/Client Education
Cardiac toxicity usually only at excessive dosing	• Obtain the client's baseline ECG and monitor ECG during treatment.
Sedation	• Usually diminishes over time • Advise clients to avoid hazardous activities such as driving if sedation is excessive. • Advise the client to take medication at bedtime to minimize daytime sleepiness and to promote sleep.
Toxicity evidenced by dysrhythmias, mental confusion, and agitation, followed by seizures and coma	• Give clients who are acutely ill only a 1-week supply of medication. • Monitor the client for signs of toxicity. • Notify the primary care provider if signs of toxicity occur.

Contraindications/Precautions

Δ   Pregnancy Risk Category C

Δ   Use cautiously in clients with seizure disorders, coronary artery disease, diabetes, liver, kidney and respiratory disorders, urinary retention and obstruction, and hyperthyroidism.

Medication/Food Interactions: Nursing Interventions and Client Education

Medication/Food Interactions	Nursing Interventions/Client Education
Monoamine oxidase inhibitors (MAOIs) – concurrent use causes hypertension	• Avoid concurrent use of TCAs and MAOIs.
Antihistamines and other anticholinergic agents – additive anticholinergic effects	• Avoid concurrent use of TCAs and antihistamines.
Epinephrine, NE (direct-acting sympathomimetics) – ↑ amounts of these medications in synaptic space because uptake is blocked by TCAs leading to ↑ intensity of their effects	• Avoid concurrent use of TCAs and these medications.
Ephedrine, amphetamine (indirect-acting sympathomimetics) – decreased responses to these medications due to the inhibition of their uptake and their inability to get to the site of action in the nerve terminal	• Avoid concurrent use of TCAs and these medications.
Alcohol, benzodiazepines, opioids, and antihistamines – additive CNS depression when used concurrently	• Advise the client to avoid other CNS depressants.

Therapeutic Nursing Interventions and Client Education

Δ   Instruct the client to take this medication as prescribed on a daily basis to establish therapeutic plasma levels.

Δ   Assist with the client's medication regimen compliance by informing the client that therapeutic effects may not be experienced for 1 to 3 weeks.

Δ   Instruct the client to continue therapy after improvement in symptoms. Sudden discontinuation of the medication can result in relapse.

Δ   Advise the client that therapy usually continues for 6 months after resolution of symptoms and may continue for a year or longer.

Δ   Suicide prevention can be facilitated by prescribing only a week's worth of medication for an acutely ill client, and then only prescribing 1 month's worth of medication at a time.

Δ   Instruct the client in ways to minimize anticholinergic side effects, which include:

  • Sipping fluids and sucking on hard candy to ↓ dry mouth.

  • Avoiding hazardous activities if visual disturbances occur.

  • Wearing sunglasses outside to prevent photophobia.

  • Voiding just before taking the medication to minimize urinary retention.

  • ↑ intake of dietary fiber and fluids to prevent constipation.

  • Not participating in strenuous exercise in warm weather due to suppression of sweating.

Nursing Evaluation of Medication Effectiveness

Δ   Depending on therapeutic intent, effectiveness may be evidenced by an:

  • Improvement in depressive state as evidenced by elevated mood, greater alertness and activity level, improved appetite, and normal sleep pattern.

  • Improvement of symptoms as evidenced by greater ability to perform ADLs, and to interact socially with peers.

  • Improvement of sleeping and eating habits.

Key Points

Medication Classification: Selective Serotonin Reuptake Inhibitors (SSRIs)

Select Prototype Medication: **fluoxetine (Prozac)**

Other Medications: citalopram (Celexa), escitalopram oxalate (Lexapro), paroxetine (Paxil), sertraline (Zoloft)

Expected Pharmacological Action

Δ   SSRIs selectively block reuptake of the monoamine neurotransmitter serotonin in the synaptic space, thereby intensifying the effects that can be produced.

Therapeutic Uses

Δ   Major depression

Δ   Obsessive compulsive disorders (OCD)

Δ   Bulimia nervosa

Δ   Premenstrual dysphoric disorders

Δ   Panic disorders

Δ   Posttraumatic disorder (PTSD)

Side/Adverse Effects: Nursing Interventions and Client Education

Side/Adverse Effects	Nursing Interventions/Client Education
Sexual dysfunction (e.g., no orgasm, impotence, decreased libido)	• Warn the client of possible side effects and to notify the primary care provider if intolerable. • Strategies to manage sexual dysfunction may include lowering dosage, discontinuing medication temporarily (medication holiday), and using adjunct medications to ↑ sexual function (e.g., sildenafil [Viagra] and buspirone [BuSpar]). • Switch to an atypical antidepressant with less sexual dysfunction side effects (e.g., bupropion [Wellbutrin] and nefazodone [Serzone]).
Weight gain	• Monitor the client's weight gain. • Encourage the client to participate in regular exercise and to follow a healthy, low-caloric diet.
Serotonin syndrome begins 2 to 72 hr after starting treatment (e.g., **mental confusion, agitation, anxiety,** hallucinations, hyperreflexia tremors).	• Advise the client to observe for symptoms. If symptoms occur, instruct the client to notify the primary care provider and stop the medication.
Withdrawal syndrome (e.g., headache, nausea, visual disturbances, anxiety)	• The medication should be discontinued gradually. • Instruct the client to taper dose gradually.
Hyponatremia – more likely in older adult clients taking diuretics	• Obtain baseline serum sodium, and monitor level periodically throughout treatment.
Rash	• Advise the client that a rash can be treated with an antihistamine or withdrawal of medication.
Sleepiness, faintness, lightheadedness	• Advise the client that these side effects are not common, but can occur. • The client should avoid driving if these side effects occur.

Contraindications/Precautions

Δ   Pregnancy Risk Category C

Δ   Contraindicated in clients taking MAOIs

Δ   Use cautiously in clients with liver and renal dysfunction, cardiac disease, seizure disorders, diabetes, ulcers, and a history of GI bleeding.

Medication/Food Interactions: Nursing Interventions and Client Education

Medication/Food Interactions	Nursing Interventions/Client Education
MAOIs – ↑ the risk of serotonin syndrome.	• The client should not be administered an MAOI while taking fluoxetine. MAOIs should be discontinued for 14 days prior to starting an SSRI. If already taking fluoxetine, the client should wait 5 weeks before starting an MAOI.
Warfarin (Coumadin) – fluoxetine can displace warfarin from bound protein and result in ↑ warfarin levels.	• Monitor the client's prothrombin time (PT) and INR levels. • Assess the client for signs of bleeding. • A dosage adjustment may be required.
Tricyclic antidepressants and lithium – Fluoxetine can ↑ the levels of these medications.	• Concurrent use is not recommended.
NSAIDs and anticoagulants – fluoxetine suppresses platelet aggregation and thus ↑ the risk of bleeding when used concurrently with these medications.	• Advise the client to monitor for signs of bleeding (e.g., bruising, hematuria) and to notify the primary care provider if they occur.

Therapeutic Nursing Interventions and Client Education

Δ   Advise the client to take the medication with meals/food.

Δ   Instruct the client to take the medication on a daily basis to establish therapeutic plasma levels.

Δ   Assist the client with medication regimen compliance by informing the client that therapeutic effects may not be experienced for 1 to 3 weeks.

Δ   Instruct the client to continue therapy after improvement in symptoms. Sudden discontinuation of medication can result in relapse.

Δ   Advise the client that therapy usually continues for 6 months after resolution of symptoms and may continue for a year or longer.

Δ   Older adult clients taking diuretics should be monitored for sodium levels. Obtain baseline sodium levels and monitor periodically.

Nursing Evaluation of Medication Effectiveness

Δ   Depending on therapeutic intent, effectiveness may be evidenced by an:

•   Improvement in depressive state as evidenced by elevated mood, greater alertness and activity level, improved appetite, and normal sleep pattern.

•   Improvement of symptoms as evidenced by greater ability to perform ADLs, and to interact socially with peers.

•   Improvement of sleeping and eating habits.

Key Points

Medication Classification: Monoamine Oxidase Inhibitors (MAOIs)

Select Prototype Medication:	**phenelzine (Nardil)**
Other Medications:	isocarboxazid (Marplan)

Expected Pharmacological Action

Δ   These medications block MAO-A in the brain, thereby increasing the amount of norepinephrine (NE) and serotonin available for transmission of impulses. An increased amount of NE and serotonin at nerve endings intensifies responses and relieves depression.

Therapeutic Uses

Δ   Atypical depression

Δ   Bulimia nervosa

Δ   Obsessive compulsive disorders (OCD)

Side/Adverse Effects: Nursing Interventions and Client Education

Side/Adverse Effects	Nursing Interventions/Client Education
CNS stimulation (e.g., anxiety, agitation, hypomania, mania)	• Advise clients to observe for symptoms. If symptoms occur, instruct the client to notify the primary care provider.
Orthostatic hypotension	• Instruct clients about the signs of postural hypotension (lightheadedness, dizziness). If these occur, advise the client to sit or lie down. Orthostatic hypotension can be minimized by getting up slowly. • Monitor the client's blood pressure and heart rate for the hospitalized client. Take orthostatic blood pressures, waiting at least 1 min between lying down and sitting or standing. If a significant change in blood pressure and HR is noted, do not administer medication, and notify the primary care provider.

Side/Adverse Effects	Nursing Interventions/Client Education
Hypertensive crisis resulting from intake of dietary tyramine – severe hypertension as a result of intensive vasoconstriction and stimulation of the heart: Client will most likely experience headache, nausea, ↑ HR and BP.	• Hypertensive crisis is managed by inducing rapid vasodilation. This is accomplished with IV phentolamine, a rapid-acting alpha-adrenergic blocker. Hypertensive crisis can also be treated with sublingual nifedipine. • Provide continuous cardiac monitoring and respiratory support as indicated.

Contraindications/Precautions

Δ Pregnancy Risk Category C

Δ Contraindicated in clients taking SSRIs, clients with pheochromocytoma, heart failure, cardiovascular and cerebral vascular disease, and severe renal insufficiency

Δ Use cautiously in clients with diabetes and seizure disorders.

Medication/Food Interactions: Nursing Interventions and Client Education

Medication/Food Interactions	Nursing Interventions/Client Education
Indirect-acting sympathomimetic medications (e.g., **ephedrine, amphetamine)** – these medications promote the release of NE and can lead to hypertensive crisis	• Advise the client not to use any medications with sympathomimetic actions. • Instruct the client that OTC decongestants and cold remedies frequently contain medications with sympathomimetic action.
Tricyclic antidepressants – concurrent use can lead to hypertensive crisis.	• Use MAOIs and TCAs cautiously.
Selective serotonin reuptake inhibitors (SSRIs) – concurrent use can lead to serotonin syndrome	• Concurrent use should be avoided.
Antihypertensives – additive hypotensive effect	• Monitor the client's blood pressure. • Notify the primary care provider if there is a significant drop in the client's blood pressure. May need to reduce the client's dosage of antihypertensive.
Meperidine (Demerol) – concurrent use can lead to hyperpyrexia	• Alternative analgesic should be used.

Medication/Food Interactions	Nursing Interventions/Client Education
Tyramine-rich foods – hypertensive crisis can occur: The client will most likely experience headache, nausea, ↑ HR and ↑ BP	• Assess the client for ability to follow strict adherence to dietary restrictions. • Inform the client of symptoms and to notify the primary care provider if they occur. • Provide the client with written instructions regarding foods and beverages to be avoided. • Tyramine-rich foods include aged cheese, salami, avocados, bananas, protein, dietary supplements, and red wine. • Advise the client to avoid taking any medications without approval of the primary care provider.
Vasopressors (e.g., **phenylethylamine, caffeine)** – concurrent use may result in hypertension	• Advise the client to avoid foods that contain these agents (e.g., caffeinated beverages, chocolate, fava beans, ginseng).

Therapeutic Nursing Interventions and Client Education

Δ   Instruct the client to take the medication on a daily basis to establish therapeutic plasma levels.

Δ   Assist with medication regimen compliance by informing the client that therapeutic effects may not be experienced for 1 to 3 weeks.

Δ   Instruct the client to continue therapy after improvement in symptoms. Sudden discontinuation of medication can result in relapse.

Δ   Advise the client that therapy usually continues for 6 months after resolution of symptoms and may continue for a year or longer.

Δ   Give clients a list of tyramine-rich food so hypertensive crises can be avoided.

Δ   Advise the client to avoid taking any other prescription or nonprescription medications unless approved by the primary care provider.

Nursing Evaluation of Medication Effectiveness

Δ   Depending on therapeutic intent, effectiveness may be evidenced by an:

• Improvement in depressive state as evidenced by elevated mood, greater alertness and activity level, improved appetite, and normal sleep pattern.

• Improvement of symptoms as evidenced by greater ability to perform ADLs, and to interact socially with peers.

• Improvement of sleeping and eating habits.

Key Points

Medication Classification: Atypical Antidepressants

Select Prototype Medication: **bupropion HCL (Wellbutrin)**

Other Medications: mirtazapine (Remeron), venlafaxine (Effexor), Reboxetine (Vestra), trazodone (Desyrel)

Expected Pharmacological Action

Δ   These medications act by inhibiting dopamine uptake.

Therapeutic Uses

Δ   Treatment of depression

Δ   Aid to quit smoking

Side/Adverse Effects: Nursing Interventions and Client Education

Side/Adverse Effects	Nursing Interventions/Client Education
Headache, dry mouth, constipation, ↑ HR, nausea, restlessness, weight loss	• Advise clients to observe for symptoms and to notify the primary care provider if intolerable. • Treat headache with mild analgesic. • Advise the client to sip on fluids to treat dry mouth and to ↑ dietary fiber to prevent constipation.
Seizures	• Avoid administering to clients at risk for seizures, such as a client with a head injury. • Monitor clients for seizures and treat accordingly.

Contraindications/Precautions

Δ   Pregnancy Risk Category B

Δ   Contraindicated in clients with a seizure disorder

Δ   Contraindicated in clients taking MAOIs

Medication/Food Interactions: Nursing Interventions and Client Education

Medication/Food Interactions	Nursing Interventions/Client Education
MAOIs such as **phenelzine (Nardil)** – ↑ the risk of toxicity	• MAOIs should be discontinued 2 weeks prior to beginning treatment with bupropion.

Therapeutic Nursing Interventions and Client Education

Δ   Instruct the client to take medication on a daily basis to establish therapeutic plasma levels.

Δ   Assist with medication regimen compliance by informing the client that therapeutic effects may not be experienced for 1 to 3 weeks.

Δ   Instruct the client to continue therapy after improvement in symptoms. Sudden discontinuation of medication can result in relapse.

Δ   Advise the client that therapy usually continues for 6 months after resolution of symptoms and may continue for 1 year or longer.

Nursing Evaluation of Medication Effectiveness

Δ   Depending on therapeutic intent, effectiveness may be evidenced by:

• Improvement in depressive state as evidenced by elevated mood, greater alertness and activity level, improved appetite, and normal sleep pattern.

• Improvement of symptoms as evidenced by greater ability to perform ADLs, and to interact socially with peers.

• Improvement of sleeping and eating habits.

• Cessation of smoking.

Key Points

Medication Classification: Mood Stabilizers

Select Prototype Medication: **lithium carbonate**
Mood stabilizing anticonvulsants:
valproic acid (Depakote), carbamazepine
(Tegretol)

Expected Pharmacological Action

Δ   Lithium produces neurochemical changes in the brain including serotonin receptor blockade

Δ   Use of lithium will show evidence of decrease in neuronal atrophy and/or increase in neuronal growth

Therapeutic Uses

Δ   These medications are used in the treatment of bipolar disorders. They control episodes of acute mania, and help to prevent the return of mania or depression.

Δ   Other uses include:

• Alcoholism.

• Bulimia.

• Schizophrenia.

Side/Adverse Effects: Nursing Interventions and Client Education

Side/Adverse Effects	Nursing Interventions/Client Education
Effects with excessive lithium levels	
Gastrointestinal effects (e.g., nausea, **diarrhea**, abdominal pain)	• Advise the client that symptoms are usually transient. • Administer medication with meals or milk.
Tremors that can interfere with fine motor skills and can be exacerbated by factors such as stress and caffeine	• Administer beta-adrenergic blocking agents such as propanolol (Inderal). • Reduce peak levels by using lowest possible dosage, giving in divided doses or using long-acting formulations.
Polyuria	• Use potassium-sparing diuretic, such as amiloride (Midamor). • Instruct the client to maintain adequate fluid intake by drinking at least 8 to 12, 8 oz glasses of water/day.
Renal toxicity	• Monitor the client's I&O. • Adjust dosage and keep dose low. • Assess baseline kidney function and monitor kidney function periodically.
Goiter and hypothyroidism	• Obtain the client's baseline T_3, T_4, and TSH levels prior to starting treatment, and then annually. • Advise the client to monitor for signs of hypothyroidism (e.g., cold, dry skin; decreased heart rate, weight gain). • Goiter and hypothyroid symptoms are reversible with discontinuation of lithium or administration of a thyroid hormone such as levothyroxine (Synthroid).
Teratogenesis	• Advise the client to avoid use during pregnancy.
Use in lactation	• Advise women to avoid breastfeeding while on lithium treatment.

Contraindications/Precautions

Δ   Pregnancy Risk Category D

Δ   Discourage clients from breastfeeding if lithium therapy is necessary.

Δ   Use cautiously in clients with renal dysfunction, heart disease, sodium depletion, and dehydration.

Medication/Food Interactions: Nursing Interventions and Client Education

Medication/Food Interactions	Nursing Interventions/Client Education
Diuretics – Sodium is excreted with the use of diuretics: With ↓ serum sodium, lithium excretion is ↓, which can lead to toxicity.	• Monitor the client for signs of toxicity. • Advise the client to observe for symptoms and to notify the primary care provider. • Encourage the client to maintain a diet adequate in sodium, and to drink 8 to 12, glasses of water/day.
NSAIDs (e.g., **ibuprofen [Motrin] and celecoxib [Celebrex]**) – concurrent use will ↑ renal reabsorption of lithium, leading to toxicity	• Avoid use of NSAIDs to prevent toxic accumulation of lithium. • Aspirin does not cause this to occur, so aspirin can be used for analgesia.
Anticholinergics (e.g., **antihistamines, tricyclic antidepressants**) – abdominal discomfort can result from anticholinergic-induced urinary retention and polyuria	• Advise the client to avoid medications with anticholinergic effects.

Therapeutic Nursing Interventions and Client Education

Δ   Monitor plasma lithium levels while undergoing treatment. At initiation of treatment, monitor levels every 2 to 3 days and then every 1 to 3 months.

- • During initial treatment of a manic episode, levels should be between 0.8 to 1.4 mEq/L.

- • Maintenance level range is between 0.4 to 1.0 mEq/L.

- • Plasma levels > 1.5 mEq/L can result in toxicity.

Δ   The client with a toxic plasma lithium level should be hospitalized and provided with supportive measures. Hemodialysis may be indicated.

Δ   Advise the client that effects begin within 5 to 7 days, but that it may take 2 to 3 weeks to achieve full benefits.

Δ   Encourage the client to maintain adequate sodium intake and to drink 8 to 12 glasses of water/day.

Δ   Advise the client to report signs of toxicity.

Δ   Advise the client to take lithium as prescribed. The medication must be taken 2 to 3 times/day.

Δ   Encourage the client to comply with laboratory appointments needed to monitor lithium effectiveness and adverse effects.

Nursing Evaluation of Medication Effectiveness

Δ   Absence or decrease of acute manic or depressive episodes

Δ   Relief of acute manic symptoms (e.g., flight of ideas, obsessive talking, agitation) or depressive symptoms (e.g., fatigue, poor appetite, psychomotor retardation)

Δ   Improvement in ability to perform ADLs

Δ   Improvement in ability to interact socially with peers

Key Points

Medication Classification: Sedative Hypnotic Medications-Benzodiazepines

Select Prototype Medication: **diazepam (Valium)**

Other Medications: alprazolam (Xanax), lorazepam (Ativan), chlordiazepoxide (Librium)

Expected Pharmacological Action

Δ These medications enhance the action of gamma-amino butyric acid (GABA) in the CNS.

Therapeutic Uses

Δ These medications are used to treat:

- Anxiety disorders.
- Seizure disorders.
- Insomnia.
- Muscle spasm.
- Alcohol withdrawal.
- Panic disorder.
- Induction of anesthesia.

Side/Adverse Effects: Nursing Interventions and Client Education

Side/Adverse Effects	Nursing Interventions/Client Education
CNS depression (e.g., lightheadedness, drowsiness, incoordination)	• Advise the client to observe for symptoms. If symptoms occur, instruct the client to notify the primary care provider. • Advise clients to avoid hazardous activities (e.g., driving, operating heavy equipment/machinery).
Anterograde amnesia	• Advise the client to observe for symptoms. If symptoms occur, instruct the client to notify the primary care provider and stop the medication.
Paradoxical response (e.g., insomnia, excitation, euphoria, anxiety, rage)	• Advise the client to observe for symptoms. If symptoms occur, instruct the client to notify the primary care provider and stop the medication.
Respiratory depression, especially with IV administration	• Monitor the client's vital signs. • Have resuscitation equipment available. • Advise the client to observe for symptoms. If symptoms occur, instruct the client to notify the primary care provider.
Teratogenesis	• Advise childbearing women to avoid becoming pregnant.
Acute toxicity; oral toxicity (e.g., drowsiness, lethargy, confusion); IV toxicity (respiratory depression)	• For oral toxicity, gastric lavage can be used, followed by the administration of activated charcoal or saline cathartics. • For IV toxicity, administer flumazenil (Romazicon) to counteract sedation and reverse side effects. • Monitor the client's vital signs, maintain patent airway, and provide fluids to maintain blood pressure. • Have resuscitation equipment available.

Contraindications/Precautions

Δ   Pregnancy Risk Category D

Δ   Contraindicated in clients with sleep apnea and/or respiratory depression

Δ   Use cautiously in clients with substance abuse.

Medication/Food Interactions: Nursing Interventions and Client Education

Medication/Food Interactions	Nursing Interventions/Client Education
CNS depressants (e.g., **alcohol, barbiturates, opioids**)	• Advise the client to observe for symptoms. If symptoms occur, instruct the client to notify the primary care provider. • Advise clients to avoid hazardous activities (e.g., driving, operating heavy equipment/machinery).

Therapeutic Nursing Interventions and Client Education

Δ Advise the client to take the medication as prescribed and to avoid abrupt discontinuation of treatment to prevent withdrawal symptoms.

Δ When discontinuing benzodiazepines, taper dose over several weeks.

Δ Administer medication with meals. Advise the client to swallow sustained-released tablets and to avoid chewing or crushing the tablet.

Δ Inform the client about possible development of dependency during and after treatment, and to notify the primary care provider if symptoms occur.

Nursing Evaluation of Medication Effectiveness

Δ Improvement of symptoms as evidenced by absence of panic attacks, decrease or absence of anxiety, normal sleep pattern, absence of seizures, absence of withdrawal symptoms from alcohol, and relaxation of muscles

Key Points

Medication Classification: Sedative Hypnotic Medications-Non-Benzodiazepines

Select Prototype Medication: **zolpidem (Ambien)**

Other Medications: zaleplon (Sonata), eszopiclone (Lunesta)
trazodone (Desyrel)

Expected Pharmacological Action

Δ   These medications only bind to benzodiazepine$_1$ subtype of receptors, thereby enhancing the action of gamma-amino butyric acid (GABA) in the CNS. This results in prolonged sleep duration and decreased awakenings. These medications **do not** function as an antianxiety, muscle relaxant, or antiepileptic agent.

Therapeutic Uses

Δ   Management of insomnia

Side/Adverse Effects: Nursing Interventions and Client Education

Side/Adverse Effects	Nursing Interventions/Client Education
Daytime sleepiness and lightheadedness	• Administer medication at bedtime. • Advise the client to take medication allowing for at least 8 hr of sleep.

Contraindications/Precautions

Δ   Pregnancy Risk Category B

Δ   Contraindicated in clients who are breastfeeding

Δ   Schedule IV-controlled substance

Δ   Use cautiously in older adult clients.

Δ   Use cautiously in clients with impaired kidney, liver, and/or respiratory function.

Medication/Food Interactions: Nursing Interventions and Client Education

Medication/Food Interactions	Nursing Interventions/Client Education
CNS depressants (e.g., **alcohol, barbiturates, opioids)** – additive CNS depression	• Advise clients to avoid alcohol and other CNS depressants.
Food – ↓ absorption when taken with food	• Advise the client to take on an empty stomach.

Therapeutic Nursing Interventions and Client Education

Δ   Advise the client to take the medication just before bedtime.

Δ   Advise the client that the medication is not associated with physical dependence and tolerance.

Nursing Evaluation of Medication Effectiveness

Δ   Monitor the client for improvement of symptoms (e.g., prolonged sleep pattern).

Key Points

Medication Classification: Anxiolytic-Non-Barbiturate

Select Prototype Medication:	**buspirone (BuSpar)**
Other Medications:	**None**

Expected Pharmacological Action

Δ   The exact antianxiety mechanism of this medication is unknown. This medication does bind to serotonin and dopamine receptors. There is no potential for abuse, and these medications do not result in sedation nor potentiate the effects of other CNS depressants.

Therapeutic Uses

Δ   Treatment of general anxiety disorder (GAD)

Side/Adverse Effects: Nursing Interventions and Client Education

Side/Adverse Effects	Nursing Interventions/Client Education
CNS effects (e.g., faintness, nausea, headache, lightheadedness, agitation)	• This medication does not interfere with activities because no sedation is caused.

Contraindications/Precautions

Δ   Pregnancy Risk Category B

Δ   Use cautiously in older adult clients and clients with liver and/or renal dysfunction.

Medication/Food Interactions: Nursing Interventions and Client Education

Medication/Food Interactions	Nursing Interventions/Client Education
Erythromycin, ketoconazole, grapefruit juice – ↑ the effects of buspirone when used concurrently	• Avoid the use of these antimicrobial agents. • Advise the client to avoid drinking grapefruit juice.

Therapeutic Nursing Interventions and Client Education

Δ   Advise the client to take the medication with meals to prevent gastric irritation.

Δ   Advise the client that effects do not occur rapidly and may take a week to start, and several more for full benefit to be felt. Should not be used when rapid results are needed or on a PRN basis.

Nursing Evaluation of Medication Effectiveness

Δ   Improvement of symptoms (e.g., decreased muscle tension, feeling rested, increased ability to concentrate and stay focused)

Δ   Improvement in ability to participate in social and occupational interactions

Key Points

Medication Classification: CNS Stimulants

Select Prototype Medication: **methylphenidate (Ritalin, Concerta)**

Other Medications: amphetamine, dextroamphetamine (Dexedrine), amphetamine/ dextroamphetamine mixture, (Adderall), Caffeine

Expected Pharmacological Action

Δ   These medications release norepinephrine and dopamine into the CNS.

Δ   These medications inhibit the reuptake of norepinephrine and dopamine in the CNS.

Therapeutic Uses

Δ   Attention deficit/hyperactivity disorders (ADHD)

Δ   Narcolepsy

Δ   Obesity

Δ   Weight reduction

Side/Adverse Effects: Nursing Interventions and Client Education

Side/Adverse Effects	Nursing Interventions/Client Education
CNS stimulation (e.g., insomnia, restlessness)	• Advise clients to observe for symptoms, and if symptoms occur, instruct the client to notify the primary care provider. • Dosage may need to be reduced.
Weight loss	• Monitor the client's weight. • Promote good nutrition in children. • Encourage children to eat at regular meal times and avoid unhealthy foods for snacks.
Cardiovascular effects (e.g., dysrhythmias, chest pain, high blood pressure) – may ↑ the risk of sudden death in clients with heart abnormalities	• Monitor the client's vital signs and ECG. • Advise clients to observe for symptoms and to notify the primary care provider if they occur.

Contraindications/Precautions

- Δ   Methylphenidate (Ritalin, Concerta)

  - •   Pregnancy Risk Category C

- Δ   Use cautiously in clients with hyperthyroidism, heart disease, glaucoma, history of drug abuse, and those clients taking MAOIs.

Medication/Food Interactions: Nursing Interventions and Client Education

Medication/Food Interactions	Nursing Interventions/Client Education
MAOIs – concurrent use may cause hypertensive crisis	• Avoid concurrent use.
Caffeine – concurrent use may cause an ↑ in CNS stimulant effects	• Instruct the client to avoid foods that contain caffeine.
Phenytoin (Dilantin), warfarin (Coumadin) and phenobarbital – methylphenidate inhibits metabolism of these medications leading to ↑ serum levels	• Monitor the client for adverse effects (e.g., CNS depression, signs of bleeding). • Concurrent use of these medications should be used cautiously.
OTC cold and decongestant medications – OTC decongestants and cold remedies frequently contain medications with sympathomimetic action that can lead to ↑ CNS stimulant effects.	• Instruct the client to avoid use of OTC medications.

Therapeutic Nursing Interventions and Client Education

- Δ   Advise clients to swallow sustained-release tablets whole and to not chew or crush tablet.

- Δ   Teach the client the importance of administering the medication on a regular schedule.

Nursing Evaluation of Medication Effectiveness

- Δ   Depending on therapeutic intent, effectiveness may be evidenced by:

  - •   Improvement of symptoms of ADHD in children and adults such as ↑ ability to focus and complete tasks and interact with peers.

  - •   Improved ability to stay awake.

Key Points

Major Drugs of Abuse and Medications to Support Withdrawal/Abstinence

Δ   Abstinence syndrome occurs when a client abruptly withdraws from a drug that he is physically dependent on.

Δ   Withdrawing from a substance that has the potential to cause an abstinence syndrome can cause distressing symptoms that may or may not lead to coma and death.

Major Drugs of Abuse

Substance	Withdrawal Symptoms
Alcohol	• The degree of symptoms is based on the degree of physical dependence. Withdrawal from a low degree of alcohol dependence will result in a mild reaction including nausea, anxiety, and tremors. Withdrawal from a high degree of alcohol dependence can be life-threatening and require hospitalization. Effects usually start within 12 to 72 hr of the last intake of alcohol and continue for 5 to 7 days. • Symptoms include abdominal cramping, vomiting, tremors, ↑ blood pressure, ↑ heart rate, ↑ temperature, and tonic-clonic seizures. Delirium tremors can occur, in which the client experiences extremely disturbing hallucinations.
Opioids	• Abstinence syndrome begins with sweating and rhinorrhea, progressing from tremors and irritability to severe weakness, nausea and vomiting, pain in the muscles and bones, and muscle spasms. Withdrawal is very unpleasant, but is not life-threatening, and it is self-limiting in 7 to 10 days.
Nicotine	• Abstinence syndrome is evidenced by irritability, nervousness, restlessness, insomnia, and difficulty concentrating.

Management of Withdrawal

Δ   Goals of withdrawal may include:

•   Limit abstinence syndrome symptoms.

•   Prevention of delirium tremens and seizures (alcohol).

•   Promote participation in a program to support abstinence.

Alcohol

Medications	Mechanism of Action	Nursing Interventions and Client Education
Benzodiazepines (e.g., chlordiazepoxide [Librium], diazepam [Valium], lorazepam [Ativan])	• Maintain the client's vital signs within normal limits • ↓ in delirium tremors and risk of seizures • ↓ in the intensity of symptoms	• May be administered when necessary or around the clock. • Obtain the client's baseline vital signs. • Monitor the client's vital signs on an ongoing basis. • Provide for seizure precautions (e.g., padded side rails, suction equipment at bedside).
Adjunct medications: carbamazepine (Tegretol), clonidine (Catapres), propranolol (Inderal)	• ↓ in seizures • ↓ in craving • Depress autonomic response – ↓ in blood pressure, heart rate, and temperature	• Obtain the client's baseline vital signs. • Monitor the client's vital signs on an ongoing basis. • Provide for seizure precautions (e.g., padded side rails, suction equipment at bedside).

Abstinence maintenance - following detox

Disulfiram (Antabuse)	• Disulfiram used concurrently with alcohol will cause acetaldehyde syndrome to occur. • Effects can be mild including nausea, extreme vomiting, weakness, and hypotension. • Acetaldehyde syndrome can progress to respiratory depression, cardiovascular suppression, seizures, and death.	• Inform the client of the potential dangers of drinking any alcohol. • Advise clients to avoid any products that contain alcohol (e.g., cough syrups, aftershave lotion). • Encourage the client to participate in an abstinence program and mental health counseling. • Encourage the client to wear a medical alert bracelet.

Medications	Mechanism of Action	Nursing Interventions and Client Education
Naltrexone (ReVia)	• Naltrexone is a pure opioid antagonist that suppresses the craving and pleasurable effects of alcohol.	• Encourage the client to participate in an abstinence program and mental health counseling. • Take the client's accurate history to determine if the client is also dependent on opioids. Use of naltrexone will initiate withdrawal syndrome. • Advise the client to take with meals to ↓ GI distress. If the client has difficulty with compliance, recommend monthly IM injections.
Acamprosate (Campral)	• Acamprosate ↓ unpleasant effects resulting from abstinence (e.g., anxiety, restlessness).	• Encourage the client to participate in an abstinence program and mental health counseling. • Inform the client that diarrhea may result. • Advise the client to maintain adequate fluid intake and to receive adequate rest. • Advise the client to avoid use in pregnancy.
Opioids		
Methadone substitution	• Methadone substitution is an oral opioid that replaces the opioid the client is addicted to. • This will prevent abstinence syndrome from occurring and remove the need for the client to obtain illegal drugs. • It is used for withdrawal and long-term maintenance. • Dependence will be transferred from the illegal opioid to methadone.	• Inform the client that the methadone dose must be slowly tapered to produce detoxification. • Provide emotional support. • Encourage the client to participate in an abstinence program and mental health counseling.

Medications	Mechanism of Action	Nursing Interventions and Client Education
Clonidine (Catapres)	• Clonidine assists with the control of symptoms related to autonomic hyperactivity (e.g., nausea, vomiting).	• Obtain baseline vital signs. • If the client experiences drowsiness, advise the client to avoid activities that require mental alertness until symptoms subside. • To treat dry mouth, encourage the client to chew on gum or hard candy, and to sip small amounts of water or ice chips.
Buprenorphine (Subutex), buprenorphine combined with naloxone (Suboxone)	• These medications are agonist-antagonist opioids used for both detoxification and maintenance.	• The client must receive medication from the approved treatment center. • Encourage the client to participate in an abstinence program and mental health counseling.
Nicotine		
Bupropion (Zyban)	• Bupropion ↓ nicotine craving and symptoms of withdrawal	• To treat dry mouth, encourage the client to chew on gum or hard candy and to take small amounts of water or ice chips. • Advise the client to avoid caffeine and other CNS stimulants to control insomnia.

Medications	Mechanism of Action	Nursing Interventions and Client Education
Nicotine replacement therapy (e.g., nicotine gum [Nicorette] and nicotine patch [Nicotrol])	• These nicotine replacements are a pharmaceutical product substitute for the nicotine in cigarettes or chewing tobacco.	• Advise the client to chew gum slowly and intermittently over 30 min. • Advise the client to avoid eating or drinking 15 min prior to and while chewing gum. • Use of chewing gum is not recommended for longer than 6 months. • Advise the client to apply a nicotine patch to an area of clean, dry skin each day. • Advise the client to follow product directions for dosage times. • Advise the client to stop using patches, and to notify the primary care provider if local skin reactions occur. • Advise the client to avoid use of any nicotine products while pregnant or breastfeeding.

Primary Reference:

Lehne, R. A. (2007). *Pharmacology for nursing care* (6th ed.). St. Louis, MO: Saunders.

Additional Resources:

Skidmore-Roth, L. (2006). *Mosby's nursing drug reference*. St. Louis, MO: Elsevier.

Wilson, B. A., Shannon, M., Shields, K., Stang, C. (2007). *Nurse's drug guide*. Upper Saddle River, NJ: Prentice Hall.

Unit 5 Medications Affecting the Nervous System

Application Exercises

1. Which of the following nursing interventions is most effective in promoting excretion of a general anesthetic agent from a postsurgical client?

>   A. Increase intravenous fluid rate.
>   B. Offer oral fluids as soon as possible.
>   C. Assist to turn, cough, and deep breathe.
>   D. Use passive range-of-motion exercises.

2. A client's plasma lithium level is 0.2 mEq/L. The nurse can expect to implement which of the following nursing interventions?

>   A. Administer an additional oral dose of lithium.
>   B. Prepare to give emergency resuscitation.
>   C. Infuse 1 L of 0.9% NS over 4 hr.
>   D. Prepare the client immediately for another laboratory draw.

3. A nurse is teaching the parents of a child taking methylphenidate (Ritalin) for ADHD how to administer the medication. Which of the following responses by the nurse is most appropriate?

>   A. "Give your child the medication at bedtime."
>   B. "Discontinue the medication when your child is feeling better."
>   C. "Administer an OTC cold medication for flu symptoms."
>   D. "Provide your child with a nutritious diet and healthy snacks between meals."

4. A client starting phenelzine (Nardil) for treatment of depression should be monitored for which of the following effects?

>   A. Orthostatic hypotension
>   B. Respiratory depression
>   C. GI bleeding
>   D. Rash

5. A nurse is providing teaching to a client who is starting amitriptyline (Elavil) for treatment of depression. Which of the following should be included? (Select all that apply.)

_____ Therapeutic effects will be felt almost immediately.

_____ Stop taking the medication after a week of improved mood.

_____ Client can minimize orthostatic hypotension by getting up slowly.

_____ Decrease dietary fiber intake to control diarrhea.

_____ Chew sugarless gum to prevent dry mouth.

6. Teaching for a client taking high doses of phenytoin (Dilantin) for a seizure disorder should include

A. taking the medication with an antacid to prevent GI upset.

B. practicing good hygiene, using a soft toothbrush, and flossing daily.

C. using an OTC sleeping aid if difficulty sleeping.

D. limiting alcohol intake to two glasses of wine.

7. A client taking valproic acid (Depakote) for seizure control tells the nurse that he drinks a 6-pack of beer a day. What priority assessment should take place?

A. Plasma levels of valproic acid

B. Brain CT scan

C. Liver function studies

D. ECG

8. Which of the following foods should be avoided by a client who is taking an MAOI?

A. Fresh vegetables

B. Cheese

C. Apples

D. Grilled steak

9. Match the following medications with the appropriate side effect and indicated treatment.

levodopa (Dopar)	A. Excessive muscarinic stimulation and respiratory depression that can be treated with atropine
fluoxetine (Prozac)	B. Malignant hyperthermia that can be treated with dantrolene to ↓ metabolic activity of skeletal muscle
neostigmine (Prostigmin)	C. Psychosis as evidenced by visual hallucinations that can be treated with antipsychotic medications, clozapine (Clozaril)
halothane (Fluothane)	D. Gingival hyperplasia managed with good oral hygiene
phenelzine (Nardil)	E. Spinal headache: Advise the client to lie flat for 12 hr postsurgery.
Lithium	F. Muscle pain in the upper body and back that can be treated with a short-term muscle relaxant, such as diazepam (Valium)
chlorpromazine (Thorazine)	G. Sexual dysfunction that can be managed with lowering the dosage, discontinuing the medication temporarily (medication holiday), and use of adjunct medications to ↑ sexual function (e.g., sildenafil [Viagra] and buspirone [BuSpar])
lidocaine (Xylocaine)	H. Hypertensive crisis that can be treated with alpha-adrenergic blocker to induce rapid vasodilation
succinylcholine (Anectine)	I. Hyperthyroidism that can be treated with administration of a thyroid hormone, such as levothyroxine (Synthroid)
phenytoin (Dilantin)	J. Early EPS that can be controlled with anticholinergic medications

Unit 5 Medications Affecting the Nervous System

Application Exercises Answer Key

1. Which of the following nursing interventions is most effective in promoting excretion of a general anesthetic agent from a postsurgical client?

   A. Increase intravenous fluid rate.

   B. Offer oral fluids as soon as possible.

   C. Assist to turn, cough, and deep breathe.

   D. Use passive range-of-motion exercises.

   General anesthetics are excreted through the lungs. Turning, coughing, and deep breathing will assist in excretion through this route. Increasing IV fluids and performing passive range-of-motion exercises do not assist the lungs to excrete a general anesthetic. Clients should not be offered oral fluids until the gag reflex returns.

2. A client's plasma lithium level is 0.2 mEq/L. The nurse can expect to implement which of the following nursing interventions?

   A. Administer an additional oral dose of lithium.

   B. Prepare to give emergency resuscitation.

   C. Infuse 1 L of 0.9% NS over 4 hr.

   D. Prepare the client immediately for another laboratory draw.

   This plasma level is subtherapeutic and the client should be given an additional dose. Emergency resuscitation may be indicated if the client's laboratory value indicates toxicity. There is no indication that the client needs supplemental fluids. There is no reason to question the laboratory result.

3. A nurse is teaching the parents of a child taking methylphenidate (Ritalin) for ADHD how to administer the medication. Which of the following responses by the nurse is most appropriate?

>   A. "Give your child the medication at bedtime."
>
>   B. "Discontinue the medication when your child is feeling better."
>
>   C. "Administer an OTC cold medication for flu symptoms."
>
>   **D. "Provide your child with a nutritious diet and healthy snacks between meals."**

Methylphenidate can depress appetite, so it is important for the client to eat a well-balanced diet to ensure adequate growth and development. The medication is a stimulant and thus should not be given at bedtime. This medication should not be stopped abruptly. Over-the-counter decongestants and cold remedies frequently contain medications with sympathomimetic action that can lead to an increase in CNS stimulant effects.

4. A client starting phenelzine (Nardil) for treatment of depression should be monitored for which of the following effects?

>   **A. Orthostatic hypotension**
>
>   B. Respiratory depression
>
>   C. GI bleeding
>
>   D. Rash

Orthostatic hypotension is a side effect of MAOIs. Clients experience CNS stimulation, not depression. GI bleeding is a side effect of aspirin and NSAIDs. Rash is a side effect of fluoxetine (Prozac).

5. A nurse is providing teaching to a client who is starting amitriptyline (Elavil) for treatment of depression. Which of the following should be included? (Select all that apply.)

> _____ Therapeutic effects will be felt almost immediately.
>
> _____ Stop taking the medication after a week of improved mood.
>
> __X__ **Client can minimize orthostatic hypotension by getting up slowly.**
>
> _____ Decrease dietary fiber intake to control diarrhea.
>
> __X__ **Chew sugarless gum to prevent dry mouth.**

Orthostatic hypotension is a side effect of amitriptyline and can be minimized by getting up slowly. Dry mouth is a side effect of amitriptyline and can be minimized by chewing sugarless gum. Therapeutic effects may take several weeks to be achieved. Medication should not be stopped abruptly and therapy will most likely last 6 to 12 months to prevent relapse. Clients should increase dietary fiber to prevent constipation.

6. Teaching for a client taking high doses of phenytoin (Dilantin) for a seizure disorder should include

    A. taking the medication with an antacid to prevent GI upset.

    B. practicing good hygiene, using a soft toothbrush, and flossing daily.

    C. using an OTC sleeping aid if difficulty sleeping.

    D. limiting alcohol intake to two glasses of wine.

Gingival hyperplasia can occur with phenytoin use. Good oral hygiene can help minimize the effects. Antacids will interfere with absorption. OTC sleeping aids can have an additive CNS depressant effect. Clients taking phenytoin for seizure control should abstain from drinking any alcohol.

7. A client taking valproic acid (Depakote) for seizure control tells the nurse that he drinks a 6-pack of beer a day. What priority assessment should take place?

    A. Plasma levels of valproic acid

    B. Brain CT scan

    C. Liver function studies

    D. ECG

Monitoring liver function studies is a priority for a client taking valproic acid to detect hepatotoxicity. Chronic alcohol use can lead to further liver damage. Obtaining plasma levels of valproic acid is important, but not the highest priority for this client. Brain CT scan and ECG are not indicated in this client.

8. Which of the following foods should be avoided by a client who is taking an MAOI?

    A. Fresh vegetables

    B. Cheese

    C. Apples

    D. Grilled steak

Cheese contains dietary tyramine that can interact with MAOIs to precipitate hypertensive crisis. Tyramine is not contained in fresh vegetables, apples, or grilled steak.

9. Match the following medications with the appropriate side effect and indicated treatment.

levodopa (Dopar)

fluoxetine (Prozac)

neostigmine
(Prostigmin)

halothane (Fluothane)

phenelzine (Nardil)

Lithium

chlorpromazine
(Thorazine)

lidocaine (Xylocaine)

succinylcholine
(Anectine)

phenytoin (Dilantin)

A. Excessive muscarinic stimulation and respiratory depression that can be treated with atropine

B. Malignant hyperthermia that can be treated with dantrolene to ↓ metabolic activity of skeletal muscle

C. Psychosis as evidenced by visual hallucinations that can be treated with antipsychotic medications, clozapine (Clozaril)

D. Gingival hyperplasia managed with good oral hygiene

E. Spinal headache: Advise the client to lie flat for 12 hr postsurgery.

F. Muscle pain in the upper body and back that can be treated with a short- term muscle relaxant, such as diazepam (Valium)

G. Sexual dysfunction that can be managed with lowering the dosage, discontinuing the medication temporarily (medication holiday), and use of adjunct medications to ↑ sexual function (e.g., sildenafil [Viagra] and buspirone [BuSpar])

H. Hypertensive crisis that can be treated with alpha-adrenergic blocker to induce rapid vasodilation

I. Hyperthyroidism that can be treated with administration of a thyroid hormone, such as levothyroxine (Synthroid)

J. Early EPS that can be controlled with anticholinergic medications

Neostigmine (Prostigmin) (A); succinylcholine (Anectine) (F); levodopa (Dopar) (C); phenytoin (Dilantin) (D); lidocaine (Xylocaine) (E); halothane (Fluothane) (B); fluoxetine (Prozac) (G); phenelzine (Nardil) (H); lithium (I); chlorpromazine (Thorazine) (J).

Unit 6	Medications Affecting the Cardiovascular System

Contributor: Leona Pie, MPH, BSN, RN

 NCLEX® Connections:

Learning Objective: Review and apply knowledge within **"Medications Affecting the Cardiovascular System"** in readiness for performance of the following nursing activities as outlined by the NCLEX® test plans:

Δ   Assess/monitor the client for expected effects of medications.

Δ   Assess/monitor the client for side/adverse effects of medications.

Δ   Assess/monitor the client for actual/potential specific food and medication interactions.

Δ   Identify contraindications, actual/potential incompatibilities, and interactions between medications, and intervene appropriately.

Δ   Identify symptoms/evidence of an allergic reaction, and respond appropriately.

Δ   Evaluate/monitor and document the therapeutic and adverse/side effects of medications.

Δ   Provide/reinforce client teaching on actions, therapeutic effects, potential side/adverse effects, and interactions of medications.

 General Key Points

Δ   Several mechanisms are involved in the regulation of **arterial pressure.**

•   The **autonomic nervous system** helps to control arterial pressure by adjustments in cardiac output and peripheral resistance.

•   The **renin-angiotensin-aldosterone system (RAAS)** helps to control arterial pressure by:

◊   Releasing the hormone **angiotensin II**, a powerful vasoconstrictor of arterioles and veins.

◊   Releasing **aldosterone,** which promotes sodium and water retention by the kidneys.

•   Sodium and water retention by the **kidneys** help maintain arterial pressure by increasing blood volume and cardiac output.

- • Decreasing blood volume and dilating the arterioles and vein help to control arterial pressure.

- • There is no identifiable cause of primary (essential) **hypertension**. Primary hypertension accounts for approximately 90% of the cases of hypertension.

Δ Untreated **hypertension** ↑ the risk of morbidity and mortality from kidney disease, stroke, myocardial infarction (MI), heart failure, and angina pectoris.

Δ **Hypertension** can be managed with pharmacological therapy, as well as **lifestyle changes** (e.g. weight loss, complying with the Dietary Approaches to Stop Hypertension [DASH] diet, maintaining adequate levels of potassium and calcium, quitting smoking, restricting alcohol and sodium intake, and participating in aerobic exercise on a regular basis).

Δ **Heart failure, cardiac failure, or pump failure** results from the inability of the heart muscle to pump enough blood to supply the whole body.

Δ The different determinants of cardiac output such as **heart rate, stroke volume, preload, and afterload** are affected in heart failure.

Δ Inability to pump sufficient blood results in:

- • ↓ **tissue perfusion** as evidenced by fatigue, weakness, and activity intolerance.

- • **Pulmonary and systemic congestion or volume overload** as evidenced by jugular venous distention, peripheral edema, and dyspnea.

Δ Medications to treat **angina** are available in different formulations. Clients need to be instructed in the proper use and administration of the formulation prescribed.

Δ **Cardiac medications** can be classified in various ways. For example, nitroglycerine (Nitrostat) is classified by its chemical composition as an aminoglycoside, by its pharmacological action as a vasodilator, and by its therapeutic effect as a medication used for the treatment of angina pectoris.

Δ When caring for clients receiving cardiac medications, it is important to know the intended therapeutic effect. For example, a nurse should know if the intended therapeutic effect for a client receiving nifedipine (Procardia) is to lower blood pressure (e.g., treatment of hypertension), or to prevent anginal attacks (e.g., treatment of angina pectoris).

Key Points

Medication Classification: Adrenergic Agonists

Select Prototype Medication: epinephrine (Adrenaline): catecholamine
dopamine (Intropin): catecholamine
dobutamine (Dobutrex): catecholamine

Other Medications: Isoproterenol: catecholamine
Terbutaline: noncatecholamine

Expected Pharmacological Action

Δ   Catecholamine adrenergic agonists cannot be taken by the oral route, do not cross the blood-brain barrier, and the duration of action is short.

Receptors	Site/Response
Alpha$_1$	• Activation of receptors in arterioles of skin, viscera and mucous membranes, and veins lead to vasoconstriction
Beta$_1$	• Heart stimulation leads to increased heart rate, increased myocardial contractility, and increased rate of conduction through the AV node • Activation of receptors in the kidney lead to the release of renin
Beta$_2$	• Activation of receptors in the arterioles of the heart, lungs, and skeletal muscles lead to vasodilation • Bronchial stimulation leads to bronchodilation • Activation of receptors in uterine smooth muscle causes relaxation • Activation of receptors in the liver cause glycogenolysis • Skeletal muscle receptor activation leads to muscle contraction
Dopamine	• Activation of receptors in the kidney cause the renal blood vessels to dilate.

Receptors	Pharmacologic Action	Therapeutic Use
epinephrine (Adrenaline)		
Alpha$_1$	• Vasoconstriction	• Slows absorption of local anesthetics • Manages superficial bleeding • ↓ congestion of nasal mucosa • ↑ **blood pressure**

Receptors	Pharmacologic Action	Therapeutic Use
Beta$_1$	• ↑ heart rate • ↑ myocardial contractility • ↑ rate of conduction through the AV node	• **Treatment of AV block and cardiac arrest**
Beta$_2$	• Bronchodilation	• Asthma
dopamine (Intropin)		
Low dose – Dopamine	• Renal blood vessel dilation	• Shock • Heart failure
Moderate dose – Dopamine Beta$_1$	• Renal blood vessel dilation • ↑ heart rate • ↑ myocardial contractility • ↑ rate of conduction through the AV node	
High dose – Dopamine Beta$_1$ Alpha$_1$	• Renal blood vessel dilation • ↑ heart rate • ↑ myocardial contractility • ↑ rate of conduction through the AV node • Vasoconstriction	
dobutamine (Dobutrex)		
Beta$_1$	• ↑ heart rate • ↑ myocardial contractility • ↑ rate of conduction through the AV node	• Heart failure

Side/Adverse Effects: Nursing Interventions and Client Education

Side/Adverse Effects	Nursing Interventions/Client Education
epinephrine (Adrenaline)	
Vasoconstriction from activation of alpha$_1$ receptors in the heart can lead to hypertensive crisis.	• Provide for continuous cardiac monitoring. • Report changes in vital signs to the primary care provider.
Beta$_1$ receptor activation in the heart can cause dysrhythmias. Beta$_1$ receptor activation also ↑ the workload of the heart and ↑ oxygen demand leading to the development of angina.	• Provide for continuous cardiac monitoring. • Monitor the client closely for dysrhythmias, change in HR and chest pain. • Notify the primary care provider of signs of dysrhythmias, ↑ heart rate and chest pain, and treat per protocol.

dopamine (Intropin)	
Beta$_1$ receptor activation in the heart can cause dysrhythmias. Beta$_1$ receptor activation also ↑ the workload of the heart and ↑ oxygen demand leading to development of angina.	• Provide for continuous cardiac monitoring. • Monitor the client closely for dysrhythmias, change in HR, and chest pain. • Notify the primary care provider of signs of dysthymias, ↑ HR, and chest pain, and treat per protocol.
Necrosis can occur from extravasation of high doses of dopamine.	• Monitor IV site carefully. • Discontinue infusion at first sign of irritation.
dobutamine (Dobutrex)	
↑ HR	• Provide for continuous cardiac monitoring. • Report changes in vital signs to the primary care provider.

Contraindications/Precautions

Δ Pregnancy Risk Category C – epinephrine, dopamine; Pregnancy Risk Category B – dobutamine

Δ These medications are contraindicated in clients with tachydysrhythmias and ventricular fibrillation.

Δ Use cautiously in clients with hyperthyroidism, angina, history of myocardial infarction, hypertension, and diabetes.

Medication/Food Interactions: Nursing Interventions and Client Education

Medication/Food Interactions	Nursing Interventions/Client Education
MAOIs – inactivates epinephrine, therefore, MAOIs will prevent this inactivation, and thereby prolong and intensify effects of epinephrine.	• Avoid use of MAOIs in clients receiving epinephrine.
Tricyclic antidepressants – block uptake of epinephrine, which will prolong and intensify effects of epinephrine.	• Clients taking these medications concurrently may need a lowered dosage of epinephrine.
General anesthetics – can cause the heart to become hypersensitive to the effects of epinephrine leading to dysthymias.	• Perform continuous ECG monitoring of client. • Notify the primary care provider of signs of chest pain, dysthymias, and ↑ heart rate.
Alpha-adrenergic blocking agents, such as phentolamine – block action at alpha receptors. No interaction with dobutamine.	• Phentolamine may be used to treat epinephrine toxicity.
Beta-adrenergic blocking agents, such as propranolol – block action at beta receptors.	• Propranolol may be used to treat chest pain and dysrhythmias.
Diuretics – promote beneficial effect of dopamine.	• Monitor for therapeutic effects.

Therapeutic Nursing Interventions and Client Education

Δ   Must be administered IV by continuous infusion.

Δ   Use IV pump to control infusion.

Δ   Dosage titrated based on blood pressure response.

Δ   Stop infusion at first evidence of infiltration. Extravasation can be treated with local injection of an alpha-adrenergic blocking agent, such as phentolamine.

Δ   Assess/monitor the client for chest pain. Notify the primary care provider if chest pain occurs.

Δ   Provide continuous ECG monitoring. Notify the primary care provider of signs of tachycardia or dysrhythmias.

Nursing Evaluation of Medication Effectiveness

Δ   Depending on therapeutic intent, effectiveness may be evidenced by:

•   Improved perfusion as evidenced by urine output of $\geq$ 30 mL/hr (with normal renal function), improved mental status, and systolic blood pressure maintained at $\geq$ 90 mm Hg.

Key Points

Medication Classification: Alpha Adrenergic Blockers (Sympatholytics)

Select Prototype Medication: prazosin (Minipress)

Other Medications: doxazosin mesylate (Cardura)

Expected Pharmacological Action

Δ   Selective alpha$_1$ blockade results in:

  • Venous and arterial dilation.

  • Smooth muscle relaxation of the prostatic capsule and bladder neck.

Therapeutic Uses

Δ   Alpha adrenergic blockers are used in the treatment of hypertension.

Δ   Doxazosin mesylate (Cardura) may be used to ↓ symptoms of benign prostatic hypertrophy (BPH) (e.g., urgency, frequency, dysuria).

Side/Adverse Effects: Nursing Interventions and Client Education

Side/Adverse Effects	Nursing Interventions/Client Education
First-dose orthostatic hypotension	• Start treatment with low dosage of medication. • First dose may be given at night. • Monitor blood pressure for 2 hr after the initiation of treatment. • Instruct the client to avoid activities requiring mental alertness for the first 12 to 24 hr. • Instruct the client to change positions slowly and to lie down if feeling dizzy, lightheaded, or faint.

Contraindications/Precautions

Δ   Pregnancy Risk Category C

Δ   Contraindicated in clients with hypersensitivity to medication

Medication/Food Interactions: Nursing Interventions and Client Education

Medication/Food Interactions	Nursing Interventions/Client Education
Antihypertensive medications – may have additive hypotensive effect	• Instruct the client to observe for signs of hypotension (e.g., dizziness, lightheadedness, faintness). • Instruct the client to lie down if feeling dizzy, lightheaded, or faint, and change positions slowly.
↓ antihypertensive effects – NSAIDs and clonidine can counteract the antihypertensive effects of prazosin	• Advise clients to avoid OTC NSAIDs.

Therapeutic Nursing Interventions and Client Education

Δ   Obtain baseline blood pressure and heart rate.

Δ   Instruct the client that the medication can be taken with food.

Δ   Recommend that the client take initial dose at bedtime to ↓ "first-dose" hypotensive effect.

Nursing Evaluation of Medication Effectiveness

Δ   Depending on therapeutic intent, effectiveness may be evidenced by:

•   ↓ in blood pressure and maintenance of normotensive blood pressure.

•   Reduction in benign prostatic hypertrophy symptoms.

Key Points

Medication Classification: Centrally Acting Alpha₂ Agonists

Select Prototype Medication: **clonidine (Catapres)**

Other Medications: guanfacine HCl (Tenex), methyldopa (Aldomet)

Expected Pharmacological Action

Δ   These medications act within the CNS to ↓ sympathetic outflow. This results in ↓ of norepinephrine (NE) released from sympathetic nerves, thereby decreasing the amount of NE that is available to stimulate the adrenergic receptors (both alpha and beta receptors) of the heart and peripheral vascular system.

•   ↓ in sympathetic outflow to the myocardium results in bradycardia and ↓ cardiac output (CO).

•   ↓ in sympathetic outflow to the peripheral vasculature results in vasodilation, which leads to ↓ blood pressure.

Therapeutic Uses

Δ   Treatment of hypertension

Δ   Severe cancer pain – administered parenterally by epidural infusion

Δ   Investigational use – migraine headache, flushing from menopause, and management of withdrawal symptoms from alcohol, tobacco, and opioids

Side/Adverse Effects: Nursing Interventions and Client Education

Side/Adverse Effects	Nursing Interventions/Client Education
Drowsiness and sedation	• Drowsiness will diminish as use of medication continues. • Advise the client to avoid activities that require mental alertness until symptoms subside.
Dry mouth	• Advise the client to be compliant with medication regimen. • Reassure the client that symptom usually resolves in 2 to 4 weeks. • Encourage the client to chew on gum or hard candy, and to take small amounts of water or ice chips.

Side/Adverse Effects	Nursing Interventions/Client Education
Rebound hypertension	• Advise the client not to discontinue treatment without consulting the primary care provider. • Clonidine should be discontinued gradually over the course of 2 to 4 days.

Contraindications/Precautions

Δ   Pregnancy Risk Category C

Δ   Avoid use during pregnancy to prevent fetal injury.

Medication/Food Interactions: Nursing Interventions and Client Education

Medication/Food Interactions	Nursing Interventions/Client Education
Antihypertensive medications – may have an additive hypotensive effect	• Instruct the client to observe for signs of hypotension (e.g., dizziness, lightheadedness, faintness). • Instruct the client to lie down if feeling dizzy, lightheaded, or faint, and change positions slowly.
Prazosin, MAOIs, and tricyclic antidepressants – concurrent use of these medications and clonidine can counteract the antihypertensive effect of clonidine	• Monitor the client for therapeutic effect.
CNS depressants – additive CNS depression can occur when used concurrently with other CNS depressants, such as alcohol	• Advise the client of additive CNS depression with alcohol, and encourage the client to avoid use.

Therapeutic Nursing Interventions and Client Education

Δ   Advise child-bearing women to rule out pregnancy before starting treatment regimen.

Δ   Medication is usually administered twice a day in divided doses. Take larger dose at bedtime to ↓ the occurrence of daytime sleepiness.

Δ   Transdermal patches are applied every seven days. Advise the client to apply patch on hairless, intact skin on torso or upper arm.

Nursing Evaluation of Medication Effectiveness

Δ   Depending on therapeutic intent, effectiveness may be evidenced by:

•   ↓ blood pressure.

•   Maintenance of normotensive state.

•   Absence of pain.

Key Points

Medication Classification: Beta Adrenergic Blockers (Sympatholytics)

Select Prototype Medication:	**Cardioselective: metoprolol (Lopressor)** **Nonselective: propranolol (Inderal)**
Other Medications:	Cardioselective: atenolol (Tenormin) metoprolol succinate (Toprol XL) Nonselective: nadolol (Corgard)

Expected Pharmacological Action and Therapeutic Uses

Δ   In cardiac conditions, the primary effects of beta-adrenergic blockers are a result of **beta$_1$-adrenergic blockade** in the myocardium and in the electrical conduction system of the heart.

- ↓ heart rate (chronotropic [rate] action)

- ↓ myocardial contractility (inotropic [force] action)

- ↓ rate of conduction through the AV node

Therapeutic Use	Pharmacological Action
Angina pectoris	• Blocking of SNS leads to ↓ HR, ↓ myocardial contractility, and ↓ rate of conduction through the AV node. These effects ↓ the workload of the heart, which results in ↓ myocardial oxygen demands. • There is also a modest ↑ in myocardial oxygen supply as a result of a slower heart allowing more time for coronary blood flow to reach the myocardium.
Hypertension	• Exact mechanism unknown: may be related to long-term use causing reduction in peripheral vascular resistance
Cardiac dysrhythmias	• Block electrical conduction through the SA and AV node
Myocardial infarction	• ↓ heart rate and ↓ contractility, which leads to ↓ oxygen demand • ↓ blood pressure further ↓ oxygen demand. • Also, a slower HR leads ↑ myocardial oxygen supply.
Heart failure	• Exact mechanism unknown: may be related to a ↓ in sympathetic stimulation and prevention of dysrhythmias.

Δ   Other uses may include:

- Treatment of hyperthyroidism, migraine headache, stage fright, pheochromocytoma, and glaucoma.

Side/Adverse Effects: Nursing Interventions and Client Education

Side/Adverse Effects	Nursing Interventions/Client Education
Beta$_1$ Blockade – metoprolol (Lopressor)	
Bradycardia	• Monitor the client's pulse if below 60 beats/min, hold medication, and notify the primary care provider. If symptomatic (e.g., with low blood pressure), administer atropine and isoproterenol to restore heart rate. • Use cautiously in clients with diabetes. This medication can mask tachycardia, an early sign of low blood glucose in clients with diabetes. Advise clients to monitor blood glucose to detect hypoglycemia.
↓ cardiac output	• Use cautiously with clients in heart failure. Doses are started very low and titrated to the desired level. • There is a delayed response, and it may take 1 to 3 months for beneficial effects to occur. • Advise the client to observe for signs of worsening heart failure (e.g., shortness of breath, edema, fatigue). • The primary care provider should be notified if symptoms occur.
AV block	• Obtain a baseline ECG and monitor. • Clients with AV block should not be administered beta-blockers.
Orthostatic hypotension	• Advise the client to sit or lie down if experiencing dizziness or faintness. • The client should avoid sudden changes of position and rise slowly.
Rebound myocardium excitation	• The myocardium becomes sensitized to catecholamines with long-term use of beta-blockers. • Advise clients not to stop taking beta-blockers abruptly, but to follow the primary care provider's instructions. • Use of beta-blockers can be discontinued over 1 to 2 weeks.
Beta$_2$ Blockade – propranolol (Inderal)	
Bronchoconstriction	• Avoid in clients with asthma. • Clients with asthma should be administered a beta$_1$ selective agent.

Side/Adverse Effects	Nursing Interventions/Client Education
Glycogenolysis is inhibited	• Clients with diabetes rely on the breakdown of glycogen into glucose to manage low blood glucose (can happen with insulin overdose). • In addition, a ↓ heart rate can further mask symptoms of impending low blood glucose level. Clients with diabetes should be administered a beta$_1$ selective agent.

Contraindications/Precautions

Δ   Beta-adrenergic blockers are contraindicated in clients with AV block and sinus bradycardia.

Δ   Nonselective beta-adrenergic blockers are contraindicated in clients with asthma, bronchospasm, and heart failure.

Δ   Use cardioselective beta-adrenergic blockers cautiously in clients with heart failure, asthma, bronchospasm, diabetes, with history of severe allergies, and depression.

Medication/Food Interactions: Nursing Interventions, and Client Education

Medication/Food Interactions	Nursing Interventions/Client Education
Beta₁ Blockade – metoprolol (Lopressor)	
Calcium channel blockers (CCB): verapamil (Calan) and diltiazem (Cardizem) – intensifies the effects of beta-blockers	• CCB intensify effects of beta-blockers • ↓ heart rate • ↓ myocardial contractility • ↓ rate of conduction through the AV node • Monitor clients closely if taking a CCB and beta-blocker concurrently.
Antihypertensive medications – concurrent use of antihypertensive medications with beta-blockers can intensify the hypotensive effect of both medications	• Monitor clients for a drop in blood pressure.
Beta₂ Blockade – propranolol (Inderal)	
Insulin – prevents glycogenolysis (Same as above)	• May need to adjust dosage of insulin when using propranolol.

Therapeutic Nursing Interventions and Client Education

Δ   Advise clients not to discontinue medication without consulting the primary care provider.

Δ   Advise clients to avoid sudden changes in position to prevent occurrence of orthostatic hypotension.

Δ   Instruct the client not to crush or chew extended release tablets.

Δ   Teach the client to self monitor heart rate and blood pressure at home on a daily basis.

Nursing Evaluation of Medication Effectiveness

Δ   Depending on therapeutic intent, effectiveness may be evidenced by:

• Absence of chest pain.

• Absence of cardiac dysrhythmias.

• Normotensive blood pressure readings.

• Control of heart failure signs and symptoms.

Key Points

Medication Classification: Angiotensin-Converting Enzyme-ACE Inhibitors

Select Prototype Medication: **captopril (Capoten)**

Other Medications: enalapril (Vasotec), fosinopril (Monopril), lisinopril (Prinivil), ramipril (Altace)

Expected Pharmacological Action

Δ   ACE inhibitors produce their effects by blocking the **production** of angiotensin II. This results in:

  • Vasodilation (mostly arteriole).

  • Excretion of sodium and water, and retention of potassium (through effects on the kidney).

  • Possible prevention of angiotensin II and aldosterone-induced pathological changes in the blood vessels and heart.

Therapeutic Uses

Δ   Heart failure

Δ   Hypertension

Δ   Myocardial infraction – ↓ mortality and ↓ risk of heart failure

Δ   Diabetic and nondiabetic nephropathy

Δ   For clients at high risk for a cardiovascular event, ramipril (Altace) can be used to prevent MI, stroke, or death.

Side/Adverse Effects: Nursing Interventions and Client Education

Side/Adverse Effects	Nursing Interventions/Client Education
First dose orthostatic hypotension	• If the client is already taking a diuretic, the medication should be stopped temporarily for 2 to 3 days prior to the start of an ACE inhibitor. • Start treatment with a low dosage of the medication. • Monitor the client's blood pressure for 2 hr after initiation of treatment. • Instruct the client to change positions slowly and to lie down if feeling dizzy, lightheaded, or faint.
Cough	• Inform the client of the possibility of experiencing a dry cough. • The client should notify the primary provider as medication will most likely be discontinued.
Hyperkalemia	• Monitor potassium levels to maintain normal range of 3.0 to 5 mEq/L. • The client should only take potassium supplements and potassium salt substitutes if prescribed by the primary care provider.
Rash and dysgeusia (altered taste)	• The client should inform the primary care provider if these effects occur. • Symptoms will stop with discontinuation of the medication.
Angioedema	• Manifested as swelling of the tongue and oral pharynx. • Treat severe effects with subcutaneous injection of epinephrine. • Symptoms will stop with discontinuation of medication.
Neutropenia – rare but serious complication of captopril (Capoten)	• Monitor the client's WBC counts every 2 weeks for 3 months, then periodically. • Reversible when detected early. • Inform the client to notify the primary care provider at the first signs of infection (e.g., fever, sore throat). • If the client develops low WBC, ACE inhibitors will most likely be discontinued.

Contraindications/Precautions

△ Pregnancy Risk Category D during second and third trimester related to fetal injury

△ Contraindicated in clients with renal stenosis when present bilaterally or in a single remaining kidney

△ Contraindicated in clients with a history of angioedema following use of ACE inhibitor

△ Use cautiously in clients with renal impairment. Dosages will most likely be reduced, except for fosinopril (Monopril).

△ Clients with renal impairment and disorders, such as systemic lupus erythematosus, are at greater risk for developing neutropenia. Closely monitor these clients for signs of infection.

Medication/Food Interactions: Nursing Interventions and Client Education

Medication/Food Interactions	Nursing Interventions/Client Education
Diuretics – can contribute to first-dose hypotension	• The client should be advised to temporarily stop taking diuretics 2 to 3 days before the start of therapy with an ACE inhibitor.
Antihypertensive medications – may have an additive effect	• Advise clients that dosage of medication may need to be adjusted if ACE inhibitors are added to the treatment regimen.
Potassium supplements and potassium-sparing diuretics – ↑ risk of hyperkalemia	• The client should only take potassium supplements and potassium salt substitutes if prescribed by the primary care provider.
Lithium – ACE inhibitors can ↑ lithium levels.	• Monitor the client's lithium levels to avoid toxicity.
NSAIDs – use of these medications may ↓ the antihypertensive effect of ACE inhibitors	• The client should inform the primary care provider of the use of these OTC medications and minimize use.

Therapeutic Nursing Interventions and Client Education

Δ   Advise the client that the medication may be prescribed as a single formulation or in combination with hydrochlorothiazide.

Δ   Advise the client that blood pressure has to be monitored after the first dose for at least 2 hr to detect hypotension.

Δ   Instruct the client that captopril should be taken at least 1 hr before meals. All other ACE inhibitors can be taken with or without food.

Δ   Advise the client to notify the primary care provider if cough, rash, dysgeusia, and/or signs of infection occur.

Nursing Evaluation of Medication Effectiveness

Δ   Depending on therapeutic intent, effectiveness may be evidenced by:

•   ↓ in blood pressure.

•   Improvement of heart failure (e.g. ability to perform activities of daily living, improved breath sounds, absence of edema).

•   Improvement in renal function as evidenced by ↓ in proteinuria.

Key Points

Medication Classification: Angiotensin II Receptor Blockers (ARBs)

Select Prototype Medication: **losartan (Cozaar)**

Other Medications: valsartan (Diovan), irbesartan (Avapro), candesartan (Atacand), olmesartan (Benicar)

Expected Pharmacological Action

Δ   Blocks the **action** of angiotensin II in the body. This results in:

- Vasodilation (mostly arteriole).

- Excretion of sodium and water, and retention of potassium (through effects on the kidney).

Δ   The major difference between ARBs and ACE inhibitors is that cough and hyperkalemia are not side effects of ARBs.

Therapeutic Uses

Δ   Reduction of hypertension (all ARBs)

Δ   Management of heart failure and prevention of mortality following MI (valsartan)

Δ   Stroke prevention (losartan)

Δ   Delay progression of diabetic nephropathy (irbesartan, losartan)

Side/Adverse Effects: Nursing Interventions and Client Education

Side/Adverse Effects	Nursing Interventions/Client Education
Angioedema	• Advise the client to observe for signs and symptoms (e.g., skin wheals, swelling of tongue). • The client should notify the primary care provider immediately if symptoms occur.
Fetal injury	• Advise women of risk during the second and third trimester of pregnancy.

Contraindications/Precautions

Δ   Contraindicated in second and third trimester related to fetal injury (Pregnancy Risk Category D)

Δ   Contraindicated in clients with renal stenosis when present bilaterally or in a single remaining kidney

Δ   Use cautiously in clients who experienced angioedema with ACE inhibitor, not an absolute contraindication

Medication/Food Interactions: Nursing Interventions and Client Education

Medication/Food Interactions	Nursing Interventions/Client Education
Antihypertensive medications – may have additive effect when used with ARBs	• Advise clients that dosage of medication may need to be adjusted if ACE inhibitors are added to the treatment regimen.

Therapeutic Nursing Interventions and Client Education

Δ   Advise the client that medication may be prescribed as a single formulation or in combination with hydrochlorothiazide.

Δ   Advise clients that ARBs can be taken with or without food.

Nursing Evaluation of Medication Effectiveness

Δ   Depending on therapeutic intent, effectiveness may be evidenced by:

•   ↓ in blood pressure.

•   Improvement of heart failure (e.g. ability to perform activities of daily living, improved breath sounds, absence of edema).

•   Improvement in renal function as evidenced by a ↓ in proteinuria.

Key Points

Medication Classification: Calcium Channel Blockers

Select Prototype Medication: **nifedipine (Adalat, Procardia)**

Other Medications: amlodipine (Norvasc), felodipine (Plendil), nicardipine (Cardene), verapamil (Calan), diltiazem (Cardizem)

Expected Pharmacological Action

Medication	Expected Pharmacological Action	Site of Action at Therapeutic Doses
Nifedipine (Adalat, Procardia)	• Blocking of calcium channels in blood vessels leads to **vasodilation** of peripheral arterioles and arteries/arterioles of the heart.	• Act primarily on arterioles • Veins not significantly affected.
Verapamil (Calan) Diltiazem (Cardizem)	• Blocking of calcium channels in blood vessels leads to **vasodilation** of peripheral arterioles and arteries/arterioles of the heart. • Blocking of calcium channels in the myocardium, the SA node, and the AV node leads to a **↓ force of contraction, a ↓ heart rate, and slowing of the rate of conduction through the AV node.**	• Act on arterioles and the heart at therapeutic doses • Veins not significantly affected.

Therapeutic Uses

Medication	Angina pectoris	Hypertension	Cardiac dysrhythmias (e.g., atrial fibrillation, atrial flutter, SVT)
Nifedipine (Adalat, Procardia)	X	X	
Amlodipine (Norvasc)	X	X	
Nicardipine (Cardene)	X	X	
Felodipine (Plendil)		X	
Verapamil (Calan) Diltiazem (Cardizem)	X	X	X

Side/Adverse Effects: Nursing Interventions and Client Education

Side/Adverse Effects	Nursing Interventions/Client Education
nifedipine (Adalat, Procardia)	
Reflex tachycardia	• Monitor the client for an ↑ heart rate. • Beta-blocker (e.g., metoprolol [Lopressor]) can be administered to counteract tachycardia.
Peripheral edema	• Inform the client to observe for swelling in lower extremities and notify the primary care provider if it occurs. • A diuretic may be prescribed to control edema.
Acute toxicity	• With excessive doses, the heart, in addition to blood vessels, is affected. • See interventions below.
verapamil (Calan) diltiazem (Cardizem)	
Orthostatic hypotension and peripheral edema	• Monitor the client's blood pressure, edema, and weigh daily. • Instruct the client to observe for swelling in lower extremities, and notify the primary care provider if it occurs. • A diuretic may be prescribed to control edema. • Instruct clients about the signs of postural hypotension (lightheadedness, dizziness). If these occur, advise the client to sit or lie down. Can be minimized by getting up slowly.
Constipation (primarily verapamil)	• Advise the client to ↑ intake of high fiber food and oral fluids, if not restricted.

Side/Adverse Effects	Nursing Interventions/Client Education
Suppression of cardiac function (e.g., bradycardia, heart failure)	• Monitor the client's ECG, pulse rate, and rhythm. • Advise the client to observe for suppression of cardiac function (e.g., slow pulse, activity intolerance), and to notify the primary care provider if these occur. • The primary care provider may discontinue the medication.
Dysrhythmias – QRS complex is widened and QT interval is prolonged	• Monitor the client's vital signs and ECG.
Acute toxicity	• Monitor the client's vital signs and ECG. Gastric lavage and cathartic may be indicated. • Administer medications to counteract toxic levels of calcium channel blocker (e.g, IV norepinephrine for hypotension, calcium to ↓ myocardial contractility, and atropine and isoproterenol for bradycardia and AV block). • IV fluids and the Trendelenburg position may be necessary to reverse hypotension. • Have equipment for cardioversion and cardiac pacer available, and lidocaine IV for dysrhythmias.

Contraindications/Precautions

Δ Pregnancy Risk Category C

Δ Use cautiously with women who are lactating.

Δ Contraindicated in clients with heart block, hypotension, bradycardia, aortic stenosis, or severe heart failure.

Δ Use verapamil and diltiazem cautiously in clients receiving digoxin and beta-blockers.

Δ Use cautiously in older adults, clients with kidney or liver disorders, and mild to moderate heart failure.

Medication/Food Interactions: Nursing Interventions and Client Education

Medication/Food Interactions	Nursing Interventions/Client Education
nifedipine (Adalat, Procardia)	
Beta-blockers (e.g. metoprolol [Lopressor]) are used to ↓ reflex tachycardia.	• Monitor the client for excessive slowing of heart rate.
Grapefruit juice – consuming grapefruit juice and nifedipine can lead to toxicity.	• Monitor the client for signs of a ↓ in blood pressure, an ↑ in heart rate, and flushing. • Advise the client to avoid drinking grapefruit juice.
verapamil (Calan) diltiazem (Cardizem)	
Digoxin – verapamil can ↑ digoxin levels increasing the risk of digoxin toxicity. Digoxin can cause an additive effect and intensify AV conduction suppression.	• Digoxin levels should be monitored to maintain therapeutic range between 0.5 to 0.8.ng/mL. • Monitor vital signs for bradycardia and for signs of AV block, such as a ↓ ventricular rate.
Beta-blockers – concurrent use can lead to heart failure, AV block, and bradycardia.	• Allow several hours between administration of IV verapamil (Calan) and beta-blockers.
Grapefruit juice – consuming grapefruit juice and verapamil or diltiazem can lead to toxicity.	• Monitor the client for signs of constipation, a ↓ in blood pressure, a ↓ in heart rate, and AV block. • Advise the client to avoid drinking grapefruit juice.

Therapeutic Nursing Interventions and Client Education

Δ   Advise clients not to chew or crush sustained release tablets.

Δ   For intravenous administration, administer injections slowly over a period of 2 to 3 min.

Δ   Advise the client with angina to record pain frequency, intensity, duration, and location. The primary care provider should be notified if attacks ↑ in frequency, intensity, and/or duration.

Δ   Advise and teach the client to monitor blood pressure and heart rate, and keep a blood pressure record.

Nursing Evaluation of Medication Effectiveness

Δ   Depending on therapeutic intent, effectiveness may be evidenced by:

• ↓ in blood pressure and maintenance of normotensive blood pressure.

• Control of angina attacks.

• Absence of dysrhythmias.

Key Points

Medication Classification: Medications for Hypertensive Crisis

Select Prototype Medication:	sodium nitroprusside
Other Medications:	labetalol (Trandate), diazoxide (Hyperstat), fenoldopam (Corlopam), trimethaphan (Arfonad)

Expected Pharmacological Action

Δ These medications are antihypertensive agents that cause direct vasodilation of arteries and veins resulting in rapid reduction of blood pressure (↓ preload and afterload).

Therapeutic Uses

Δ Hypertensive emergencies

Δ ↓ in bleeding during surgery by producing controlled hypotension.

Side/Adverse Effects: Nursing Interventions and Client Education

Side/Adverse Effects	Nursing Interventions/Client Education
Excessive hypotension	• Administer medication slowly as rapid administration will cause blood pressure to go down rapidly. • Monitor the client's blood pressure and ECG.
Cyanide poisoning	• Signs of cyanide poisoning can include headache and drowsiness, and may lead to cardiac arrest. • ↑ risk in clients with liver dysfunction. • Administer medication slowly at a rate of 5 mcg/kg/min, and give thiosulfate concurrently. Thiosulfate is needed to deactivate cyanide. Stop nitroprusside infusion if cyanide toxicity occurs.
Thiocyanate poisoning	• Can be manifested as altered mental status and psychotic behavior. • Avoid prolonged use of nitroprusside. If used for > 3 days, plasma thiocyanate should be monitored. Level should be < 0.1 mg/mL.

Contraindications/Precautions

Δ   Pregnancy Risk Category C

Δ   Use cautiously in clients with liver and kidney disease, clients with fluid and electrolyte imbalances, and older adults.

Therapeutic Nursing Interventions and Client Education

Δ   Solutions of nitroprusside may have a slight brown coloration. Discard solutions that are dark blue, red, or green.

Δ   Solutions of sodium nitroprusside should be protected from light to prevent degradation.

Δ   Do not mix other medications with nitroprusside.

Δ   When administering the medication to the client, continuously monitor the client's blood pressure and ECG.

Nursing Evaluation of Medication Effectiveness

Δ   Return and maintenance of blood pressure to baseline

Key Points

Medication Classification: Organic Nitrates

Select Prototype Medication: **nitroglycerine (Nitrol, Nitrostat)**

Other Medications: isosorbide dinitrate (Imdur)

Expected Pharmacological Action

Δ   In stable angina, nitroglycerine (NTG) ↓ cardiac oxygen demand by dilating veins and decreasing venous return (preload).

Δ   In variant angina, nitroglycerine relaxes or prevents spasm in coronary arteries, thus **increasing** oxygen supply.

Therapeutic Uses

Δ   Treatment of angina

•   Acute attack and prophylaxis of stable angina

•   Variant angina

Δ   IV administration

•   Control of angina not responding to other medications

•   Perioperatively to control blood pressure or produce hypotension

•   Heart failure resulting from acute MI

Side/Adverse Effects: Nursing Interventions and Client Education

Side/Adverse Effects	Nursing Interventions/Client Education
Headache	• Advise the client of symptoms and instruct the client to use aspirin or acetaminophen to relieve pain. • The client should notify the primary care provider if symptoms do not resolve in a few weeks. Dosage may need to be reduced.
Orthostatic hypotension	• Advise the client to sit or lie down if experiencing dizziness or faintness. • The client should avoid sudden changes of position and rise slowly.
Reflex tachycardia	• Monitor the client's vital signs. • Administer a beta-blocker such as metoprolol (Lopressor) if symptoms occur.
Tolerance	• All long-acting forms of nitroglycerine should be taken with a medication free period each day.

Contraindications/Precautions

Δ   Pregnancy Risk Category C

Δ   Contraindicated in clients with hypersensitivity to nitrates

Δ   Contraindicated in clients with traumatic head injury because medication can ↑ intracranial pressure

Δ   Use cautiously in clients taking antihypertensive medications.

Δ   Use cautiously in clients who have renal or liver dysfunction.

Medication/Food Interactions: Nursing Interventions and Client Education

Medication/Food Interactions	Nursing Interventions/Client Education
Alcohol – use of alcohol can contribute to hypotensive effect of nitroglycerine	• Advise the client to avoid use of alcohol.
Antihypertensive medications, (e.g. beta-blockers) such as **atenolol (Tenormin)**; calcium channel blockers, such as **nifedipine (Procardia)**; and diuretics, such as **hydrochlorothiazide** – used concurrently with nitroglycerine can contribute to hypotensive effect	• Use nitroglycerine cautiously in clients receiving these medications.

Medication/Food Interactions	Nursing Interventions/Client Education
Sildenafil (Viagra)	• Use of sildenafil and nitroglycerine can result in life-threatening hypotension. • Instruct the client not to take sildenafil if prescribed nitroglycerine.

Therapeutic Nursing Interventions and Client Education

Route	Use	Client Education
Sublingual tablet • Rapid onset • Short duration	**Treat** acute attack **Prophylaxis** of acute attack	• Client should use this rapid-acting nitrate at the first sign of chest pain. Instruct the client not to wait until pain is severe. • Instruct the client to use prior to activity that is known to cause chest pain, such as climbing a flight of stairs. • The client should place the tablet under the tongue and allow it to dissolve. • Tablets should be stored in original bottles, and in a cool, dark place. • Instruct the client to discard tablets after 24 months unless indicated on package.
Translingual spray • Rapid onset • Short duration	**Treat** acute attack **Prophylaxis** of acute attack	• Client should use this rapid-acting nitrate at the **first sign** of chest pain. Instruct the client not to wait until pain is severe. • Instruct the client to use prior to activity that is known to cause chest pain, such as climbing a flight of stairs. • The medication should be sprayed against oral mucosa and not inhaled.

Route	Use	Client Education
Transmucosal • Rapid onset • Long duration	**Treat** acute attack **Prophylaxis** of acute attack **Long-term prophylaxis** against anginal attacks	• Client should use this rapid-acting nitrate at the **first sign** of chest pain. Instruct the client not to wait until pain is severe. • Instruct the client to use prior to activity that is known to cause chest pain, such as climbing a flight of stairs. • Instruct the client not to chew the tablet, but to place the tablet between the upper lip and gum, or between the cheek and gum to be dissolved.
Sustained-release oral capsules • Slow onset • Long duration	**Long-term prophylaxis** against anginal attacks	• The client should swallow capsules without crushing or chewing.
Transdermal • Slow onset • Long duration	**Long-term prophylaxis** against anginal attacks	• To prevent underdosing or overdosing, patches should not be cut. • Instruct the client to place the patch on a hairless area of skin (e.g., chest, back, or abdomen) and rotate sites to prevent skin irritation. • The client should wash skin with soap and water and dry thoroughly before applying new patch. • The client should be instructed to remove the patch at night to reduce the risk of developing tolerance to nitroglycerin. The client should be medication free a minimum of 8 hr each day; preferably at night.

Route	Use	Client Education
Topical ointment • Slow onset • Long duration	**Long-term prophylaxis** against anginal attacks	• Ointment is prescribed in inches and is measured using specific applicator paper. • Advise the client to remove prior dose before new dose is applied. • Medication should be spread 2.5 to 3.5 in over paper, applied to a clean, hairless area of the body, and covered with clear plastic wrap. • Follow same guidelines for site selection as for transdermal patch. • Advise the client to avoid touching ointment with hands.
Intravenous	• Control of angina not responding to other medications • Perioperatively to control blood pressure or produce hypotension • Heart failure resulting from acute MI	• Administer with IV tubing supplied by manufacturer using a glass IV bottle. • Due to short duration of action, IV infusions must be administered continuously. • Start at a slow rate, usually 5 mcg/min, and titrate gradually until desired response. • Provide continuous monitoring of heart rate and blood pressure during administration.

Δ   Nitroglycerine is administered in different formulations. Instruct the client in the proper use of formulation prescribed by the primary care provider.

Δ   Treatment of anginal attack

- Instruct the client to stop activity.

- The client should take dose of rapid-acting nitroglycerine immediately.

- If pain is unrelieved in 5 min, the client should call 9-1-1 or be driven to an emergency department.

- Client can take up to two more doses at 5 min intervals.

Δ   Advise the client not to stop taking long-acting nitroglycerine abruptly. The client should follow the primary care provider's instructions.

Nursing Evaluation of Medication Effectiveness

Δ   Depending on therapeutic intent, effectiveness may be evidenced by:

- Prevention of acute anginal attacks.

- Long-term management of stable angina.

- Control of perioperative blood pressure.

- Control of heart failure following acute MI.

Key Points

Medication Classification: Cardiac Glycosides

Select Prototype Medication: **digoxin (Lanoxin, Lanoxicaps, and Digitek)**

Other Medications: none

Expected Pharmacological Action

Δ   (+) inotropic effect = ↑ force of myocardial contraction

- ↑ force and efficiency of myocardial contraction → improves the heart's effectiveness as a pump – improving SV and CO.

Δ   (-) chronotropic effect = ↓ heart rate

- At therapeutic levels, digoxin slows the rate of SA node depolarization and the rate of impulses through the conduction system of the heart.
- A ↓ heart rate gives the ventricles more time to fill with blood coming from the atria, which leads to ↑ SV and ↑ CO.

Therapeutic Uses

Δ   Treatment of heart failure

Δ   Dysrhythmias – atrial fibrillation

Side/Adverse Effects: Nursing Interventions and Client Education

Side/Adverse Effects	Nursing Interventions/Client Education
Dysrhythmias (caused by interfering with the electrical conduction in the myocardium); cardiotoxicity leading to bradycardia	• Conditions that ↑ the risk of developing digoxin-induced dysrhythmias include hypokalemia, ↑ serum digoxin levels, and heart disease. • Monitor serum levels of K+ to maintain level between 3.0 to 5.0 mEq/L. • Instruct the client to report signs of hypokalemia (e.g., nausea/vomiting, general weakness). Potassium supplements may be prescribed if the client is concurrently taking a diuretic. • Teach the client to consume high potassium foods (e.g., bananas, potatoes). • Monitor the client's digoxin level to maintain therapeutic range between 0.5 to 0.8 ng/mL. • Teach the client to monitor pulse rate, and recognize and report changes. The rate may be irregular with early or extra beats noted.
GI effects include anorexia (usually the first sign) nausea, vomiting, and abdominal pain	• Teach the client to monitor for these effects and instruct the client to report to the primary care provider.
CNS effects to include fatigue, weakness, vision changes – diplopia, blurred vision, yellow-green or white halos around objects	• Teach the client to monitor for these effects and instruct the client to report to primary care provider.

Contraindications/Precautions

Δ Pregnancy Risk Category C

Δ Contraindicated in clients with disturbances in ventricular rhythm including ventricular fibrillation, ventricular tachycardia, and second and third-degree heart block

Δ Use cautiously in clients with hypokalemia, partial AV block, advanced heart failure, and renal insufficiency.

Medication/Food Interactions: Nursing Interventions and Client Education

Medication/Food Interactions	Nursing Interventions/Client Education
Thiazide diuretics, such as hydrochlorothiazide (HCTZ) and loop diuretics, such as furosemide (Lasix) – these medications ↑ the risk of digoxin-induced dysrhythmias	• Monitor K+ level and maintain between 3.5 to 5.0 mEq/L • Hypokalemia can be treated with potassium supplements or a potassium-sparing diuretic.
ACE inhibitors and ARBs – ↑ the risk of hyperkalemia, which can lead to ↓ therapeutic effects of digoxin	• Use cautiously if these medications are also used with potassium supplements or a potassium-sparing diuretic.
Sympathomimetic medications such as dopamine (Intropin) – these medications complement the inotropic action of digoxin	• ↑ the rate and force of heart muscle contraction. May be beneficial, but also may ↑ the risk of tachydysrhythmias.
Quinidine ↑ the risk of digoxin toxicity when used concurrently.	• Use of quinidine and digoxin should be avoided.
Verapamil (Calan) – verapamil ↑ plasma levels of digoxin	• If used concurrently, digoxin dose should be ↓. Usually avoided due to verapamil cardiosuppression action counteracting action of digoxin.

Therapeutic Nursing Interventions and Client Education

Δ   Advise clients to take the medication as prescribed and not to double the dose when a dose is not taken at the prescribed time.

Δ   Check pulse rate and rhythm before administration of digoxin and record, notify the primary care provider if heart rate is < 60 beats/min in an adult, < 70 beats/min in children, and < 90 beats/min in infants.

Δ   Administer digoxin at the same time daily.

Δ   Monitor digoxin levels periodically while on treatment and maintain therapeutic levels between 0.5 to 2.0 ng/mL to prevent digoxin toxicity.

Δ   Avoid taking OTC medications to prevent adverse side effects and medication interactions.

Δ   Instruct clients to observe symptoms of hypokalemia, such as muscle weakness, and to notify the primary care provider if symptoms occur.

Δ   Instruct clients to observe symptoms of digoxin toxicity (e.g., anorexia, fatigue, weakness), and to notify the primary care provider if symptoms occur.

Δ   Management of digoxin toxicity

  •   Digoxin and potassium-sparing medication should be stopped immediately.

  •   Monitor K+ levels. For levels < 3.5 mEq/L, potassium should be administered intravenously or by mouth. Do not give any further K+ if level > 5.0 mEq/L.

  •   Treat dysrhythmias with phenytoin or lidocaine.

  •   Treat bradycardia with atropine.

  •   For excessive overdose, activated charcoal, cholestyramine, or Digibind can be used to bind digoxin and prevent absorption.

Nursing Evaluation of Medication Effectiveness

Δ   Depending on therapeutic intent, effectiveness may be evidenced by:

  •   Control of heart failure signs and symptoms.

  •   Absence of cardiac dysrhythmias.

Key Points

Medication Classification: Antidysrhythmic Medications

Select Prototype Medication:	**Class IA sodium channel blockers: procainamide (Pronestyl, Procanbid)** **Class IB sodium channel blockers: lidocaine (Xylocaine)** **Class IV calcium channel blockers: verapamil (Calan), diltiazem (Cardizem)** **Class III potassium channel blockers: amiodarone (Cordarone, Pacerone)** **Endogenous glucoside: adenosine (Adenocard)**
Other Medications:	**Class III potassium channel blockers:** bretylium, sotalol (Betapace), dofetilide (Tikosyn) **Endogenous glucoside:** ibutilide (Corvert)

Classifications	Expected Pharmacologic Action	Therapeutic Uses
Class IA sodium channel blockers procainamide (Pronestyl, Procanbid) quinidine sulfate (Quinidex Extentabs) disopyramide (Norpace) tocainide (Tonocard) propafenone (Rythmol)	• ↓ electrical conduction • ↑ automaticity • ↓ rate of repolarization	• Supraventricular tachycardia • Ventricular tachycardia • Atrial flutter • Atrial fibrillation
Class IB sodium channel blocker lidocaine (Xylocaine)	• ↓ electrical conduction • ↓ automaticity • ↑ rate of repolarization	• Short-term use only for ventricular dysrhythmias
Class IV calcium channel blockers verapamil (Calan) diltiazem (Cardizem)	• ↓ force of contraction • ↓ heart rate • Slowing of rate of conduction through the AV node	• Atrial fibrillation and flutter • SVT

Classifications	Expected Pharmacologic Action	Therapeutic Uses
Class III potassium channel blockers Amiodarone (Cordarone, Pacerone) bretylium, sotalol (Betapace), dofetilide (Tikosyn)	• ↓ rate of repolarization • ↓ electrical conduction • ↓ contractility • ↓ automaticity	• Conversion of atrial fibrillation – oral route • Recurrent ventricular fibrillation • Recurrent ventricular tachycardia
Endogenous glucoside Adenosine (Adenocard) ibutilide (Corvert)	• ↓ electrical conduction through AV node	• Paroxysmal SVT • Wolff-Parkinson-White syndrome

Side/Adverse Effects: Nursing Interventions and Client Education

Side/Adverse Effects	Nursing Interventions/Client Education
procainamide (Pronestyl)	
Systemic lupus syndrome (e.g., painful, inflamed joints)	• Symptoms will resolve with discontinuation of medication. • If no alternative can be used, symptoms can be controlled with NSAIDs. • Clients should be monitored for nuclear antibody titers (ANA). If levels ↑, therapy might be discontinued.
Blood dyscrasias, such as neutropenia	• Monitor the client's weekly complete blood counts for the first 12 weeks; then periodically. • Monitor clients for signs of infection and bleeding. Medication should be stopped if evidence of bone marrow suppression.
Cardiotoxicity – of particular note is that the QRS complex is widened and the QT interval is prolonged	• Monitor the client's vital signs and ECG. • If dysrhythmias occur, hold medication and contact the primary care provider.
lidocaine (Xylocaine)	
CNS effects (e.g., drowsiness, altered mental status, paresthesias, seizures)	• Carefully monitor the client and notify the primary care provider if symptoms occur. • Administer phenytoin (Dilantin) to control seizure activity.
Respiratory arrest	• Monitor the client's vital signs and ECG. • Ensure resuscitation equipment ready at bedside.

Side/Adverse Effects	Nursing Interventions/Client Education
amiodarone (Cordarone, Pacerone)	
Pulmonary toxicity	<ul><li>Obtain the client's baseline chest x-ray and pulmonary function tests.</li><li>Continue to monitor pulmonary function through course of therapy.</li><li>Advise the client to observe for symptoms of dyspnea, cough, and chest pain.</li><li>Notify the primary care provider if symptoms occur.</li></ul>
Cardiac effects lead to sinus bradycardia and AV block related to: ↓ electrical conduction. ↓ contractility. ↓ automaticity. May cause heart failure to develop	<ul><li>Monitor blood pressure and ECG</li><li>Monitor client for signs of heart failure (e.g., dyspnea, cough, chest pain, neck vein distention, crackles).</li><li>Notify the primary care provider if evidence of heart failure.</li></ul>
IV – primarily affects AV node Hypotension	<ul><li>If AV block occurs, medication should be discontinued and possible insertion of pacemaker.</li><li>Medication may be discontinued.</li></ul>
Visual disturbances (e.g., photophobia, blurred vision, may lead to blindness)	<ul><li>Advise the client to report visual disturbances.</li></ul>
Other effects may include liver and thyroid dysfunction; GI disturbances, CNS effects.	<ul><li>Obtain baseline liver and thyroid function, and monitor periodically.</li><li>Advise the client to observe for symptoms, and report to the primary care provider if they occur.</li></ul>
Phlebitis with IV administration	<ul><li>Use of central venous catheter is indicated.</li></ul>
Hypotension, bradycardia, AV block	<ul><li>Monitor cardiac status</li></ul>
adenosine (Adenocard)	
Sinus bradycardia (↓ conduction through AV node), dyspnea (bronchoconstriction), flushing of face (vasodilation)	<ul><li>Effects usually last 1 min or less</li><li>Monitor the client for signs and symptoms, and notify the primary care provider if symptoms occur.</li></ul>

Contraindications/Precautions

Procainamide (Pronestyl)	<ul><li>Pregnancy Risk Category C</li><li>Contraindicated in clients with hypersensitivity to quinidine, with complete heart block, and systemic lupus erythematous</li><li>Use cautiously in clients with partial AV block, liver disorders, heart failure, and digoxin toxicity.</li></ul>
Lidocaine (Xylocaine)	<ul><li>Pregnancy Risk Category B</li><li>Contraindicated in clients with Stokes-Adams syndrome, Wolff-Parkinson-White syndrome, and severe heart block</li><li>Use cautiously in clients with liver and renal dysfunction, and heart failure.</li></ul>
Amiodarone (Cordarone, Pacerone)	<ul><li>**Pregnancy Risk Category D**</li><li>Contraindicated in clients with AV block and bradycardia, newborns, and infants.</li><li>Use cautiously in clients with liver, thyroid, respiratory dysfunction, heart failure, and fluid and electrolyte imbalances.</li></ul>
Adenosine (Adenocard)	<ul><li>Pregnancy Risk Category C</li><li>Contraindicated in clients with second and third degree heart block, AV block, atrial flutter, and atrial fibrillation</li><li>Use cautiously in clients with asthma and older adults.</li></ul>

Medication/Food Interactions: Nursing Interventions and Client Education

Medication/Food Interactions	Nursing Interventions/Client Education
procainamide (Pronestyl)	
Antidysrhythmics – ↑ in therapeutic or potential for toxic effects	<ul><li>Monitor heart rate and rhythm.</li><li>Notify the primary care provider of change or start of new dysrhythmia.</li></ul>
Anticholinergic medications – ↑ anticholinergic effects (e.g., dry mouth, urinary retention, constipation, and tachycardia).	<ul><li>Monitor heart rate.</li><li>Sucking on hard candy or chewing gum can help relieve dry mouth.</li><li>Administer stool softeners, such as docusate sodium (Colace) to prevent constipation.</li></ul>
Antihypertensives – additive hypotensive effect	<ul><li>Monitor the client's blood pressure.</li><li>Notify the primary care provider if there is a significant drop in the client's blood pressure.</li></ul>

Medication/Food Interactions	Nursing Interventions/Client Education
lidocaine (Xylocaine)	
Cimetidine, beta-blockers, phenytoin – ↑ the effects of lidocaine	• Monitor the client for side effects, such as drowsiness.
amiodarone (Cordarone, Pacerone)	
Quinidine, procainamide, digoxin, diltiazem, and warfarin – amiodarone ↑ plasma levels of these medications.	• Dosages of these medications should be lowered.
Cholestyramine ↓ levels of amiodarone.	• Monitor for therapeutic effects.
Diuretics, other antidysrhythmics, antibiotics (e.g., erythromycin, azithromycin [Zithromax]) – ↑ the risk of dysrhythmias	• Use cautiously with clients taking these medications.
Beta-blockers, verapamil, diltiazem – concurrent use can lead to bradycardia	• Monitor client closely.
Grapefruit juice – consuming grapefruit juice can lead to toxicity.	• Advise the client to avoid drinking grapefruit juice.
adenosine (Adenocard)	
Methylxanthines, such as theophylline and caffeine. Receptors for adenosine are blocked.	• Clients with asthma may need higher doses or a different medication.
Dipyridamole (Persantine) – cellular uptake is blocked leading to intensification of effects	• Monitor the client for signs of excessive dosage, and notify the primary care provider if these occur.

Therapeutic Nursing Interventions and Client Education

Procainamide (Pronestyl)	• Advise clients to take medications as prescribed. • Advise clients not crush or chew sustained-released preparations.
Lidocaine (Xylocaine)	• Intravenous administration is usually started with a loading dose, followed by a maintenance dose of 1 to 4 mg/min. • Adjust the rate according to cardiac response. • Usually used for no more than 24 hr. • Never administer lidocaine preparation that contains epinephrine (usually in lidocaine used for local anesthesia). Severe hypertension or dysrhythmias may occur.
Amiodarone (Cordarone, Pacerone)	• Amiodarone is highly toxic; therefore, monitor the client closely for adverse side effects. • Inform the client that adverse effects may continue for an extended period of time after the medication is discontinued. • Provide client with written information regarding potential toxicities
Adenosine (Adenocard)	• Adenosine has a very short half-life, so adverse reactions are mild and last for less than 1 min. • Administration should be by intravenous bolus, flushed with saline following administration.

Nursing Evaluation of Medication Effectiveness

Δ Depending on therapeutic intent, effectiveness may be evidenced by:

• Improvement of symptoms (e.g. chest pain, shortness of breath, bradycardia, or tachycardia).

• Absence of dysrhythmias.

• Return to baseline ECG, pulse rate, and regular rhythm.

Key Points

Medication Classification: Antilipemics-HMG CoA Reductase Inhibitors (Statins)

Select Prototype Medication: **atorvastatin (Lipitor)**

Other Medications: simvastatin (Zocor), lovastatin (Mevacor), pravastatin sodium (Pravachol), rosuvastatin (Crestor)

Expected Pharmacological Action

Δ   LDL cholesterol levels are ↓ by a complex mechanism

- By suppressing cholesterol synthesis, the liver ↑ the number of low density lipid (LDL) receptors in the liver cells.

- This ↑ in the number of low density lipid (LDL) receptors in the liver cells allows the body to remove a greater amount of LDL from the blood.

Δ   Production of very low-density lipoproteins (VLDL) is ↓

Δ   ↑ of high-density lipoproteins (HDL) levels

Δ   Besides affecting lipid levels, other beneficial effects include: promotion of vasodilation, ↓ in plaque site inflammation, and ↓ risk of thromboembolism.

Therapeutic Uses

Δ   Primary hypercholesterolemia

Δ   Prevention of coronary events – primary and secondary

Δ   Protection against MI and stroke for clients with diabetes

Δ   Raise levels of HDL in clients with primary hypercholesterolemia

Side/Adverse Effects: Nursing Interventions and Client Education

Side/Adverse Effects	Nursing Interventions/Client Education
Hepatotoxicity, evidenced by ↑ in serum transaminase	• Obtain the client's baseline liver function. • Monitor liver function tests after 12 weeks and then every 6 months. • Advise the client to observe for symptoms of liver dysfunction (e.g., anorexia, vomiting, nausea, jaundice), and notify the primary care provider if symptoms occur. • Advise the client to avoid alcohol. • Stop the medication if liver function tests are abnormal.
Myopathy, evidenced by muscle aches, pain, and tenderness	• Obtain baseline creatine kinase (CK) level. • Monitor CK levels while on treatment periodically. • Monitor symptoms of muscle aches, pain, and tenderness, and notify the primary care provider if symptoms occur. • Stop medication if results of CK levels are elevated.
Peripheral neuropathy, as evidenced by weakness, numbness, tingling, and pain in the hands and feet	• Advise the client to observe for signs and symptoms, and to notify the primary care provider if symptoms occur.

Contraindications/Precautions

Δ Pregnancy Risk Category X

Δ Contraindicated in clients with hepatitis induced by viral infection or alcohol

Δ Contraindicated in pregnant women

Δ Rosuvastatin should be avoided in clients of Asian descent.

Δ Use cautiously in clients taking fibrates and medications that inhibit CYP3A4, such as ketoconazole.

Medication/Food Interactions: Nursing Interventions and Client Education

Medication/Food Interactions	Nursing Interventions/Client Education
Fibrates (e.g., gemfibrozil, fenofibrate) – ↑ the risk of myopathy	• Obtain baseline creatine kinase (CK) level. • Monitor the client's CK levels while on treatment periodically. • Monitor symptoms of muscle aches, pain, and tenderness, and notify the primary care provider if symptoms occur. • Stop medication if results of CK levels are elevated.
Medications that suppress CYP3A4, such as **erythromycin** – levels of statins can be ↑ when taken concurrently with these medications	• Level of statin may need to be ↓. • Client may be switched to pravastatin. • Advise the client to inform the primary care provider of all medications currently taken.
Grapefruit juice – drinking grapefruit juice while taking lovastatin or simvastatin can lead to toxicity.	• Advise the client to limit the amount of grapefruit juice consumed each day. The client should not drink more than 1 qt a day.

Therapeutic Nursing Interventions and Client Education

Δ   Administer lovastatin with evening meal; other statins can be taken without food intake.

Δ   Atorvastatin or fluvastatin should be used in clients with renal insufficiency. For other statins, dosages will be reduced.

Δ   Advise the client to obtain baseline cholesterol levels, HDL, LDL, and triglycerides, and monitor periodically while on medication.

Δ   Advise the client to obtain baseline liver, renal function tests, and monitor periodically while on treatment.

Nursing Evaluation of Medication Effectiveness

Δ   Depending on therapeutic intent, effectiveness may be evidenced by:

•   Normal cholesterol levels.

•   ↑ HDL levels.

•   ↓ LDL levels.

•   Absence of cardiovascular events.

Key Points

Medication Classification: Antilipemics: Fibrates

Select Prototype Medication:	**gemfibrozil (Lopid)**
Other Medications:	fenofibrate (Tricor, Lofibra)

Expected Pharmacological Action

Δ ↓ in triglyceride levels – very low density lipoprotein (VLDL) by increasing the rate of VLDL excretion.

Δ ↑ in HDL levels by promoting production of precursors to HDLs

Therapeutic Uses

Δ Reduction of plasma triglycerides (VLDL)

Δ ↑ levels of HDL

Side/Adverse Effects: Nursing Interventions and Client Education

Side/Adverse Effects	Nursing Interventions/Client Education
Gall bladder stones	• Advise clients to observe for symptoms of gall bladder disease (e.g., right upper quadrant pain, fat intolerance, bloating). • Advise the client to notify the primary care provider if symptoms occur.
Myopathy (e.g., muscle tenderness, pain)	• Obtain baseline creatine kinase (CK) level. • Monitor CK levels while on treatment periodically. • Monitor symptoms of muscle aches, pain, and tenderness, and notify the primary care provider if symptoms occur. • Stop medication if results of CK levels are elevated.
Hepatotoxicity	• Obtain baseline liver function tests and monitor periodically. • Advise the client to observe for symptoms of liver dysfunction (e.g., anorexia, vomiting, nausea, jaundice), and notify the primary care provider if symptoms occur. • Stop medication if liver function tests are abnormal.

Contraindications/Precautions

Δ Pregnancy Risk Category C

Δ Contraindicated in clients with liver disorders, severe renal dysfunction, and gallbladder disease

Δ Use cautiously with clients taking statins

Medication/Food Interactions: Nursing Interventions and Client Education

Medication/Food Interactions	Nursing Interventions/Client Education
Warfarin (Coumadin) – with concomitant use, ↑ the risk of bleeding	• Obtain the client's baseline prothrombin time (PT) and INR, and perform periodic monitoring. • Advise the client to monitor for signs of bleeding (e.g. bruising, bleeding gums), and notify the primary care provider if symptoms occur.
Statins – ↑ the risk of myopathy	• Obtain baseline creatine kinase (CK) level. • Monitor CK levels while on treatment periodically. • Monitor symptoms of muscle aches, pain, and tenderness, and notify the primary care provider if symptoms occur. • Stop medication if results of CK levels are elevated.
Bile acid sequestrants such as **cholestyramine** – interferes with absorption	• Advise the client to take gemfibrozil 1 hr before or 4 hr after taking bile sequestrants.

Therapeutic Nursing Interventions and Client Education

Δ Advise the client to obtain baseline cholesterol levels, HDL, LDL, and triglyceride, and monitor periodically while on medication.

Δ Advise the client to obtain baseline liver, renal function tests, and monitor periodically while on treatment.

Δ Advise the client to take medication 30 min prior to breakfast and dinner.

Nursing Evaluation of Medication Effectiveness

Δ Depending on therapeutic intent, effectiveness may be evidenced by:

• ↓ in triglyceride (VLDL) levels.

• ↑ in HDL levels.

Key Points

Medication Classification: Antilipemics-Cholesterol Absorption Inhibitor

Select Prototype Medication:	**ezetimibe (Zetia)**
Other Medications:	None

Expected Pharmacological Action

Δ   These medications inhibit absorption of cholesterol secreted in the bile and from food.

Therapeutic Uses

Δ   Clients with modified diets can use this medication as an adjunct to help lower LDL cholesterol.

Δ   Medication can be used alone or in combination with a statin medication.

Side/Adverse Effects: Nursing Interventions and Client Education

Side/Adverse Effects	Nursing Interventions/Client Education
Medication is well-tolerated	• None

Contraindications/Precautions

Δ   Pregnancy Risk Category X

Δ   Use cautiously in women who are breastfeeding.

Δ   Contraindicated in clients with renal dysfunction

Medication/Food Interactions: Nursing Interventions and Client Education

Medication/Food Interactions	Nursing Interventions/Client Education
Bile acid sequestrants, such as **cholestyramine** – interferes with absorption	Advise the client to take ezetimibe 1 hr before or 4 hr after taking bile sequestrants.
Statins, such as atorvastatin can ↑ the risk of liver dysfunction and/or myopathy.	• Obtain baseline liver function tests and monitor periodically. Advise the client to observe for signs of liver damage (e.g., anorexia, vomiting, nausea). The primary care provider should be notified and the medication will most likely be discontinued. • Monitor CK levels. Advise the client of signs to observe for (e.g. muscle aches, pain, tenderness). The primary care provider should be notified and the medication will most likely be discontinued.
Concurrent use with **fibrates,** such as gemfibrozil, ↑ the risk of gallstone development and myopathy	It is not recommended to use ezetimibe with fibrates.
Cyclosporine – levels of ezetimibe can be ↑ with concurrent use of cyclosporine	Monitor the client for side effects (e.g., liver damage, myopathy)

Therapeutic Nursing Interventions and Client Education

Δ Advise the client to obtain baseline cholesterol levels, HDL, LDL, and triglyceride, and monitor periodically while on the medication.

Δ Advise the client to obtain baseline liver, renal function tests, and monitor periodically while on treatment.

Δ Medication is taken once a day without regard to food.

Δ Advise the client to follow a low fat/low cholesterol diet and to get involved in a regular exercise regimen.

Δ Clients can take this medication in a fixed-dose combination with simvastatin as Vytorin.

Nursing Evaluation of Medication Effectiveness

Δ Depending on therapeutic intent, effectiveness may be evidenced by:

• Normal cholesterol levels.

• ↓ in LDL levels.

Key Points

Medication Classification: Antilipemics-Bile-Acid Sequestrants

Select Prototype Medication: **cholestyramine (Questran)**

Other Medications: colestipol (Colestid)

Expected Pharmacological Action

Δ   A process that involves increasing LDL receptors on liver cells, which in turn, take up serum cholesterol, which results in lowered LDL levels.

Therapeutic Uses

Δ   Medications are used as adjunct with a HMG CoA reductase inhibitor such as atorvastatin and dietary measures to lower cholesterol levels.

Side/Adverse Effects: Nursing Interventions and Client Education

Side/Adverse Effects	Nursing Interventions/Client Education
No systemic effects	• The GI tract does not absorb this medication.
Constipation	• Advise the client to ↑ the intake of high fiber food and oral fluids, if not restricted.

Contraindications/Precautions

Δ   Contraindicated in clients with biliary disease

Δ   Should not be used in clients with elevated VLDL.

Medication/Food Interactions: Nursing Interventions and Client Education

Medication/Food Interactions	Nursing Interventions/Client Education
Digoxin, warfarin, thiazides, and tetracyclines – form complexes with these medications that interfere with absorption	• Advise the client to take other medications 1 hr before or 4 hr after taking bile sequestrants.

Therapeutic Nursing Interventions and Client Education

Δ   Medication is supplied in a powder formulation. Advise the client to use adequate amount of fluid, 4 to 8 oz of water or applesauce to dissolve the medication. This will prevent irritation or impaction of the esophagus.

Nursing Evaluation of Medication Effectiveness

Δ   Depending on therapeutic intent, effectiveness may be evidenced by:

- Normal cholesterol levels.
- ↓ in LDL levels

Primary Reference:

Lehne, R. A. (2007). *Pharmacology for nursing care* (6th ed.). St. Louis, MO: Saunders.

Additional Resources:

Ignatavicius, D. D. (2006). *Medical-surgical nursing* (5th ed.). St. Louis, MO: Saunders.

Wilson, B. A., Shannon, M., Shields, K. Stang, C. (2007). *Nurse's drug guide*. Upper Saddle River, NJ: Prentice Hall.

Unit 6 Medications Affecting the Cardiovascular System

Application Exercises

1. A nurse is providing discharge teaching to a client who is prescribed nitroglycerin to control anginal pain. The client is prescribed the following medications: Nitroglycerine (Nitrostat) 0.4 mg sublingual as necessary for chest pain; Nitroglycerine (Nitro-Dur) 0.4 mg every morning; remove at bedtime. What information should the nurse include in the client's discharge teaching regarding these medications?

2. What is the most common cause of dysrhythmias in clients receiving digoxin?

3. A client has been diagnosed with hypertension. Propranolol (Inderal) would be contraindicated in which condition?

      A. Asthma

      B. Diabetes

      C. Angina

      D. Dementia

4. A client is prescribed clonidine (Catapres) orally once a day for hypertension. Which of the following client statements indicates effective teaching? (Select all that apply.)

    _____   "I will sit at the side of the of the bed in the morning before getting up."

    _____   "I will increase my intake of foods high in potassium like bananas."

    _____   "I will take the clonidine at bedtime because it may make me drowsy."

    _____   "I will chew gum or use hard candy to keep my mouth moist."

    _____   "I will change the medication patch every day."

5. When providing teaching to a client taking verapamil (Calan) for control of dysrhythmias, which of the following should the nurse include?

      A. Increase the amount of dietary fiber and fluid in diet.

      B. Drink at least one glass of grapefruit juice each day.

      C. Decrease the amount of calcium in the diet.

      D. Withhold food for 1 hr after the medication is taken.

6. A client receiving captopril (Capoten) and a spironolactone (Aldactone), a potassium-sparing diuretic, should be monitored for which of the following adverse effects? (Select all that apply.)

_____ Hyperkalemia

_____ Hypotension

_____ Reflex tachycardia

_____ Headache

_____ Drowsiness

7. Client teaching to prevent first-dose hypotension should include which of the following?

A. Taking the medication with a full glass of water

B. Taking the medication at bedtime

C. Taking the medication right before driving to work

D. Taking the medication at the same time as a diuretic

8. Which of the following statements made by a client receiving atorvastatin (Lipitor) indicates a need for further teaching?

A. "I should take my medication with dinner."

B. "I will limit my alcohol intake to 1 or 2 drinks per day."

C. "I will maintain a steady intake of green leafy vegetables."

D. "I will limit fluid intake to one-and-a-half to two liters daily."

9. Which of the following is correct regarding toxicity associated with amiodarone?

A. Visual impairment resolves when the medication is withdrawn

B. Ototoxicity is irreversible

C. Lung damage can persist for months after the medication is discontinued

D. Myopathy is a common manifestation of toxicity

10. Dopamine (Intropin) is used to treat shock for which of the following pharmacologic actions? (Select all that apply.)

_____ Vasoconstriction of blood vessels

_____ Renal blood vessel dilation

_____ Inhibition of renin release

_____ Decrease in heart rate

_____ Decrease in the rate of conduction through the AV node

Unit 6 Medications Affecting the Cardiovascular System

Application Exercises Answer Key

1. A nurse is providing discharge teaching to a client who is prescribed nitroglycerin to control anginal pain. The client is prescribed the following medications: Nitroglycerine (Nitrostat) 0.4 mg sublingual as necessary for chest pain; Nitroglycerine (Nitro-Dur) 0.4 mg every morning; remove at bedtime. What information should the nurse include in the client's discharge teaching regarding these medications?

Nitroglycerine

Side Effects	Management
Dizziness or faintness	• Sit or lie down. • Avoid sudden changes of position and rise slowly when standing up.
Headache	• Take aspirin or acetaminophen to relieve pain. If the headache does not subside in a few weeks, the client should contact the primary care provider. • The dosage may need to be reduced.
Tolerance	• Take the patch off before bed and reapply the next patch the following morning. Being nitrate free for 8 to 12 hr will help prevent tolerance to the medication.
Instructions For Proper Use of Medication	
Care of medication	• Always carry Nitrostat, the fast-acting nitroglycerine. • Keep the medication in original bottle, mark date when opened, and discard after 24 months.
Application of patch	• Place the patch on a hairless area of skin (e.g., chest, back, abdomen), and rotate sites to prevent skin irritation. • Wash skin with soap and water and dry thoroughly before applying new patch
Prophylaxis prior to strenuous activity	• Use a dose of Nitrostat, the fast-acting nitroglycerine before activities known to cause pain.
Anginal attack	• Stop activity. • Take a dose of Nitrostat, the fast-acting nitroglycerine immediately. • If pain is unrelieved in 5 min, the client should call 9-1-1 or be driven to an emergency department. • Take up to 2 more doses at 5 min intervals.
Discontinuation of medications	• Do not stop applying the Nitro-Dur patch without consulting the primary care provider.

2. What is the most common cause of dysrhythmias in clients receiving digoxin?

Hypokalemia secondary to the use of diuretics. Digoxin works by binding to and inhibiting the enzyme Na+K+-ATPase. Potassium and digoxin compete for the same binding sites on this enzyme. With hypokalemia, digoxin has more opportunity to bind to Na+K+-ATPase and leads to an increased risk of toxicity.

3. A client has been diagnosed with hypertension. Propranolol (Inderal) would be contraindicated in which condition?

      A. Asthma
      B. Diabetes
      C. Angina
      D. Dementia

Inderal is a nonselective beta-adrenergic blocker and blocks both beta$_1$ and beta$_2$ receptors. Blockade of beta$_2$ receptors in the lungs causes bronchoconstriction, so it is contraindicated in clients with asthma. Use propranolol cautiously with client's who have diabetes, but it is not contraindicated. Inderal can be used to treat angina. It is not contraindicated in dementia.

4. A client is prescribed clonidine (Catapres) orally once a day for hypertension. Which of the following client statements indicates effective teaching? (Select all that apply.)

_____	"I will sit at the side of the bed in the morning before getting up."
_____	"I will increase my intake of foods high in potassium like bananas."
X	**"I will take the clonidine at bedtime because it may make me drowsy."**
X	**"I will chew gum or use hard candy to keep my mouth moist."**
_____	"I will change the medication patch every day."

Clients taking clonidine experience drowsiness and sedative effect. Clonidine causes dry mouth; and orthostatic hypotension with clonidine is minimal. This intervention is for potassium-sparing diuretics. Clonidine patches are applied every 7 days.

5. When providing teaching to a client taking verapamil (Calan) for control of dysrhythmias, which of the following should the nurse include?

> **A. Increase the amount of dietary fiber and fluid in diet.**
>
> B. Drink at least one glass of grapefruit juice each day.
>
> C. Decrease the amount of calcium in the diet.
>
> D. Withhold food for 1 hr after the medication is taken.

CCBs can cause constipation. Clients should avoid drinking grapefruit juice when taking verapamil because concurrent use can lead to toxicity. There is no restriction on calcium intake when taking a CCB, and verapamil can be taken without regard to food.

6. A client receiving captopril (Capoten) and a spironolactone (Aldactone), a potassium-sparing diuretic, should be monitored for which of the following adverse effects? (Select all that apply.)

> __X__   **Hyperkalemia**
>
> __X__   **Hypotension**
>
> _____   Reflex tachycardia
>
> _____   Headache
>
> _____   Drowsiness

ACE inhibitors can lead to hyperkalemia. Using a potassium-sparing diuretic with an ACE inhibitor can lead to hyperkalemia. Captopril can lead to hypotension, and Aldactone may have an additive hypotensive effect. Reflex tachycardia is a side effect of calcium channel blockers; headache is a side effect of nitroglycerine; and drowsiness is a side effect of clonidine.

7. Client teaching to prevent first-dose hypotension should include which of the following?

> A. Taking the medication with a full glass of water
>
> **B. Taking the medication at bedtime**
>
> C. Taking the medication right before driving to work
>
> D. Taking the medication at the same time as a diuretic

Taking the medication at bedtime will help avoid position changes that exacerbate the symptoms of hypotension. Taking the medication with a full glass of water does not decrease first-dose hypotension. Clients should avoid activities that require mental alertness after the first dose of the medication. Taking a diuretic at the same time will intensify hypotensive effects.

8. Which of the following statements made by a client receiving atorvastatin (Lipitor) indicates a need for further teaching?

> A. "I should take my medication with dinner."
> **B. "I will limit my alcohol intake to 1 or 2 drinks per day."**
> C. "I will maintain a steady intake of green leafy vegetables."
> D. "I will limit fluid intake to one-and-a-half to two liters daily."

Alcohol should be avoided to reduce the risk of hepatotoxicity; atorvastatin should be taken in the evening with food; eating green leafy vegetables are a concern with warfarin. There is no need for fluid restriction with statins.

9. Which of the following is correct regarding toxicity associated with amiodarone?

> A. Visual impairment resolves when the medication is withdrawn
> B. Ototoxicity is irreversible
> **C. Lung damage can persist for months after the medication is discontinued**
> D. Myopathy is a common manifestation of toxicity

Because of a long half-life, symptoms persist for months after discontinuation. Ototoxicity is not a sign of amiodarone toxicity; and myopathy is seen in clients who are receiving statins and fibrates.

10. Dopamine (Intropin) is used to treat shock for which of the following pharmacologic actions? (Select all that apply.)

> __X__   **Vasoconstriction of blood vessels**
> __X__   **Renal blood vessel dilation**
> _____   Inhibition of renin release
> _____   Decrease in heart rate
> _____   Decrease in the rate of conduction through the AV node

Dopamine is used in the treatment of shock to cause renal blood vessel dilation and vasoconstriction of blood vessels. Dopamine does not affect renin release. Dopamine increases heart rate and the rate of conduction through the AV node.

Unit 7	Medications Affecting the Blood

Contributor: Havovi Patel, MS, MBBS

 NCLEX® Connections:

Learning Objective: Review and apply knowledge within **"Medications Affecting the Blood"** in readiness for performance of the following nursing activities as outlined by the NCLEX® test plans:

Δ Assess/monitor the client for expected effects of medications.

Δ Assess/monitor the client for side/adverse effects of medications.

Δ Assess/monitor the client for actual/potential specific food and medication interactions.

Δ Identify contraindications, actual/potential incompatibilities, and interactions between medications, and intervene appropriately.

Δ Identify symptoms/evidence of an allergic reaction, and respond appropriately.

Δ Evaluate/monitor and document the therapeutic and adverse/side effects of medications.

Δ Provide/reinforce client teaching on actions, therapeutic effects, potential side/ adverse effects and interactions of medications.

 General Key Points

Δ Medications affecting blood:

• Prevent the **formation of blood clots** or thrombi.

• Prevent **clumping of platelets** (aggregation).

• **Dissolve clots** or thrombi that have formed

• **Replace blood loss** to maintain homeostasis.

• Prevent **anemia.**

Δ Many of these medications increase a client's risk of bleeding.

Δ The formation of coagulation factors (VII, IX, X, and prothrombin) require vitamin K. Consequently, medications such as warfarin (Coumadin) that antagonize vitamin K, impact the production and the available quantities of these factors.

Δ   Medications in this category are classified as:

- **Anticoagulants** – heparin, enoxaparin (Lovenox), and warfarin. Anticoagulants prevent clots and the formation of fibrin. Anticoagulants are effective against venous thrombosis.

- **Antiplatelets** – aspirin, ticlopidine (Ticlid), and abciximab (Reo Pro). Antiplatelets prevent platelets from clumping together. Antiplatelets are effective against arterial thrombosis.

- **Thrombolytic agents** – streptokinase (Streptase) and alteplase (Activase). Thrombolytic agents dissolve clots that have already formed.

- **Hematopoietic growth factors** – epoetin alfa (erythropoietin), filgrastim (Neupogen), sargramostim (Leukine), and oprelvekin (Neumega). These medications promote the production of specific bone marrow cells.

- **Anti-anemic agents** – ferrous sulfate, cyanocobalamin, and folic acid replace the deficient factor (e.g., iron, vitamin B_{12}, folic acid) causing a specific anemia.

- **Blood replacement agents** – packed red blood cells (PRBCs), whole blood, fresh frozen plasma, platelets, and albumin.

Key Points

Medication Classification: Anticoagulants/Parenteral

Select Prototype Medication: **Heparin**

Other Medications: enoxaparin (Lovenox), Tinzaparin (Innohep)

Expected Pharmacological Action

Δ   Parenteral anticoagulants prevent bleeding by inactivation of thrombin formation and factor Xa, resulting in inhibition of the formation of fibrin.

Therapeutic Uses

Δ   Parenteral anticoagulants are used:

- In conditions necessitating prompt anticoagulant activity (e.g., evolving stroke, pulmonary embolism, massive deep **venous** thrombosis).

- As an anticoagulant during pregnancy.

- As an adjunct for clients having open heart surgery or renal dialysis.

- As low-dose therapy for prophylaxis against postoperative venous thrombosis (e.g., hip/knee replacement surgery, abdominal surgery).

- In disseminated intravascular coagulation.

- In conjunction with thrombolytic therapy when treating an acute myocardial infarction.

Side/Adverse Effects: Nursing Interventions and Client Education

Side/Adverse Effects	Nursing Interventions/Client Education
Hemorrhage secondary to heparin overdose	• Monitor vital signs. • Advise the client to observe for signs and symptoms of bleeding (e.g., ↑ heart rate, ↓ blood pressure, bruising, petechiae, hematomas, black tarry stools). • In the case of heparin overdose, stop heparin, administer protamine sulfate, and avoid aspirin. • Monitor activated partial thromboplastin time (aPTT). Keep value at < 2 times the baseline.
Heparin-induced thrombocytopenia, as evidenced by low platelet count and ↑ development of thrombi – mediated by antibody development	• Monitor the client's platelet count periodically throughout treatment, especially in the first month. • Stop heparin if platelet count is < 100,000/mm³. Nonheparin anticoagulants, such as lepirudin (Refludan) or argatroban (Acova), can be used as a substitute if anticoagulation is still needed.
Hypersensitivity reactions (e.g., chills, fever, urticaria)	• Administer a small test dose prior to the administration of heparin.

Contraindications/Precautions

Δ   Parenteral anticoagulants are contraindicated in clients with low platelet counts (thrombocytopenia) or uncontrollable bleeding.

Δ   These medications should not be used during or following surgeries of the eye(s), brain, or spinal cord; lumbar puncture; or regional anesthesia.

Δ   Use cautiously in clients with hemophilia, increased capillary permeability, dissecting aneurysm, peptic ulcer disease, severe hypertension, or threatened abortion.

Medication/Food Interactions: Nursing Interventions and Client Education

Medication/Food Interactions	Nursing Interventions/Client Education
Anti-platelet agents such as **aspirin** – additive risk of bleeding with concurrent use	• Avoid concurrent use when possible. • Monitor carefully for evidence of bleeding. • Take precautionary measures to avoid injury (e.g., limit venipunctures and injections).

Therapeutic Nursing Interventions and Client Education

Δ   Obtain the client's baseline vital signs.

Δ   Periodically obtain and monitor complete blood count (CBC), platelet count, and hematocrit levels.

Δ   Heparin cannot be absorbed by the intestinal tract and must be given by a deep subcutaneous injection or IV infusion.

Δ   Heparin is dispensed in units and has different concentrations. Read label carefully.

Δ   Dosages should be checked by another nurse before administration.

Δ   For continuous IV administration, use an infusion pump. Rate of infusion must be monitored every 30 to 60 min.

Δ   Monitor aPPT every 4 to 6 hr until appropriate dose is determined, and then monitor daily.

Δ   For subcutaneous injections, use a 20 to 22 gauge needle to withdraw heparin solution from the vial. Then, change the needle to a small needle (e.g., gauge 25 or 26, 1/2 to 5/8 in length).

Δ   Deep subcutaneous injections should be administered in the abdomen ensuring a distance of 2 in from the umbilicus. Do not aspirate.

Δ   Apply pressure for 1 to 2 min after the injection. Rotate and record injection sites.

Nursing Evaluation of Medication Effectiveness

Δ   aPTT levels of 60 to 80 sec

Δ   No development or no further development of venous thrombi

Key Points

Medication Classification: Treatment of Heparin Overdose

Select Prototype Medication: Protamine sulfate

Expected Pharmacological Action

Δ   Protamine sulfate binds with heparin and forms a heparin-protamine complex
that has no anticoagulant properties.

Therapeutic Uses

Δ   Antidote to severe heparin overdose

Δ   Reversal of heparin administered during procedures

Therapeutic Nursing Interventions and Client Education

Δ   Protamine sulfate should be administered slowly intravenously, no faster than
20 mg/min, or 50 mg in 10 min.

Nursing Evaluation of Medication Effectiveness

Δ   Decrease or absence of bleeding episodes

Δ   aPTT levels of 60 to 80 sec

Key Points

Medication Classification: Anticoagulant/Oral

Select Prototype Medication: **warfarin (Coumadin)**

Expected Pharmacological Action

Δ   Oral anticoagulants antagonize vitamin K, thereby preventing the synthesis of four coagulation factors: factor VII, IX, X, and prothrombin.

Therapeutic Uses

Δ   Oral anticoagulants are used in the prevention of:

- Venous thrombosis

- Thrombus formation in clients with atrial fibrillation

- Thrombus formation in clients with prosthetic heart valves

Side/Adverse Effects: Nursing Interventions and Client Education

Side /Adverse Effects	Nursing Interventions/Client Education
Hemorrhage	• Monitor the client's vital signs. • Advise the client to observe for signs and symptoms of bleeding (e.g., ↑ heart rate, ↓ blood pressure, bruising, petechiae, hematomas, black or tarry stools). • Obtain baseline prothrombin time (PT) and monitor levels of PT and International Normalized Ratio (INR) periodically. • In the case of a warfarin overdose, discontinue administration of warfarin, and administer vitamin K.

Contraindications/Precautions

Δ   Oral anticoagulants fall into Pregnancy Risk Category X due to high risk of fetal hemorrhage, fetal death, and CNS defects. Advise the client to notify the provider if she becomes pregnant while on warfarin therapy. If anticoagulation is needed during pregnancy, heparin can be safely used.

Δ   Use is contraindicated in clients with low platelet counts (thrombocytopenia) or uncontrollable bleeding.

Δ   Use is contraindicated during or following surgeries of the eye(s), brain, or spinal cord; lumbar puncture; or regional anesthesia.

Δ   Use is contraindicated in clients with vitamin K deficiencies, liver disorders, and alcoholism due to the additive risk of bleeding.

Δ   Use cautiously in clients with hemophilia, dissecting aneurysm, peptic ulcer disease, severe hypertension, or threatened abortion.

Medication/Food Interactions: Nursing Interventions and Client Education

Medication/Food Interactions	Nursing Interventions/Client Education
Heparin, aspirin, and glucocorticoids – promote bleeding with concurrent use	• Avoid concurrent use if possible. • Instruct the client to observe for inclusion of aspirin in over-the-counter medications. • If used concurrently, monitor the client carefully for signs of bleeding, and ↑ prothrombin time (PT), INR, and aPPT levels. • Medication dosage should be adjusted accordingly.
Acetaminophen, sulfonamides, parenteral cephalosporins, and aspirin – ↑ effects of warfarin **leading to the** ↑ risk for bleeding with concurrent use	• Avoid concurrent use if possible. • If used concurrently, monitor the client carefully for signs of bleeding and ↑ PT and INR. • Medication dosage should be adjusted accordingly.
Phenobarbital, carbamazepine (Tegretol), phenytoin (Dilantin), oral contraceptives, and vitamin K – ↓ anticoagulant effects with concurrent use	• Avoid concurrent use if possible. • If used concurrently, monitor the client carefully for ↓ PT and INR levels. • Medication dosage should be adjusted accordingly.
Foods high in vitamin K (e.g., dark green leafy vegetables, cabbage, cauliflower, soybeans) – ↓ anticoagulant effects with excessive intake	• Supply the client with a list of foods high in vitamin K. • Instruct the client to avoid eating excessive amounts of foods high in vitamin K.

Therapeutic Nursing Interventions and Client Education

Δ   Obtain the client's baseline vital signs.

Δ   Monitor PT levels (therapeutic level 18 to 24 sec) and INR levels (therapeutic levels 2 to 3). INR levels are the most accurate. Hold dose and notify the primary care provider if these levels exceed therapeutic ranges.

Δ   Periodically obtain and monitor CBC, platelet count, and hematocrit levels.

Δ   Clients do not experience anticoagulant effects from warfarin for 8 to 12 hr with full therapeutic effect being achieved in 3 to 5 days. Explain to hospitalized clients the need for continued heparin infusion when started on oral warfarin.

Δ   Advise clients that anticoagulation effects can persist for up to 5 days following discontinuation of medication due to long half-life.

Δ   Advise the client to avoid alcohol, over-the-counter and non-prescription medications to prevent adverse side effects and medication interactions, such as ↑ risk of bleeding.

Δ   Advise the client to employ non-medication measures to avoid development of thrombi, including avoiding sitting for prolonged periods of time, not wearing tight constricting clothing, and elevating and moving legs when sitting.

Δ   Advise the client to wear a medical alert bracelet indicating warfarin use.

Δ   Be prepared to administer vitamin K for warfarin overdose.

Δ   Teach the client to self-monitor PT and INR at home as appropriate.

Δ   Advise the client to record dosage, route, and time of warfarin administration on a daily basis.

Δ   Clients may need to be placed on medications that interact with warfarin. When the interacting medication is being deleted or added is when the client is at greatest risk for harm. Frequent PT monitoring will allow for dosage adjustments as necessary.

Δ   Advise the client to notify her healthcare providers regarding warfarin use.

Δ   Advise the client to use a soft-bristle toothbrush to prevent gum bleeding.

Nursing Evaluation of Medication Effectiveness

Δ   PT 1.5 to 2 times control

Δ   INR of 2 to 3

Δ   No development or no further development of venous thrombi

Key Points

Medication Classification: Treatment of Warfarin Overdose

Select Prototype Medication: **vitamin K (Phytonadione, Aquamephyton)**

Expected Pharmacological Action

Δ   Vitamin K promotes synthesis of coagulation factors VII, IX, X, and prothrombin.

Therapeutic Uses

Δ   Reversal of hypoprothrombinemia and bleeding due to warfarin overdose

Δ   Vitamin K deficiency

Side/Adverse Effects: Nursing Interventions and Client Education

Side/Adverse Effects	Nursing Interventions/Client Education
Anaphylactoid-type reaction (e.g., flushing, hypotension, urticaria, cardiovascular collapse)	• Administer IV vitamin K slowly and in a diluted solution to prevent reaction. • Use other routes of administration whenever possible.

Therapeutic Nursing Interventions and Client Education

Δ   Administer small doses of vitamin K (e.g., 2.5 mg by mouth, 0.5 to 1 mg IV) to prevent development of resistance to warfarin (Coumadin).

Δ   If vitamin K cannot control bleeding, administer fresh frozen plasma or whole blood.

Nursing Evaluation of Medication Effectiveness

Δ   Decrease or absence of bleeding episodes

Δ   PT 1.5 to 2 times control

Δ   INR of 2 to 3

Key Points

Medication Classification: Antiplatelets

Select Prototype Medication: **aspirin (Ecotrin)**

Other Medications: ticlopidine (Ticlid), clopidogrel (Plavix),
dipyridamole (Persantine),
abciximab (Reo Pro), tirofiban (Aggrastat)

Expected Pharmacological Action

Δ   Antiplatelets prevent platelets from clumping together by inhibiting enzymes and factors that normally lead to **arterial** clotting.

Therapeutic Uses

Δ   Antiplatelets are used for:

- Primary prevention of acute myocardial infarction

- Prevention of reinfarction in clients following an acute MI

- Prevention of stroke

- Acute coronary syndromes (abciximab [ReoPro], tirofiban [Aggrastat])

Side/Adverse Effects: Nursing Interventions and Client Education

Side/Adverse Effects	Nursing Interventions/Client Education
GI effects such as bleeding	• Advise the client to use enteric-coated tablets and to take aspirin with food. • Concurrent use of a proton pump inhibitor, such as omeprazole (Prilosec), may be appropriate.
Hemorrhagic stroke	• Advise the client to observe for signs of weakness, dizziness, and headache, and to notify the primary care provider if symptoms occur.

Contraindications/Precautions

      Δ   Antiplatelets fall into Pregnancy Risk Category D in the third trimester.

      Δ   Use is contraindicated in clients with bleeding disorders and thrombocytopenia

      Δ   Use cautiously in clients with peptic ulcer disease and severe renal and/or hepatic disorders.

Medication/Food Interactions: Nursing Interventions and Client Education

Medication/Food Interactions	Nursing Interventions/Client Education
Other medications that enhance bleeding (e.g., **NSAIDs, heparin, warfarin**) – additive risk for bleeding with concurrent use	• Advise the client to avoid concurrent use. • If used concurrently, monitor the client carefully for signs of bleeding.

Therapeutic Nursing Interventions and Client Education

      Δ   Advise the client that prevention of strokes, myocardial infarctions, and reinfarctions can be accomplished with low dose aspirin (81 mg).

      Δ   Aspirin 325 mg should be taken during initial acute episode of MI.

      Δ   Advise the client to notify their healthcare providers regarding aspirin use.

Nursing Evaluation of Medication Effectiveness

      Δ   No development of arterial thrombosis

Key Points

Medication Classification: Thrombolytic Medications

Select Prototype Medication:	**streptokinase (Streptase)**
Other Medications:	alteplase (Activase, tPA), tenecteplase (TNKase), reteplase (Retavase)

Expected Pharmacological Action

Δ   Thrombolytic medications act by **dissolving clots that have already formed.** Dissolution of clots is accomplished by conversion of plasminogen to plasmin, which in turn, destroys fibrinogen and other clotting factors.

Therapeutic Uses

Δ   Thrombolytic medications are used to treat:

- Acute myocardial infarction

- Deep vein thrombosis (DVT)

- Massive pulmonary emboli

- Ischemic stroke (alteplase)

Side/Adverse Effects: Nursing Interventions and Client Education

Side/Adverse Effects	Nursing Interventions/Client Education
Serious risk of bleeding from different sites (e.g., within brain, needle puncture sites, wounds)	• Limit venipunctures and injections. • Apply pressure dressings to recent wounds. • Monitor the client for changes in vital signs, alterations in level of consciousness, weakness, and signs of intracranial bleeding. • Notify the primary care provider if symptoms occur.
streptokinase (Streptase)	
Hypotension	• Monitor the client's blood pressure. • Give streptokinase infusion slowly to prevent hypotension.
Allergic reaction (e.g., urticaria, itching, flushing) – may also cause severe anaphylactic reaction	• Monitor the client for symptoms of allergy, and notify the primary care provider if symptoms occur. • Be prepared with life support equipment at bedside.

Contraindications/Precautions

Δ   Because of the additive risk for serious bleeding, use is contraindicated in clients with any prior intracranial hemorrhage (hemorrhagic stroke), known structural cerebral vascular lesion (arteriovenous malformation), suspected aortic dissection, active internal bleeding, history of significant closed head or facial trauma in the past 3 months, acute pericarditis, and brain tumors.

Δ   Use cautiously in clients with severe hypertension, a recent episode of ischemic stroke (6 months prior to start of treatment), or clients who have had major surgery within 2 to 4 weeks before the start of treatment.

Medication/Food Interactions: Nursing Interventions and Client Education

Medication/Food Interactions	Nursing Interventions/Client Education
Other medications that enhance bleeding (e.g., **NSAIDs, heparin, warfarin**) – additive risk for bleeding with concurrent use	• Advise the client to avoid concurrent use. • If used concurrently, monitor the client carefully for signs of bleeding.

Therapeutic Nursing Interventions and Client Education

Δ   Use of thrombolytic agents must take place within 4 to 6 hr of onset of symptoms.

Δ   Clients receiving a thrombolytic agent should be monitored in a setting that provides for close supervision and continuous monitoring during and after administration of the medication.

Δ   Obtain baseline platelet counts, hemoglobin (Hgb), hematocrit (Hct), aPTT, PT, INR, and fibrinogen levels, and monitor periodically.

Δ   Obtain baseline vital signs (e.g., heart rate, blood pressure) and monitor periodically.

Δ   Nursing care includes continuous monitoring of hemodynamic status to assess for therapeutic and adverse effects of thrombolytic (e.g., relief of chest pain, signs of bleeding). Follow agency protocol.

Δ   Provide for client safety per agency protocol.

Δ   Ensure adequate IV access for administration of emergency medications and availability of emergency equipment.

Δ   Do not mix any medications in IV with thrombolytic agents.

Δ   Minimize bruising by limiting venipunctures, and subcutaneous/intramuscular injections.

Δ   Discontinue thrombolytic therapy if life-threatening bleeding occurs. Treat blood loss with whole blood, packed red blood cells, and/or fresh frozen plasma. IV aminocaproic acid (Amicar) should be available for administration in the event of excessive fibrinolysis.

Δ   Following thrombolytic therapy, administer heparin or aspirin as prescribed to decrease the risk of rethrombosis.

Δ   Following thrombolytic therapy, administer beta-blockers as prescribed to ↓ myocardial oxygen consumption and to ↓ the incidence and severity of reperfusion arrhythmias.

Δ   Administer H$_2$ antagonists such as ranitidine (Zantac), or proton pump inhibitors, such as omeprazole (Prilosec), as prescribed to prevent GI bleeding.

Nursing Evaluation of Medication Effectiveness

Δ   Evidence of thrombus lysis and restoration of circulation (e.g., relief of chest pain, reduction of initial ST segment injury pattern as shown on ECG 60 to 90 min after start of therapy).

Key Points

Medication Classification: Iron Preparations

Select Prototype Medication:	**ferrous sulfate (Feosol)**
Other Medications:	**Iron Dextran (INFeD)**

Expected Pharmacological Action

Δ   Iron preparations provide iron needed for RBC development and oxygen transport to cells.

Therapeutic Uses

Δ   Iron preparations are used to treat:

•   Iron deficiency anemia

Δ   Iron preparations are used to prevent:

•   Iron deficiency anemia for clients who are at an increased risk, such as pregnant women, infants, and children

Side/Adverse Effects: Nursing Interventions and Client Education

Side/Adverse Effects	Nursing Interventions/Client Education
GI distress (e.g., nausea, constipation, heartburn)	• If intolerable, administer medication with food, but this greatly reduces absorption. • May need to ↓ dosage. • Monitor the client's bowel pattern and intervene as appropriate. This side effect usually resolves with continued use.
Teeth staining (liquid form)	• Teach the client to dilute liquid iron with water or juice, drink with a straw, and rinse mouth after swallowing.
Anaphylaxis risk with parenteral administration	• IV route is safer. • Administer a test dose and observe client closely. • Give IM doses deep IM using Z track technique. • Give initial IV dose slowly. Observe client closely for 60 min following first dose. • Be prepared with life-support equipment.

Contraindications/Precautions

Δ Contraindicated for clients with previous hypersensitivity to iron

Δ Contraindicated in clients with hemolytic anemia, peptic ulcer disease, and severe liver disease

Medication/Food Interactions: Nursing Interventions and Client Education

Medication/Food Interactions	Nursing Interventions/Client Education
Reduced absorption of iron with coadministration of **antacids** or **tetracyclines**	• Separate use by at least 2 hr.
Vitamin C – ↑ absorption, but ↑ side effects	• Avoid vitamin C intake when taking medication.

Therapeutic Nursing Interventions and Client Education

Δ Instruct the client to take iron on an empty stomach (e.g., 1 hr before meals to maximize absorption). Stomach acid increases absorption.

Δ Inform the client to anticipate a harmless dark green or black color stool.

Δ Instruct the client to increase water and fiber intake (unless contraindicated), and to maintain an exercise program to counter the constipation effects.

Δ Encourage concurrent intake of appropriate quantities of foods high in iron (e.g., liver, egg yolks, muscle meats, yeast).

Nursing Evaluation of Medication Effectiveness

Δ Increase in reticulocyte count, hemoglobin, and hematocrit levels

Key Points

Medication Classification: Vitamin B$_{12}$-Cyanocobalamin

Select Prototype Medication: **vitamin B$_{12}$**

Expected Pharmacological Action

Δ   Vitamin B$_{12}$ is necessary to convert folic acid from its inactive form to its active form. All cells rely on folic acid for DNA production.

Therapeutic Uses

Δ   Treatment of vitamin B$_{12}$ deficiency

Δ   Megaloblastic (macrocytic) anemia related to vitamin B$_{12}$ deficiency

Side/Adverse Effects: Nursing Interventions and Client Education

Side/Adverse Effects	Nursing Interventions/Client Education
Hypokalemia secondary to the ↑ RBC production effects of vitamin B$_{12}$	• Monitor the client's potassium levels during the start of treatment. • Observe the client for symptoms of potassium deficiency (e.g., muscle weakness, abnormal cardiac rhythm). • Client may require potassium supplements.

Medication/Food Interactions: Nursing Interventions and Client Education

Medication/Food Interactions	Nursing Interventions/Client Education
Masking of signs of vitamin B$_{12}$ deficiency with concurrent administration of **folic acid**	• Make sure that the client receives adequate doses of vitamin B$_{12}$ when using folic acid.

Therapeutic Nursing Interventions and Client Education

Δ   Obtain baseline vitamin B$_{12}$, Hgb, Hct, RBC, and reticulocyte counts. Monitor periodically.

Δ   Monitor the client for signs of vitamin B$_{12}$ deficiency (e.g., beefy red tongue, pallor, neuropathy).

Δ   Cyanocobalamin may be administered intranasally, orally, or by IM or SC injection. Injections are painful and are usually reserved for individuals with significant reduced ability to absorb vitamin B$_{12}$ (e.g., lack of intrinsic factor [pernicious anemia], enteritis, and partial removal of stomach).

Δ   Clients with malabsorption syndrome can use intranasal preparation or parenteral preparation.

Δ   Clients with irreversible malabsorption syndrome (e.g., parietal cell atrophy, total gastrectomy) will need lifelong treatment, usually parenterally.

Δ   Encourage concurrent intake of appropriate quantities of foods high in vitamin B_{12}, such as dairy products.

Δ   Perform Schillings test to determine vitamin B_{12} absorption in the gastrointestinal tract.

Δ   Advise clients to be compliant with laboratory tests. Blood counts and vitamin B_{12} levels should be monitored every 3 to 6 months.

Nursing Evaluation of Medication Effectiveness

Δ   Improvement of megaloblastic anemia as evidenced by ↑ reticulocyte count, absence of megaloblasts, and normal Hgb and Hct levels.

Δ   Improvement of neurologic symptoms (e.g., absence of tingling sensation of hands and feet, numbness of extremities). Improvement may take months, and some clients will never attain full recovery.

Key Points

Medication Classification: Folic Acid

Select Prototype Medication: **Folic acid**

Expected Pharmacological Action

Δ   **Folic acid** is essential in the production of DNA and erythropoiesis (RBC, WBC, and platelets).

Therapeutic Uses

Δ   Folic acid is used:

- In the treatment of megaloblastic (macrocytic) anemia secondary to folic acid deficiency

- In the prevention of neural tube defects during pregnancy

- For malabsorption syndrome such as sprue

Side/Adverse Effects: Nursing Interventions and Client Education

Side/Adverse Effects	Nursing Interventions/Client Education
None	

Contraindications/Precautions

Δ   Indiscriminate use of folic acid is inappropriate due to the risk of masking signs of vitamin B_{12} deficiency.

Medication/Food Interactions: Nursing Interventions and Client Education

Medication/Food Interactions	Nursing Interventions/Client Education
↓ folate levels with concurrent use of **sulfonamides, sulfasalazine, or methotrexate**	• Avoid concurrent use of these medications.

Therapeutic Nursing Interventions and Client Education

Δ   Assess the client for signs and symptoms of megaloblastic anemia (e.g., pallor, easy fatigability, palpitations).

Δ   Obtain the client's baseline folic acid levels, RBC and reticulocyte counts, Hgb, and Hct levels. Monitor periodically.

Δ   Advise clients with folic acid deficiency to concurrently increase intake of food sources of folic acid, such as green leafy vegetables and liver.

Nursing Evaluation of Medication Effectiveness

Δ   Folate level 6 to 15 mcg/mL

Δ   Return of RBC, reticulocyte count, and Hgb and Hct to normal levels

Δ   Monitor the client for improvement of anemia symptoms (e.g., absence of pallor, dyspnea, easy fatigability).

Δ   Absence of neural tube defects in newborns

Key Points

Medication Classification: Hematopoietic Growth Factors

Select Prototype Medication: **epoetin alfa (Epogen, Procrit)**

Other Medications: darbepoetin alfa (Aranesp)

Expected Pharmacological Action

Δ   Hematopoietic growth factors act on the bone marrow to increase production of red blood cells

Therapeutic Uses

Δ   Epoetin is used for

• Anemia of chronic renal failure

• HIV-infected clients taking zidovudine (Retrovir)

• Anemia induced by chemotherapy

• Anemia in clients scheduled for elective surgery

Side/Adverse Effects: Nursing Interventions and Client Education

Side/Adverse Effects	Nursing Interventions/Client Education
Hypertension secondary to elevations in hematocrit level	• This side effect occurs due to the elevation of hematocrit levels. • Monitor the client's hematocrit levels and blood pressure, and if elevated, administer antihypertensive medications.
Increased risk for a cardiovascular event (e.g., MI, stroke, cardiac arrest) with an ↑ in Hgb > 12 g/dL or > 1 g in 2 weeks	• ↓ dosage when these limits are reached.

Contraindications/Precautions

Δ   This medication is contraindicated in clients with uncontrolled hypertension.

Δ   Use cautiously in clients with cancers of the bone marrow.

Therapeutic Nursing Interventions and Client Education

Δ   Monitor the client's iron levels and take measures to ensure a normal iron level. RBC growth is dependent upon adequate quantities of iron, folic acid, and vitamin B_{12}. Without adequate levels of these, erythropoietin is significantly less effective.

Δ   Monitor the client's Hgb and Hct twice a week until target range is reached.

Δ   Obtain the client's baseline blood pressure.

Δ   In clients with chronic renal failure, control hypertension before the start of treatment.

Δ   Epoetin alfa should not be agitated and should not be combined with other medications.

Nursing Evaluation of Medication Effectiveness

Δ   Hemoglobin level of 10 to 12 g/dL and hematocrit of 40%

Δ   Increased reticulocyte count

Key Points

Medication Classification: Hematopoietic Growth Factors/Granulocyte Colony Stimulating Factor

Select Prototype Medication: **filgrastim (Neupogen)**

Other Medications: pegfilgrastim (Neulasta)

Expected Pharmacological Action

Δ These medications stimulate the bone marrow to increase production of neutrophils.

Therapeutic Uses

Δ Decreases the risk of infection in clients with neutropenia, such as cancer

Side/Adverse Effects: Nursing Interventions and Client Education

Side/Adverse Effects	Nursing Interventions/Client Education
Bone pain	• Monitor the client for symptoms and notify the primary care provider. • Administer acetaminophen.
Leukocytosis	• Monitor CBC two times per week during treatment. • ↓ dose or interrupt treatment, if WBC >50,000 mm^3, absolute neutrophil count (ANC) >20,000 mm^3, or platelets >500,000 mm^3.

Contraindications/Precautions

Δ This medication is contraindicated in clients who are sensitive to *Escherichia coli* protein.

Δ Use cautiously in clients with cancer of the bone marrow.

Therapeutic Nursing Interventions and Client Education

Δ   Filgrastim should not be agitated and should not be combined with other medications.

Δ   Monitor CBC two times per week.

Nursing Evaluation of Medication Effectiveness

Δ   Absence of infection

Δ   In chemotherapy for cancer treatment, an absolute neutrophil count increase to greater than 10,000/mm^3 after the chemotherapeutic induced nadir (the peak of chemotherapeutic cell destruction usually occurring 10 to 14 days after administration).

Key Points

Medication Classification: Hematopoietic Growth Factors / Granulocyte Macrophage Colony Stimulating Factor

Select Prototype Medication: **sargramostim (Leukine)**

Expected Pharmacological Action

Δ   This medication acts on the bone marrow to increase production of white blood cells (e.g., neutrophils, monocytes, macrophages, eosinophils).

Therapeutic Uses

Δ   Sargramostim:

- Facilitates recovery of the bone marrow after bone marrow transplant.

- Is used in the treatment of failed bone marrow transplant.

Side/Adverse Effects: Nursing Interventions and Client Education

Side/Adverse Effects	Nursing Interventions/Client Education
Diarrhea, weakness, rash, malaise, and bone pain	• Monitor the client for symptoms, and notify the primary care provider if they occur. • Administer acetaminophen.
Leukocytosis, thrombocytosis	• Monitor CBC two times per week during treatment. • Reduce dose or interrupt treatment, if WBC >50,000 mm^3, absolute neutrophil count >20,000 mm^3, or platelets >500,000 mm^3.

Contraindications/Precautions

Δ   Use is contraindicated in clients allergic to yeast products

Δ   Use cautiously in clients with heart disease, hypoxia, peripheral edema, pleural and pericardial effusion.

Δ   Use cautiously in clients with cancer of the bone marrow.

Therapeutic Nursing Interventions and Client Education

Δ Obtain baseline CBC, differential and platelet count, and monitor periodically while on treatment.

Δ Sargramostim should not be agitated and should not be combined with other medications.

Nursing Evaluation of Medication Effectiveness

Δ Absence of infection

Δ WBC and differential within normal ranges

Key Points

Medication Classification: Thrombopoietic Growth Factors

Select Prototype Medication: **oprelvekin (Interleukin 11, Neumega)**

Expected Pharmacological Action

Δ   This medication increases the production of platelets.

Therapeutic Uses

Δ   Decreases thrombocytopenia in clients receiving myelosuppressive chemotherapy

Side/Adverse Effects: Nursing Interventions and Client Education

Side/Adverse Effects	Nursing Interventions/Client Education
Fluid retention (e.g., peripheral edema, dyspnea on exertion)	• Use cautiously in clients with heart failure and pleural effusion. • Monitor the client's I&O. • If symptoms occur, stop the medication and notify the primary care provider.
Cardiac dysrhythmias (e.g., tachycardia, atrial fibrillation, atrial flutter)	• Use cautiously in clients with a history of cardiac dysrhythmias. • Monitor the client's vital signs, heart rate and rhythm. • If symptoms occur, stop the medication and notify the primary care provider.
Conjunctival injection, transient blurring of vision, and papilledema	• Advise the client to observe for symptoms, and if symptoms occur, stop the medication and notify the primary care provider.

Contraindications/Precautions

Δ   Use cautiously in clients with cancer of the bone marrow.

Therapeutic Nursing Interventions and Client Education

Δ   Obtain the client's baseline CBC, platelet count, and electrolytes.

Δ   Oprelvekin should not be agitated and should not be combined with other medications.

Δ   Administer oprelvekin once daily, and start administration 4 to 6 hr after starting chemotherapy. Continue treatment for 21 days or until platelet counts increase to 50,000/ mm^3.

Nursing Evaluation of Medication Effectiveness

Δ   Platelet count > 50,000 mm^3

Key Points

Medication Classification: Blood and Blood Products

Select Prototype Medication: **Whole blood**

Expected Pharmacological Action

Δ   Administration of whole blood increases circulating blood volume

Therapeutic Uses

Δ   Whole blood is used as replacement therapy

- To treat acute blood loss secondary to traumatic injuries or surgical procedures.

- To induce volume expansion in clients with extensive burn injury, dehydration, shock.

Side/Adverse Effects: Nursing Interventions and Client Education

Side/Adverse Effects	Nursing Interventions/Client Education
Acute hemolytic reaction (e.g., chills, fever, low back pain, tachycardia, tachypnea, hypotension)	• Upon initiation of the transfusion, obtain baseline vital signs, stay with the client, and monitor vital signs every 5 min for 15 min. • Stop transfusion immediately if symptoms occur, and notify the primary care provider.
Febrile nonhemolytic reaction, most common (e.g., sudden chills); fever (e.g., ↑ of temperature greater than 1° from baseline); headache	• Upon initiation of the transfusion, obtain baseline vital signs, stay with client, and monitor vital signs every 5 min for 15 min. • Observe for signs and symptoms of a reaction and stop the transfusion if they occur. • Notify the primary care provider immediately and follow parameters regarding resumption or discontinuation of transfusion. • Administer acetaminophen.
Anaphylactic reactions (e.g., anxiety, urticaria, wheezing, shock, cardiac arrest)	• Upon initiation of the transfusion, obtain baseline vital signs, stay with the client, and monitor vital signs every 5 min for 15 min. • If symptoms occur, stop the transfusion and notify the primary care provider immediately. • Initiate CPR if necessary. • Have epinephrine ready for IM or IV injection. • Do not restart transfusion.

Side/Adverse Effects	Nursing Interventions/Client Education
Mild allergic reactions (e.g., flushing, itching, urticaria)	• Upon initiation of the transfusion, stay with the client, and monitor vital signs every 5 min for 15 min. • If symptoms occur, stop the transfusion and notify the primary care provider immediately. • If symptoms are very mild and there is no respiratory compromise, antihistamines may be prescribed and the transfusion restarted slowly.
Circulatory overload (e.g., cough, shortness of breath, crackles, hypertension, tachycardia, distended neck veins)	• Observe the client for signs and symptoms of fluid volume excess. • If symptoms occur, stop the transfusion and notify the primary care provider immediately. • Place the client upright with feet down. • Administer diuretics and oxygen as appropriate. • Monitor I&O. • A slower rate of infusion may be indicated.
Sepsis (e.g., rapid onset of chills and fever, vomiting, diarrhea, hypotension, shock)	• Observe the client for signs and symptoms during and following transfusion. • Notify the primary care provider immediately if symptoms occur. • Obtain blood culture, send blood transfusion bag for analysis for possible contaminants, and treat sepsis with antibiotics, IV fluids, vasopressors, and steroids.

Contraindications/Precautions

Δ Contraindicated in clients with hypersensitivity reactions

Δ Observe culturally sensitive (religious) issues regarding blood transfusion, such as Jehovah's Witness.

Therapeutic Nursing Interventions and Client Education

Δ Before starting a whole blood transfusion, verify the primary care provider's orders, the client's blood typing, obtain consent for transfusion, and check the client's blood transfusion history.

Δ A second person is necessary to check identification of donor blood and recipient, blood compatibility, and expiration date.

Δ Assess the client before, during, and after administration.

Δ Obtain the client's baseline vital signs and assessment of urinary output, document on the client's medical record, record start and completion times of transfusion, total volume of transfusion, and the client's response to the transfusion.

Δ Assess infusion site for infection or infiltration.

Δ Assess patency of IV line and prime IV tubing with 0.9% normal saline (NS).

Δ Do not administer blood along with any IV solution other than 0.9% NS. IV solutions containing dextrose cause hemolysis of red blood cells.

Δ Administer blood using a gauge 19 or larger intravenous needle (to avoid breakage of cells and blockage of needle lumen), a blood filter (to remove particles and possible contaminants within old blood) and use a Y tubing connection (so that 0.9% NS can be infused by piggyback).

Δ Observe universal precautions during handling and administration of blood products.

Δ Do not administer blood products with any other medications.

Δ Complete transfusion within 2 to 4 hr.

Δ In the event a blood transfusion reaction is noted:

- Stop transfusion immediately and notify the primary care provider immediately.

- Do not turn on IV fluids that are connected to the Y tubing because the remaining blood in the Y tubing will be infused and aggravate the client's reaction. Administer a new IV solution of 0.9% NS.

- Stay with the client and monitor vital signs and urinary output.

- Notify blood bank, recheck identification tag and numbers on the blood bag, and send blood bag and IV tubing to blood bank for analysis.

- Obtain urine specimen and send to laboratory to determine for RBC hemolysis.

- Complete transfusion log sheet, which includes complete record of baseline vital signs, ongoing monitoring, and client's response to transfusion. Incorporate in client's medical record.

Nursing Evaluation of Medication Effectiveness

Δ Increase in hemoglobin of 1 to 2 g/dL per unit of blood administered

Δ Blood pressure above shock parameters

Key Points

Medication Classification: Blood and Blood Products

Select Prototype Medication: **Packed red blood cells**

Expected Pharmacological Action

Δ   Administration of packed red blood cells increases the number of red blood cells.

Therapeutic Uses

Δ   Packed red blood cells (RBCs) are used to treat:

- Severe symptomatic anemia (Hgb < 6 g/dL).

- Hemoglobinopathies.

- Medication-induced hemolytic anemia.

- Erythroblastosis fetalis.

Side/Adverse Effects: Nursing Interventions and Client Education

Side/Adverse Effects	Nursing Interventions/Client Education
Acute hemolytic reaction (e.g., chills, fever, low back pain, tachycardia, tachypnea, hypotension)	• Upon initiation of the transfusion, obtain baseline vital signs, stay with the client, and monitor vital signs every 5 min for 15 min. • Stop transfusion immediately if symptoms occur, and notify the primary care provider.
Febrile nonhemolytic reaction, most common (e.g., sudden chills); fever (e.g., increase of temperature greater than 1° from baseline); headache	• Upon initiation of the transfusion, obtain baseline vital signs, stay with client, and monitor vital signs every 5 min for 15 min. • Observe for signs and symptoms of a reaction and stop the transfusion if they occur. • Notify the primary care provider immediately and follow parameters regarding resumption or discontinuation of transfusion. • Administer acetaminophen.

Side/Adverse Effects	Nursing Interventions/Client Education
Anaphylactic reactions (e.g., anxiety, urticaria, wheezing, shock, cardiac arrest)	• Upon initiation of the transfusion, obtain baseline vital signs, stay with the client, and monitor vital signs every 5 min for 15 min. • If symptoms occur, stop the transfusion and notify the primary care provider immediately. • Initiate CPR if necessary. • Have epinephrine ready for IM or IV injection. • Do not restart transfusion.
Mild allergic reactions (e.g., flushing, itching, urticaria)	• Upon initiation of the transfusion, stay with the client, and monitor vital signs every 5 min for 15 min. • If symptoms occur, stop the transfusion and notify the primary care provider immediately. • If symptoms are very mild and there is no respiratory compromise, antihistamines may be prescribed and the transfusion restarted slowly.
Sepsis (e.g., rapid onset of chills and fever, vomiting, diarrhea, hypotension, shock)	• Observe for signs and symptoms during and following transfusion. • Notify the primary care provider immediately if symptoms occur. • Obtain blood culture, send blood transfusion bag for analysis for possible contaminants, and treat sepsis with antibiotics, IV fluids, vasopressors, and steroids.

Contraindications/Precautions

Δ   Contraindicated in clients with hypersensitivity reactions

Δ   Observe culturally sensitive (religious) issues regarding blood transfusion, such as Jehovah's Witness.

Therapeutic Nursing Interventions and Client Education

Δ   Before starting a packed RBC transfusion, verify the primary care provider's orders, client's blood typing, obtain consent for transfusion, and check client's blood transfusion history.

Δ   A second person is necessary to check identification of donor blood and recipient, blood compatibility, and expiration date.

Δ   Assess the client before, during, and after administration.

Δ   Obtain baseline vital signs and assessment of urinary output, document on client's medical record, record start and completion times of transfusion, total volume of transfusion, and client's response to transfusion.

Δ   Assess infusion site for infection or infiltration.

Δ   Assess patency of IV line.

Δ   Do not administer blood along with any IV solution other than 0.9% NS. IV solutions containing dextrose cause hemolysis of red blood cells.

Δ   Administer blood using a gauge 19 or larger intravenous needle (to avoid breakage of cells and blockage of needle lumen), a blood filter (to remove particles and possible contaminants within old blood), and use a Y tubing connection (so that 0.9% NS can be infused by piggyback).

Δ   Observe universal precautions during handling and administration of blood products.

Δ   Do not administer blood products with any other medications.

Δ   Complete transfusion within 2 to 4 hr.

Δ   In the event a blood transfusion reaction is noted:

•   Stop transfusion immediately and notify the primary care provider immediately.

•   Do not turn on IV fluids that are connected to the Y tubing because the remaining blood in the Y tubing will be infused and aggravate the client's reaction. Administer a new IV solution of 0.9% NS.

•   Stay with the client and monitor vital signs and urinary output.

•   Notify blood bank, recheck identification tag and numbers on the blood bag, and send blood bag and IV tubing to blood bank for analysis.

•   Obtain urine specimen and send to laboratory to determine for RBC hemolysis.

•   Complete transfusion log sheet, which includes complete record of baseline vital signs, ongoing monitoring, and client's response to transfusion. Incorporate in client's medical record.

Nursing Evaluation of Medication Effectiveness

Δ   Increase in Hgb level of 1 to 2 g/dL per unit administered

Key Points

Medication Classification: Blood and Blood Products

Select Prototype Medication: **Platelet concentrate**

Expected Pharmacological Action

Δ   Administration of platelet concentrate increases platelet counts.

Therapeutic Uses

Δ   Platelet concentrate is used to treat:

- Thrombocytopenia (platelet count < 20,000/mm^3) (e.g., aplastic anemia, chemotherapy-induced bone marrow suppression)

- Active bleeding (platelet count < 80,000 mm^3)

Side/Adverse Effects: Nursing Interventions and Client Education

Side/Adverse Effects	Nursing Interventions/Client Education
Febrile reaction, most common (e.g., sudden chills or rigors); fever (e.g., increase of temperature greater than 1° from baseline); headache	• Upon initiation of the transfusion, obtain baseline temperature, stay with client, and monitor vital signs every 5 min for 15 min. • Observe for signs and symptoms of a reaction and stop the transfusion if they occur. • Notify the primary care provider immediately, and follow parameters regarding resumption or discontinuation of transfusion. • Administer acetaminophen.
Mild allergic reactions (e.g., flushing, itching, urticaria)	• Upon initiation of the transfusion, stay with the client, and monitor vital signs every 5 min for 15 min. • If symptoms occur, stop the transfusion and notify the primary care provider immediately. If symptoms are very mild and there is no respiratory compromise, antihistamines may be prescribed and the transfusion restarted slowly.

Side/Adverse Effects	Nursing Interventions/Client Education
Sepsis (e.g., rapid onset of chills and fever, vomiting, diarrhea, hypotension, shock)	• Observe for signs and symptoms during and following transfusion. • Notify the primary care provider immediately if symptoms occur. • Obtain blood culture, send blood transfusion bag for analysis for possible contaminants, and treat sepsis with antibiotics, IV fluids, vasopressors, and steroids.

Contraindications/Precautions

Δ   Contraindicated in clients with hypersensitivity reactions

Therapeutic Nursing Interventions and Client Education

Δ   Before starting a platelet concentrate transfusion, verify the primary care provider's orders, client's blood typing, obtain consent for transfusion, and check the client's blood transfusion history.

Δ   A second person is necessary to check identification of donor platelet concentrate and recipient, compatibility, and expiration date.

Δ   Assess the client before, during, and after administration of platelet concentrate.

Δ   Obtain baseline vital signs, document on client's medical record, record start and completion times of platelet concentrate transfusion, total volume of transfusion, and client's response to transfusion.

Δ   Assess infusion site for infection or infiltration.

Δ   Use special platelet transfusion tubing set (smaller filter, shorter tubing).

Δ   Administer any prescribed premedications (e.g., meperidine, to minimize reactions such as fever and rigors).

Δ   Administer at rate prescribed by primary care provider/hospital policy (e.g., 15 to 30 min/unit).

Δ   Do not administer with any other medications.

Δ   Obtain baseline bleeding time and monitor periodically.

Nursing Evaluation of Medication Effectiveness

Δ   Reduced bleeding

Δ   Increase in platelet count

Key Points

Medication Classification: Blood and Blood Products

Select Prototype Medication: **Fresh frozen plasma**

Expected Pharmacological Action

Δ   Administration of fresh frozen plasma replaces coagulation factors.

Therapeutic Uses

Δ   Fresh frozen plasma is used to treat:

- Active bleeding or massive hemorrhage.

- Extensive burns.

- Shock.

- Disseminated intravascular coagulation.

- Antithrombin III deficiency.

- Thrombotic thrombocytopenic purpura.

Δ   Fresh frozen plasma is used to reverse:

- Anticoagulation effects of warfarin.

Δ   Fresh frozen plasma is used as:

- Replacement therapy for coagulation factors II, V, VII, IX, X, and XI.

Side/Adverse Effects: Nursing Interventions and Client Education

Side/Adverse Effects	Nursing Interventions/Client Education
Acute hemolytic reaction (e.g., chills, fever, low back pain, tachycardia, tachypnea, hypotension)	• Upon initiation of the transfusion, obtain baseline vital signs, stay with the client, and monitor vital signs every 5 min for 15 min. • Stop transfusion immediately if symptoms occur, and notify the primary care provider.

Side/Adverse Effects	Nursing Interventions/Client Education
Febrile nonhemolytic reaction, most common (e.g., sudden chills); fever (e.g., increase of temperature greater than 1° from baseline); headache	• Upon initiation of the transfusion, obtain baseline vital signs, stay with the client, and monitor vital signs every 5 min for 15 min. • Observe for signs and symptoms of a reaction and stop the transfusion if they occur. • Notify the primary care provider immediately, and follow parameters regarding resumption or discontinuation of transfusion. • Administer acetaminophen.
Anaphylactic reactions (e.g., anxiety, urticaria, wheezing, shock, cardiac arrest)	• Upon initiation of the transfusion, obtain baseline vital signs, stay with client, and monitor vital signs every 5 min for 15 min. • If symptoms occur, stop the transfusion and notify the primary care provider immediately. • Initiate CPR if necessary. • Have epinephrine ready for IM or IV injection. • Do not restart transfusion.
Mild allergic reactions (e.g., flushing, itching, urticaria)	• Upon initiation of the transfusion, stay with client, and monitor vital signs every 5 min for 15 min. • If symptoms occur, stop the transfusion and notify the primary care provider immediately. If symptoms are very mild and there is no respiratory compromise, antihistamines may be prescribed and the transfusion restarted slowly.
Circulatory overload (e.g., cough, shortness of breath, crackles, hypertension, tachycardia, distended neck veins)	• Observe client for signs and symptoms of fluid volume excess. If symptoms occur, stop the transfusion and notify the primary care provider immediately. • Place the client upright with feet down. • Administer diuretics and oxygen as appropriate. • Monitor I&O. • A slower rate of infusion may be indicated.
Sepsis (e.g., rapid onset of chills and fever, vomiting, diarrhea, hypotension, shock)	• Observe for signs and symptoms during and following transfusion. • Notify the primary care provider immediately if symptoms occur. • Obtain blood culture, send blood transfusion bag for analysis for possible contaminants, and treat sepsis with antibiotics, IV fluids, vasopressors, and steroids.

Contraindications/Precautions

Δ   Contraindicated in clients with hypersensitivity reactions

Therapeutic Nursing Interventions and Client Education

Δ   Before starting fresh frozen plasma transfusion, verify the primary care provider's orders, client's blood typing, obtain consent for transfusion, and check the client's blood transfusion history.

Δ   A second person is necessary to check identification of donor fresh frozen plasma and recipient, compatibility, and expiration date.

Δ   Assess the client before, during, and after administration of fresh frozen plasma.

Δ   Obtain baseline vital signs, document on client's medical record, record start and completion times of fresh frozen plasma transfusion, total volume of transfusion, and client's response to transfusion.

Δ   Assess patency of IV line.

Δ   Assess infusion site for infection or infiltration.

Δ   Administer at rate prescribed by primary care provider/hospital policy (e.g., 30 to 60 min/unit).

Δ   Do not administer with any other medications.

Δ   Obtain baseline bleeding time and monitor periodically.

Nursing Evaluation of Medication Effectiveness

Δ   Reduced bleeding

Δ   Prothrombin or activated partial thromboplastin time < 1.5 times normal

Key Points

Medication Classification: Blood and Blood Products

Select Prototype Medication: **Pheresed granulocytes**

Expected Pharmacological Action

△   Pheresed granulocytes replace neutrophils/granulocytes.

Therapeutic Uses

△   Pheresed granulocytes are used to treat:

•   Severe neutropenia (ANC < 500).

•   Life-threatening bacterial/fungal infection not responding to antibiotic therapy.

•   Neonatal sepsis.

•   Neutrophil dysfunction.

Side/Adverse Effects: Nursing Interventions and Client Education

Side/Adverse Effects	Nursing Interventions/Client Education
Acute hemolytic reaction (e.g., chills, fever, low back pain, tachycardia, tachypnea, hypotension)	• Upon initiation of the transfusion, obtain baseline vital signs, stay with the client, and monitor vital signs every 5 min for 15 min. • Stop transfusion immediately if symptoms occur, and notify the primary care provider.
Febrile nonhemolytic reaction, most common (e.g., sudden chills); fever (e.g., increase of temperature greater than 1° from baseline); headache	• Upon initiation of the transfusion, obtain baseline vital signs, stay with the client, and monitor vital signs every 5 min for 15 min. • Observe for signs and symptoms of a reaction, and stop the transfusion if they occur. • Notify the primary care provider immediately, and follow parameters regarding resumption or discontinuation of transfusion. • Administer acetaminophen.

Side/Adverse Effects	Nursing Interventions/Client Education
Anaphylactic reactions (e.g., anxiety, urticaria, wheezing, shock, cardiac arrest)	• Upon initiation of the transfusion, obtain baseline vital signs, stay with the client, and monitor vital signs every 5 min for 15 min. • If symptoms occur, stop the transfusion and notify the primary care provider immediately. • Initiate CPR if necessary. • Have epinephrine ready for IM or IV injection. • Do not restart transfusion.
Mild allergic reactions (e.g., flushing, itching, urticaria)	• Upon initiation of the transfusion, stay with the client, and monitor vital signs every 5 min for 15 min. • If symptoms occur, stop the transfusion and notify the primary care provider immediately. • If symptoms are very mild and there is no respiratory compromise, antihistamines may be prescribed and the transfusion restarted slowly.
Circulatory overload (e.g., cough, shortness of breath, crackles, hypertension, tachycardia, distended neck veins)	• Observe the client for signs and symptoms of fluid volume excess. • If symptoms occur, stop the transfusion and notify the primary care provider immediately. • Place the client upright with feet down. • Administer diuretics and oxygen as appropriate. • Monitor I&O. A slower rate of infusion may be indicated.
Sepsis (e.g., rapid onset of chills and fever, vomiting, diarrhea, hypotension, shock)	• Observe for signs and symptoms during and following transfusion. • Notify the primary care provider immediately if symptoms occur. • Obtain blood culture, send blood transfusion bag for analysis for possible contaminants, and treat sepsis with antibiotics, IV fluids, vasopressors, and steroids.

Contraindications/Precautions

Δ   Contraindicated in clients with hypersensitivity reactions

Therapeutic Nursing Interventions and Client Education

Δ   Before starting neutrophil/pheresed granulocyte transfusion, verify the primary care provider's orders, client's blood typing, obtain consent for transfusion, and check the client's transfusion history.

Δ   A second person is necessary to check identification of donor pheresed granulocyte and recipient, compatibility, and expiration date.

Δ   Assess the client before, during, and after administration of granulocyte concentrate. Some institutions require a primary care provider to monitor the client due to the higher risk of serious antibody-antigen reactions to granulocyte infusion.

Δ   Obtain baseline vital signs, document on client's medical record, record start and completion times of granulocyte, total volume of transfusion, and client's response to transfusion.

Δ   Assess patency of IV line.

Δ   Assess infusion site for infection or infiltration.

Δ   Administer at rate prescribed by primary care provider/hospital policy (e.g., 45 to 60 min/unit).

Δ   Do not administer with any other medications.

Δ   Observe universal precaution during handling and administration of blood products.

Δ   Stay with the client and respond promptly to any noted reactivity.

Nursing Evaluation of Medication Effectiveness

Δ   Increased granulocyte count

Key Points

Medication Classification: Hypoproteinemia/Hypoalbuminemia

Select Prototype Medication: **Albumin**

Expected Pharmacological Action

     Δ   Albumin expands circulating blood volume by exerting oncotic pressure.

Therapeutic Uses

     Δ   Albumin is used to treat:

- Hypovolemia.
- Hypoalbuminemia.
- Burns.
- Adult respiratory distress.
- Severe nephrosis.
- Cardiopulmonary bypass surgery.
- Hemolytic disease of the newborn.

Side/Adverse Effects: Nursing Interventions and Client Education

Side/Adverse Effects	Nursing Interventions/Client Education
Risk for fluid volume excess such as pulmonary edema	• Monitor central venous pressure, vital signs, and for any signs of circulatory overload (e.g., shortness of breath, crackles, distended neck veins, frothy blood-tinged sputum).

Contraindications/Precautions

     Δ   Albumin is contraindicated in clients with congestive heart failure or renal insufficiency due to additive risk for fluid volume excess.

Therapeutic Nursing Interventions and Client Education

Δ   Underlying cause of hypoalbuminemia should be treated to completely reverse client's condition.

Δ   Albumin must be administered by intravenous route. Administer slowly using an infusion pump.

Δ   Albumin solutions can be administered with whole blood, plasma, saline solutions, or glucose.

Δ   Obtain baseline Hgb, Hct, total protein, albumin levels, and continue monitoring the client during the duration of treatment.

Δ   Ensure adequate hydration prior to and following treatment.

Nursing Evaluation of Medication Effectiveness

Δ   Increased blood pressure

Δ   Increased serum albumin levels

Δ   Decreased edema

Primary Reference:

Lehne, R. A. (2007). *Pharmacology for nursing care* (6th ed.). St. Louis, MO: Saunders.

Additional Resources:

Grodner, M., Long, S., & DeYoung, S. (2004). *Foundations and clinical applications of nutrition.* St. Louis, MO: Mosby.

Skidmore-Roth, L. (2006). *Mosby's nursing drug reference.* St. Louis, MO: Elsevier.

Unit 7 Medications Affecting the Blood

Application Exercises

The management of the acute phase of myocardial infarction (MI) is accomplished by using thrombolytic medications. Answer the following questions regarding thrombolytic medications.

1. The nurse knows that the main action of thrombolytic medications is to

    A. prevent thrombus formation.

    B. suppress platelet aggregation.

    C. suppress the action of vitamin K.

    D. remove the thrombus that has already formed.

2. The goal of thrombolytic therapy is to restore blood flow through the blocked coronary artery. The nurse knows that for this therapy to be most effective, this treatment must be initiated within what time of symptom onset?

    A. 4 to 6 hr

    B. 8 to 10 hr

    C. 12 to 24 hr

    D. 48 to 96 hr

3. Which of the following reversal agents should the nurse have available in the event of a streptokinase overdose?

    A. Protamine sulfate

    B. Phytonadione (vitamin K)

    C. Aminocaproic acid (Amicar)

    D. Epinephrine (Adrenaline)

4. In which of the following clinical situations is the initiation of IV heparin therapy appropriate? (Select all that apply.)

_____   Obese client with swollen painful lower right calf postoperative abdominal surgery

_____   Client scheduled for a below-the-knee amputation

_____   Client with multiple small pulmonary emboli

_____   Client with an acute myocardial infarction

_____   Client with DVT who is 5 months pregnant

_____   Client with a platelet count of 80,000/mm^3

5. A client taking warfarin (Coumadin) should be instructed to avoid eating excessive amounts of which of the following foods? (Select all that apply.)

_____   Red meat

_____   Milk products

_____   Yellow and orange fruits

_____   Dark green leafy vegetables

_____   Cabbage

6. Which of the following client findings pose a concern for the administration of a daily dose of warfarin? (Select all that apply.)

_____   aPTT 75 sec

_____   PT 18 sec

_____   Hgb 12 g/dL

_____   INR 5.6

_____   WBC 9,800/mm^3

_____   Angina unrelieved by rest

_____   Nosebleed

_____   Melena

7. Which of the following client findings suggest a need to call the primary care provider for a possible reduction in a client's ferrous sulfate dose? (Select all that apply.)

_____   Client's stool is greenish black in color.

_____   Client reports constipation.

_____   Client takes iron along with Mylanta.

_____   Client has a Hgb level of 9 g/dL.

_____   Client takes his iron with first bite of breakfast.

_____   Client reports intolerable nausea and heartburn.

8. Match the following prescribed medications/blood products with the appropriate therapeutic use. Each therapeutic use may be selected more than once.

Folic acid

Cyanocobalamin (vitamin B_{12})

Epoetin Alfa (Erythropoietin)

Filgrastim (Neupogen)

Oprelvekin (Interleukin-11)

Whole blood

Packed red blood cells

Albumin

Platelet concentration

A. Hypovolemia secondary to third spacing

B. Iron deficiency anemia

C. Reduce the risk of infection for a client receiving chemotherapy

D. Anemia in client with chronic renal failure

E. Client with hemoglobin 6 g/dL and blood pressure of 70/40 mm Hg due to sustained massive trauma

F. Client with hemoglobin 8.9 g/dL on second day postoperative total hip replacement

G. Pernicious anemia

H. Treatment of thrombocytopenia

I. Client with megaloblastic anemia with a normal B_{12} level

Unit 7 Medications Affecting the Blood

Application Exercises Answer Key

The management of the acute phase of myocardial infarction (MI) is accomplished by using thrombolytic medications. Answer the following questions regarding thrombolytic medications.

1. The nurse knows that the main action of thrombolytic medications is to

        A. prevent thrombus formation.

        B. suppress platelet aggregation.

        C. suppress the action of vitamin K.

        D. remove the thrombus that has already formed.

    Thrombolytic medications act by dissolving clots that have already formed. Dissolution of clots is accomplished by conversion of plasminogen to plasmin, which in turn destroys fibrinogen and other clotting factors. Anticoagulants (e.g., heparin, warfarin) prevent venous thrombus formation. The actions of warfarin are related to suppression of vitamin K. Aspirin suppresses platelet aggregation.

2. The goal of thrombolytic therapy is to restore blood flow through the blocked coronary artery. The nurse knows that for this therapy to be most effective, this treatment must be initiated within what time of symptom onset?

        A. 4 to 6 hr

        B. 8 to 10 hr

        C. 12 to 24 hr

        D. 48 to 96 hr

    Thrombolytic therapy is most effective within 4 to 6 hr of onset of symptoms.

3. Which of the following reversal agents should the nurse have available in the event of a streptokinase overdose?

> A. Protamine sulfate
>
> B. Phytonadione (vitamin K)
>
> **C. Aminocaproic acid (Amicar)**
>
> D. Epinephrine (Adrenaline)

IV aminocaproic acid (Amicar) should be available for administration in the event of excessive fibrinolysis. Protamine sulfate is the reversal agent for a heparin overdose. Vitamin K is the reversal agent for a warfarin overdose. Epinephrine is used to treat anaphylaxis. A streptokinase overdose results in excessive bleeding, and administration of aminocaproic acid will rapidly reverse fibrinolysis.

---

4. In which of the following clinical situations is the initiation of IV heparin therapy appropriate? (Select all that apply.)

> **__X__** **Obese client with swollen painful lower right calf postoperative abdominal surgery**
>
> _____ Client scheduled for a below-the-knee amputation
>
> **__X__** **Client with multiple small pulmonary emboli**
>
> **__X__** **Client with an acute myocardial infarction**
>
> **__X__** **Client with DVT who is 5 months pregnant**
>
> _____ Client with a platelet count of 80,000/mm^3

These are therapeutic uses of heparin that prevent the formation of additional venous thrombi and the associated risks. A client scheduled for surgery is not a candidate for IV heparin therapy because of the additive risk for intraoperative blood loss. Clients may be given low-dose heparin just prior to surgery and then following surgery to prevent postoperative venous thrombi. Heparin is contraindicated for clients with thrombocytopenia.

5. A client taking warfarin (Coumadin) should be instructed to avoid eating excessive amounts of which of the following foods? (Select all that apply.)

_____	Red meat
_____	Milk products
_____	Yellow and orange fruits
X	**Dark green leafy vegetables**
X	**Cabbage**

Dark green leafy vegetables, cabbage, cauliflower, and soybeans are high in vitamin K. Excessive intake may decrease the effects of warfarin.

6. Which of the following client findings pose a concern for the administration of a daily dose of warfarin? (Select all that apply.)

_____	aPTT 75 sec
_____	PT 18 sec
_____	Hgb 12 g/dL
X	**INR 5.6**
_____	**WBC 9,800/mm³**
_____	Angina unrelieved by rest
X	**Nosebleed**
X	**Melena**

An INR of 5.6 is too high and poses a concern regarding a risk for serious bleeding. In general, an INR of 2 to 3 is the therapeutic target for warfarin therapy. Nosebleeds (epistaxis) and melena (blood in stool) are possible signs of bleeding. An aPTT of 75 sec suggests a therapeutic heparin level. A PT of 18 sec indicates a therapeutic warfarin level. A Hgb of 12 g/dL and WBC of 9,800/mm³ are normal values. Angina unrelieved by rest could indicate a myocardial infarction, which is a reason that heparin therapy might be initiated.

7. Which of the following client findings suggest a need to call the primary care provider for a possible reduction in a client's ferrous sulfate dose? (Select all that apply.)

     _____   Client's stool is greenish black in color.

     _____   Client reports constipation.

     _____   Client takes iron along with Mylanta.

     _____   Client has a Hgb level of 9 g/dL.

     _____   Client takes his iron with first bite of breakfast.

     X   **Client reports intolerable nausea and heartburn.**

Intolerable nausea and heartburn are reasons for possible reduction in dosage. An alternative to dosage reduction is to have the client take iron with food, even though this reduces absorption. A change in stool color and constipation are expected findings. Encourage fluid intake and exercise to counter constipation. A hemoglobin of 9 g/dL supports continued therapy.

8. Match the following prescribed medications/blood products with the appropriate therapeutic use. Each therapeutic use may be selected more than once.

Folic acid	A. Hypovolemia secondary to third spacing
Cyanocobalamin (vitamin B$_{12}$)	B. Iron deficiency anemia
Epoetin Alfa (Erythropoietin)	C. Reduce the risk of infection for a client receiving chemotherapy
Filgrastim (Neupogen)	D. Anemia in client with chronic renal failure
Oprelvekin (Interleukin-11)	E. Client with hemoglobin 6 g/dL and blood pressure of 70/40 mm Hg due to sustained massive trauma
Whole blood	F. Client with hemoglobin 8.9 g/dL on second day postoperative total hip replacement
Packed red blood cells	G. Pernicious anemia
Albumin	H. Treatment of thrombocytopenia
Platelet concentration	I. Client with megaloblastic anemia with a normal B$_{12}$ level

Folic Acid (I); Whole blood (E); Cyanocobalamin (Vitamin B$_{12}$) (G); Packed red blood cells (F); Epoetin Alfa (Erythropoietin) (D); Platelet concentrate (H); Filgrastim (Neupogen) (C); Albumin (A); Oprelvekin (Interleukin-11) (H)

Unit 8	Medications Affecting the Respiratory System

Contributor: Havovi Patel, MS, MBBS

 NCLEX® Connections:

Learning Objective: Review and apply knowledge within **"Medications Affecting the Respiratory System"** in readiness for performance of the following nursing activities as outlined by the NCLEX® test plans:

∆ Assess/monitor the client for expected effects of medications.

∆ Assess/monitor the client for side/adverse effects of medications.

∆ Assess/monitor the client for actual/potential specific food and medication interactions.

∆ Identify contraindications, actual/potential incompatibilities, and interactions between medications, and intervene appropriately.

∆ Identify symptoms/evidence of an allergic reaction, and respond appropriately.

∆ Evaluate/monitor and document the therapeutic and adverse/side effects of medications.

∆ Provide/reinforce client teaching on actions, therapeutic effects, potential side/ adverse effects, and interactions of medications.

 General Key Points

∆ Medications to treat asthma are classified into two main groups:

Bronchodilators including:	Anti-inflammatory agents including:
Beta₂-adrenergic agonists – **Inhaled, short-acting medications:** albuterol (Proventil, Ventolin) **Inhaled, long-acting medications:** formoterol (Foradil Aerolizer); salmeterol (Serevent) **Oral, long-acting medications:** albuterol (Proventil, Volmax); terbutaline (Brethine) **Methylxanthines –** Oral, long-acting medications: theophylline (Theolair-SR) **Anticholinergics –** maintenance therapy: ipratropium, inhaled (Atrovent)	**Glucocorticoids –** **Inhaled medications:** beclomethasone dipropionate (QVAR); budesonide (Pulmicort Turbuhaler); fluticasone propionate (Flovent, Flovent Rotadisk, Flovent Diskus); triamcinolone acetonide (Azmacort) **Oral medications:** prednisone (Deltasone); prednisolone **Cromolyn and nedocromil:** cromolyn, inhaled (Intal); nedocromil, inhaled (Tilade) **Leukotriene modifiers:** montelukast, oral (Singulair); zafirlukast, oral (Accolate); zileuton, oral (Zyflo)
Bronchodilators can be given orally and by inhalation. They may be used for **short-term** prophylaxis, **relief** of acute attacks, and **long-term** control.	Anti-inflammatory agents are used for **long-term** prophylaxis, not for aborting ongoing asthmatic attacks.

Δ   Antiasthmatic medications can be administered by inhalation. Inhalation facilitates delivering the medication directly to the site of action. This ↑ the therapeutic effects, minimizes levels of medication in the blood, and promotes rapid relief of asthmatic episodes.

Δ   Three kinds of devices are used for inhalation therapy: MDI (metered dose inhaler), DPI (dry powder inhaler), and nebulizers. The client should be instructed on the proper use of these devices.

Key Points

Medication Classification: Beta$_2$-Adrenergic Agonists

Select Prototype Medication:	**albuterol (Proventil, Ventolin)**
Other Medications:	formoterol (Foradil Aerolizer) salmeterol (Serevent), terbutaline (Brethine)

Expected Pharmacological Action

Δ   Beta$_2$-adrenergic agonists act by selectively activating the beta$_2$-receptors in the bronchial smooth muscle resulting in bronchodilation. As a result of this:

- Bronchospasm is relieved.

- Histamine release is inhibited.

- Ciliary motility is ↑.

Medication	Route	Therapeutic Uses
Albuterol (Proventil, Ventolin)	Inhaled, short-acting Oral, long-acting	• Prevention of asthma attack (exercise-induced) • Treatment for ongoing asthma attack • Long-term control of asthma
Formoterol (Foradil Aerolizer) Salmeterol (Serevent)	Inhaled, long-acting	• Long-term control of asthma
Terbutaline (Brethine)	Oral, long-acting	• Long-term control of asthma

Side/Adverse Effects: Nursing Interventions and Client Education

Side/Adverse Effects	Nursing Interventions/Client Education
Inhaled agents – short and long acting	• Minimal adverse effects
Oral agents – tachycardia and angina due to activation of alpha$_1$ receptors in the heart	• Advise the client to observe for signs and symptoms, and to notify the primary care provider if they occur. • Dosage may need to be lowered.
Tremors due to activation of beta$_2$ receptors in skeletal muscle	• Tremors usually resolve with continued medication use. • Dosage may need to be reduced.

Contraindications/Precautions

Δ   Pregnancy Risk Category C

Δ   Contraindicated in clients with tachydysrhythmias

Δ   Use cautiously in clients with diabetes, hyperthyroidism, heart disease, hypertension, and angina.

Medication/Food Interactions: Nursing Interventions and Client Education

Medication/Food Interactions	Nursing Interventions/Client Education
Use of beta-adrenergic blockers, such as propranolol can negate effects of both.	• Beta-adrenergic blockers should not be used concurrently.
MAOIs and tricyclic antidepressants can ↑ the risk of tachycardia and angina.	• Instruct the client to report changes in heart rate and chest pain.

Therapeutic Nursing Interventions and Client Education

Δ   Beta$_2$-agonists are administered by inhalation using MDI, DPI, and nebulizer.

Δ   Clients should be instructed on how to use the different devices used in inhalation treatments.

Δ   Clients using MDI (metered dose inhaler) should:

•   Remove the cap from the inhaler.

•   Hold the inhaler with the mouthpiece at the bottom.

•   **Shake** the inhaler.

•   Hold the mouth piece at ½ to 2 inches in front of the mouth.

•   Tilt head back slightly and open mouth wide.

•   Breathe gently.

•   Press the inhaler and, at the same time, begin a slow, deep breath. Continue to breathe slowly and deeply for 3 sec to facilitate delivery to the air passages.

•   Hold breath for 10 sec to allow medication to deposit in the airways.

•   Resume normal breathing.

•   Wait 1 full min before administering the second puff.

•   Repeat steps 3 through 9 when more than one puff is needed.

•   Clean the plastic case and cap by rinsing thoroughly with warm water.

Δ   Steps for using a spacer with MDI include:

•   Inserting the inhaler/canister into spacer and shaking.

- Breathing out.

- Putting the spacer mouthpiece into the mouth.

- Pressing down on the inhaler once.

- Breathing in slowly for 3 to 5 sec.

- Holding breath for 10 sec.

Δ When the client is prescribed an inhaled **beta$_2$-agonist** and an inhaled glucocorticoid, advise the client to inhale the **beta$_2$-agonist** before inhaling the glucocorticoid. The **beta$_2$-agonist** promotes bronchodilation and enhances absorption of the glucocorticoid.

Δ Advise the client not to exceed prescribed dosages.

Δ Ensure that the client knows the appropriate dosage schedule (e.g., if the medication is to be taken on a fixed or a when necessary schedule).

Δ Formoterol (Foradil Aerolizer) and salmeterol (Serevent) are both **long-acting** beta$_2$-agonist inhalers. These inhalers are used every 12 hr for long-term control and are NOT to be used to abort an asthma attack. A short-acting beta$_2$-agonist should be used if the client needs to treat an acute attack.

Δ Advise the client to observe for signs of an impending asthma attack and to keep a log of attacks by recording how often they occur and how intense the attacks are.

Δ Instruct the client to notify the primary care provider if there is an ↑ in the frequency and intensity of asthma attacks.

Nursing Evaluation of Medication Effectiveness

Δ Depending on therapeutic intent, effectiveness may be evidenced by:

- Long-term control of asthma attacks.

- Prevention of exercise-induced asthma attack.

- Resolution of asthma attack as evidenced by absence of shortness of breath, clear breath sounds, absence of wheezing, return of respiratory rate to baseline.

Key Points

Medication Classification: Methylxanthines

Select Prototype Medication: **theophylline (Theolair)**

Expected Pharmacological Action

Δ Theophylline causes relaxation of bronchial smooth muscle results in bronchodilation.

Therapeutic Uses

Δ Theophylline is used for long-term control of chronic asthma.

Side/Adverse Effects: Nursing Interventions and Client Education

Side/Adverse Effects	Nursing Interventions/Client Education
Mild toxicity reaction may include GI distress and restlessness: More severe reactions can occur with higher therapeutic levels and can include dysrhythmias and seizures	• Monitor theophylline serum levels to keep within therapeutic range. Side effects are unlikely to occur at levels < 20 mcg/mL. • If symptoms occur, stop the medication. If necessary, activated charcoal can be used to ↓ absorption, lidocaine can be used to treat dysrhythmias, and diazepam can be used to control seizures.

Contraindications/Precautions

Δ Pregnancy Risk Category C

Δ Use cautiously in clients with heart disease, hypertension, liver and renal dysfunction, and diabetes.

Δ Use cautiously in children and older adults.

Medication/Food Interactions: Nursing Interventions and Client Education

Medication/Food Interactions	Nursing Interventions/Client Education
Caffeine ↑ CNS and cardiac adverse effects of theophylline. Caffeine can also ↑ theophylline levels.	• Advise the client to avoid consuming caffeinated beverages (e.g., coffee, caffeinated drinks).
Phenobarbital and phenytoin ↓ theophylline levels.	• When theophylline is used concurrently with these medications, ↑ the dosage of theophylline.

Medication/Food Interactions	Nursing Interventions/Client Education
Cimetidine (Tagamet) and ciprofloxacin (Cipro), and other fluoroquinolone antibiotics ↑ theophylline levels.	• When theophylline is used concurrently with these medications, ↓ the dosage of theophylline.

Therapeutic Nursing Interventions and Client Education

Δ   Advise clients to take the medication as prescribed, and if a dose is missed, the following dose should not be doubled.

Δ   Advise the client to observe for signs of an impending asthma attack and to keep a log of attacks by recording how often they occur and how intense the attacks are.

Δ   Instruct the client to notify the primary care provider if there is an ↑ in frequency and intensity of asthma attacks.

Δ   Instruct the client not to chew or crush sustained-release preparations. These medications should be swallowed whole.

Nursing Evaluation of Medication Effectiveness

Δ   Long-term control of asthma attacks

Key Points

Medication Classification: Inhaled Anticholinergics

Select Prototype Medication:	**ipratropium, inhaled (Atrovent)**
Other Medications:	tiotropium, inhaled (Spiriva)

Expected Pharmacological Action

Δ   These medications block muscarinic receptors on bronchi resulting in bronchodilation.

Therapeutic Uses

Δ   These medications are used to relieve bronchospasm associated with chronic obstructive pulmonary disease.

Δ   These medications are used for allergen-induced and exercise-induced asthma.

Side/Adverse Effects: Nursing Interventions and Client Education

Side/Adverse Effects	Nursing Interventions/Client Education
Systemic effects	Minimal
Local anticholinergic effects (dry mouth, hoarseness)	Advise the client to slp fluids and suck on hard candies to control dry mouth.

Contraindications/Precautions

Δ   Pregnancy Risk Category B

Δ   Contraindicated in clients with an allergy to peanuts because the medication preparations may contain soy lecithin

Δ   Use cautiously in clients with narrow-angle glaucoma and benign prostatic hypertrophy (due to anticholinergic effects).

Therapeutic Nursing Interventions and Client Education

Δ   Advise the client to rinse mouth after inhalation to ↓ unpleasant taste.

Δ   Usual adult dosage is two puffs. Instruct the client to wait at least 1 min between puffs.

Δ   If the client is prescribed two inhaled medications, instruct the client to wait at least 5 min between medications.

Nursing Evaluation of Medication Effectiveness

Δ   Control of bronchospasm in clients with chronic obstructive pulmonary disease

Δ   Prevention of allergen-induced and exercise-induced asthma attack

Key Points

Medication Classification: Glucocorticoids

Select Prototype Medication:	**beclomethasone dipropionate (QVAR)**
Other Medications:	budesonide (Pulmicort Turbuhaler), fluticasone propionate (Flovent), triamcinolone acetonide (Azmacort), prednisone (Deltasone)

Expected Pharmacological Action

Δ   These medications prevent inflammation, suppression of airway mucus production, and promote responsiveness of beta$_2$ receptors in the bronchial tree.

Δ   The use of glucocorticoids does not provide immediate effects, but rather promotes decreased frequency and severity of exacerbations and acute attacks.

Therapeutic Uses

Δ   Inhaled agents are used for long-term prophylaxis of asthma.

Δ   Short-term oral therapy is used to treat symptoms following an acute asthma attack.

Δ   Long-term oral therapy is used to treat chronic asthma.

Δ   Replacement therapy is used for primary adrenocortical insufficiency.

Δ   Promote lung maturity and decrease respiratory distress in fetuses at risk for preterm birth.

Side/Adverse Effects: Nursing Interventions and Client Education

Side/Adverse Effects	Nursing Interventions/Client Education
Inhaled glucocorticoids – difficulty speaking, hoarseness, and candidiasis	• Advise the client to use a spacer with MDI. • Advise the client to rinse mouth and gargle after use. If candidiasis develops, treat with mycostatin oral suspension.
Oral glucocorticoids when used for ≥ 10 days can result in:	
Suppression of adrenal gland function, such as a ↓ ability of the adrenal cortex to produce glucocorticoids: Can occur with inhaled agents and oral agents	• Administer oral glucocorticoid on an alternate day dosing schedule. • Monitor the client's blood glucose levels. • Taper the client's dose.

Side/Adverse Effects	Nursing Interventions/Client Education
Bone loss: Can occur with inhaled agents and oral agents	• Advise the client to perform weight-bearing exercises. • Advise the client to consume a diet with sufficient calcium and vitamin D intake. • Use lowest dose possible to control symptoms. • Oral medications should be given every other day.
Hyperglycemia and glucosuria	• Clients with diabetes should have their blood glucose monitored. • Clients may need an ↑ in insulin dosage.
Myopathy as evidenced by muscle weakness	• Instruct the client to report signs of muscle weakness. • Medication dosage should be decreased.
Peptic ulcer disease	• Advise the client to avoid NSAIDs. • Advise the client to report black, tarry stools. Check stool for occult blood periodically. • Administer with food or meals.
Infection	• Advise the client to notify the primary care provider if early signs of infection occur (e.g., sore throat, weakness, malaise).
Disturbances of fluid and electrolytes (e.g., fluid retention as evidenced by weight gain, and edema and hypokalemia as evidenced by muscle weakness)	• Instruct the client to observe for symptoms and report to the primary care provider.

Contraindications/Precautions

Δ   Contraindicated in clients who have received a live virus vaccine

Δ   Contraindicated in clients with systemic fungal infections

Δ   Use cautiously in children, clients with diabetes, hypertension, peptic ulcer disease, and/or renal dysfunction.

Δ   Use cautiously in clients taking NSAIDs.

Medication/Food Interactions: Nursing Interventions and Client Education

Medication/Food Interactions	Nursing Interventions/Client Education
prednisone (Deltasone)	
Potassium-depleting diuretics – concurrent use ↑ the risk of hypokalemia	• Monitor potassium level and administer supplements as needed.

Medication/Food Interactions	Nursing Interventions/Client Education
NSAID – concurrent use ↑ the risk of GI ulceration	• Advise the client to avoid use of NSAIDs. If GI distress occurs, instruct the client to notify the primary care provider.
Concurrent use of glucocorticoids will counteract the effects of insulin and oral hypoglycemics	• Client should notify primary care provider if hyperglycemia occurs. The client may need ↑ dosage of insulin or oral hypoglycemics.

Therapeutic Nursing Interventions and Client Education

Δ Instruct the client to use glucocorticoid inhalers on a regular, fixed schedule for long-term therapy of asthma. Glucocorticoids are not to be used to treat an acute attack.

Δ Administer using an MDI device, DPI, or nebulizer.

Δ The client should use a spacer with all preparations except budesonide (QVAR).

Δ When the client is prescribed an inhaled beta$_2$-agonist and an inhaled glucocorticoid, advise the client to inhale the beta$_2$-agonist before inhaling the glucocorticoid. The **beta$_2$-agonist** promotes bronchodilation and enhances absorption of the glucocorticoid.

Δ **Oral glucocorticoids are used short-term, 3 to 10 days following an acute asthma attack.**

Δ If client is on long-term oral therapy, additional dosages of oral glucocorticoids are required in times of stress (e.g., infection, trauma).

Δ Clients who discontinue oral glucocorticoid medications or switch from oral to inhaled agents require additional doses of glucocorticoids during periods of stress.

Nursing Evaluation of Medication Effectiveness

Δ Long-term control of asthma attacks

Δ Resolution of acute attack as evidenced by absence of shortness of breath, clear breath sounds, absence of wheezing, and return of respiratory rate to baseline

Key Points

Medication Classification: Mast Cell Stabilizers

Select Prototype Medication: **cromolyn sodium (Intal)**

Other Medications: nedocromil sodium (Tilade)

Expected Pharmacological Action

Δ   **Anti-inflammatory action**

- These medications stabilize mast cells, which inhibits the release of histamine and other inflammatory mediators.

- These medications suppress inflammatory cells (e.g., eosinophils, macrophages).

Therapeutic Uses

Δ   Management of **chronic asthma**

Δ   Prophylaxis of **exercise-induced** asthma

Δ   Prevention of **allergen-induced** attack

Δ   Allergic rhinitis by intranasal route

Side/Adverse Effects: Nursing Interventions and Client Education

Side/Adverse Effects	Nursing Interventions/Client Education
Safest of all asthma medications	• Safe to use for children.

Contraindications/Precautions

Δ   Pregnancy Risk Category B

Δ   Fluorocarbons in aerosols make this medication contraindicated for clients with coronary artery disease, dysrhythmias, and status asthmaticus.

Δ   Use cautiously in clients with liver and kidney impairment.

Therapeutic Nursing Interventions and Client Education

Δ   Advise the client to take medication 15 min before exercise or exposure to allergen.

Δ   Advise the client that long-term prophylaxis may take several weeks for full therapeutic effects to be established.

Δ   Advise the client that this is not a bronchodilator and is not intended for aborting an asthmatic attack.

Δ   Instruct the client in the proper use of administration devices (e.g., nebulizer, MDI).

Nursing Evaluation of Medication Effectiveness

Δ   Prevention of exercise- or allergen-induced bronchospasm

Δ   Decreased episodes of allergic rhinitis

Δ   Long-term control of asthma

Key Points

Medication Classification: Leukotriene Modifiers

Select Prototype Medication: **montelukast (Singulair)**

Other Medications: zileuton (Zyflo), zafirlukast (Accolate)

Expected Pharmacological Action

Δ Leukotriene modifiers prevent the effects of leukotrienes, thereby suppressing inflammation, bronchoconstriction, airway edema, and mucus production.

Therapeutic Uses

Δ Leukotriene modifiers are used for long-term therapy of asthma in adults and children 12 years and older.

Side/Adverse Effects: Nursing Interventions and Client Education

Side/Adverse Effects	Nursing Interventions/Client Education
Liver injury with use of zileuton (Zyflo) and zafirlukast (Accolate)	• Obtain baseline liver function tests and monitor periodically. • Advise the client to monitor for signs of liver damage (e.g., nausea, anorexia, abdominal pain). • Instruct the client to notify the primary care provider if symptoms occur.

Contraindications/Precautions

Δ Use cautiously in clients with liver dysfunction.

Medication/Food Interactions: Nursing Interventions and Client Education

Medication/Food Interactions	Nursing Interventions/Client Education
Warfarin (Coumadin) levels ↑ with concurrent use of zileuton (Zyflo) and zafirlukast (Accolate) by inhibiting metabolism of warfarin. ↑ levels of warfarin can ↑ the risk of bleeding.	• Advise the client to observe for signs of bleeding, and to notify the primary care provider. • Monitor prothrombin time (PT) and INR levels.

Medication/Food Interactions	Nursing Interventions/Client Education
Theophylline levels ↑ with concurrent use of zileuton (Zyflo) and zafirlukast (Accolate) by inhibition of metabolism of theophylline. ↑ levels of theophylline can ↑ risk for toxicity.	• Monitor theophylline levels. • Advise the client to observe for signs of theophylline toxicity (e.g., nausea, vomiting, seizures), and to notify the primary care provider.

Therapeutic Nursing Interventions and Client Education

Δ   Advise the client to take Zyflo as prescribed. Zyflo can be given with or without food.

Δ   Advise the client that Accolate should not be given with food, and to administer it 1 hr before or 2 hr after meals.

Δ   Advise the client to take Singulair once daily at bedtime.

Nursing Evaluation of Medication Effectiveness

Δ   Long-term control of asthma

Key Points

Medication Classification: Antitussive-Opioids

Select Prototype Medication:	**codeine**
Other Medications:	hydrocodone

Expected Pharmacological Action

Δ   Codeine suppresses cough.

Therapeutic Uses

Δ   Codeine is used for chronic **non-productive** cough.

Side/Adverse Effects: Nursing Interventions and Client Education

Side/Adverse Effects	Nursing Interventions/Client Education
CNS effects (e.g., dizziness, lightheadedness, drowsiness, respiratory depression)	• Obtain the client's baseline vital signs. • Monitor the client when ambulating. • Advise the client to lie down if feeling lightheaded. • Observe for signs of respiratory depression such as respiratory rate less than 12/min. Stimulate the client to breathe if respiratory depression occurs. May need to stop medication and administer naloxone (Narcan). • Advise the client to avoid driving while taking codeine.
GI distress (e.g., nausea, vomiting, constipation)	• Advise the client to take oral codeine with food. • Advise client to ↑ fluids and dietary fiber.
Potential for abuse Schedule II	• Advise the client of the potential for abuse. • Use for short duration.

Contraindications/Precautions

Δ   Pregnancy Category Risk C

Δ   Contraindicated in clients with acute asthma, head trauma, liver and renal dysfunction, and acute alcoholism

Δ   Use cautiously in children, older adults, and clients with a drug abuse history.

Therapeutic Nursing Interventions and Client Education

Δ   Advise the client to avoid hazardous activities, such as driving while taking codeine.

Δ   Advise the client to change positions slowly and to lie down if feeling dizzy.

Δ   Advise the client to avoid alcohol and other CNS depressants while taking codeine.

Nursing Evaluation of Medication Effectiveness

Δ   Absence or decreased episodes of coughing

Key Points

Medication Classification: Mucolytics

Select Prototype Medication: **acetylcysteine (Mucomyst)**

Other Medications: hypertonic saline

Expected Pharmacological Action

△   Mucolytics enhance the flow of secretions in the respiratory passages.

Therapeutic Uses

△   Mucolytics are used in clients with acute and chronic pulmonary disorders exacerbated by large amounts of secretions.

△   Mucolytics are used in clients with cystic fibrosis.

△   Acetylcysteine (Acetadote) is the antidote for poisoning with acetaminophen (nonrespiratory disorder).

Side/Adverse Effects: Nursing Interventions and Client Education

Side/Adverse Effects	Nursing Interventions/Client Education
Aspiration and bronchospasm	• Monitor the client for signs of aspiration and bronchospasm. Stop medication immediately and notify the primary care provider.

Contraindications/Precautions

△   Pregnancy Risk Category B

△   Should not be used in clients at risk for GI hemorrhage

△   Use cautiously in clients with peptic ulcer disease, esophageal varices, and severe liver disease.

Therapeutic Nursing Interventions and Client Education

△   Advise the client that acetylcysteine has an odor that smells like rotten eggs.

△   Advise the client to dilute medication in fruit juice or other beverage.

△   Advise the client that the medication will make the nasal and bronchial secretions watery and will facilitate coughing.

Δ   IV infusion started with loading dose, followed by next dose to be infused over 4 hr, followed by last dose infused over 16 hr.

Δ   Be prepared to suction the client if aspiration occurs.

Nursing Evaluation of Medication Effectiveness

Δ   Improvement of symptoms as evidenced by regular respiratory rate, lung sounds clear, and ↑ ease of expectoration.

Key Points

Medication Classification: Decongestants

Select Prototype Medication: **phenylephrine**

Other Medications: ephedrine, naphazoline, phenylpropanolamine

Expected Pharmacological Action

Δ   Decongestants stimulate alpha$_1$-adrenergic receptors causing reduction in the inflammation of the nasal membranes.

Therapeutic Uses

Δ   This medication can be used to treat allergic rhinitis by relieving nasal stuffiness.

Δ   This medication acts as a decongestant for clients with sinusitis and the common cold.

Side/Adverse Effects: Nursing Interventions and Client Education

Side/Adverse Effects	Nursing Interventions/Client Education
Rebound congestion secondary to prolonged use of topical agents	• Advise the client to use for short-term therapy, no more than 3 to 5 days. • Taper use and discontinue medication using one nostril at a time.
CNS stimulation (e.g., agitation, nervousness, uneasiness)	• CNS stimulation is rare with the use of topical agents • Advise the client to observe for signs of CNS stimulation, and to notify the primary care provider if symptoms occur. • Stop medication.
Vasoconstriction	• Advise clients with hypertension and coronary artery disease to avoid using these medications.

Contraindications/Precautions

Δ   Contraindicated in clients with chronic rhinitis

Δ   Use cautiously in clients with coronary artery disease and hypertension.

Therapeutic Nursing Interventions and Client Education

Δ   Instruct the client to be in the lateral head low position to prevent swallowing the medication.

Δ   Drops are preferred for children.

Δ   Educate the client in the differences between topical and oral agents.

- Topical agents are usually more effective and work faster.

- Topical agents have a shorter duration.

- Vasoconstriction and CNS stimulation are uncommon with topical agents, but are a concern with oral agents.

- Oral agents do not lead to rebound congestion.

Δ   Advise the client to use topical decongestions for 3 to 5 days to avoid rebound congestion.

Δ   Instruct the client not to exceed recommended doses.

Nursing Evaluation of Medication Effectiveness

Δ   Improvement of symptoms (e.g., relief of congestion, ↑ ease of breathing, ability to sleep comfortably)

Primary Reference:

Lehne, R. A. (2007). *Pharmacology for nursing care* (6th ed.). St. Louis, MO: Saunders.

Additional Resources:

Ignatavicius, D. D. (2006). *Medical-Surgical Nursing* (5th ed.). St. Louis, MO: Saunders.

Wilson, B. A., Shannon, M., Shields, K., Stang, C. (2007). *Nurse's drug guide*. Upper Saddle River, NJ: Prentice Hall.

Unit 8 Medications Affecting the Respiratory System

Application Exercises

1. A nurse is providing teaching to a client with asthma about how to use cromolyn (Intal). Which of the following should the nurse include in her teaching? (Select all that apply.)

_____ Take the medication 15 min before exercising.

_____ Follow a fixed-dosage schedule for long-term control of asthma.

_____ Expect to lose weight while taking this medication.

_____ Observe for adverse effects such as tremors, restlessness, and palpitations.

_____ Do not crush or chew tablets.

2. What information should the nurse provide to a client who is starting beclomethasone dipropionate (QVAR) for long-term management of asthma?

3. Which of the following instructions should be given to a client who has been prescribed albuterol (Proventil) and beclomethasone dipropionate (QVAR) inhalers for the control of asthma?

   A. Alternate which inhaler is used so that both are not taken the same time of day.

   B. Use the albuterol inhaler 5 min before using the beclomethasone inhaler.

   C. Only use beclomethasone if experiencing an acute attack.

   D. Use the albuterol inhaler first and immediately follow with the beclomethasone inhaler.

4. Albuterol (Proventil) is used in the treatment of asthma to

   A. decrease inflammation.

   B. promote bronchodilation.

   C. decrease airway mucus production.

   D. suppress the effects of leukotriene compounds.

5. Which of the following statements made by the client indicates that she has understood discharge teaching in the proper use of salmeterol (Serevent)?

   A. "I will use this medication every 6 hours."

   B. "I will take a dose of this medicine when I notice I am wheezing."

   C. "I will take this medication regularly every 12 hours."

   D. "I will use this medication when I am having an asthma attack."

6. A client starting oral prednisone for treatment of chronic asthma should report signs of

    A. weight gain and fluid retention.
    B. nervousness and insomnia.
    C. chest pain and tachycardia.
    D. drowsiness and activity intolerance.

7. Identify the two major classes of medications that are used to treat asthma.

8. A client taking triamcinolone acetonide (Azmacort) is instructed to use a spacer. What is the rationale for using a spacer with an MDI?

9. Match the following pharmacologic agents with the type of action they have.

    Theophylline   A. Advise the client to take this short-acting beta$_2$-agonist to abort
                             an acute asthma attack.
    Albuterol   B. Advise the client to take this medication once daily at bedtime.
    Salmeterol   C. Client should avoid caffeine when using this oral medication.
    Montelukast   D. Client can take this inhaled beta$_2$-agonist every 12 hr.

Unit 8 Medications Affecting the Respiratory System

Application Exercises Answer Key

1. A nurse is providing teaching to a client with asthma about how to use cromolyn (Intal). Which of the following should the nurse include in her teaching? (Select all that apply.)

    __X__   **Take the medication 15 min before exercising.**

    __X__   **Follow a fixed-dosage schedule for long-term control of asthma.**

    _____   Expect to lose weight while taking this medication.

    _____   Observe for adverse effects such as tremors, restlessness, and palpitations.

    _____   Do not crush or chew tablets.

Cromolyn can be used to abort an asthma attack. For long-term control, cromolyn should be taken on a fixed-dose schedule. Cromolyn does not promote weight loss, has no significant side effects, and is only given by inhalation.

2. What information should the nurse provide to a client who is starting beclomethasone dipropionate (QVAR) for long-term management of asthma?

Inhaled glucocorticoids are generally safe. Use a spacer during administration by MDI. Rinse mouth and gargle after inhaling the dose (prevents oropharyngeal candidiasis). Engage in weight-bearing exercises and ensure adequate intake of calcium and vitamin D (inhaled glucocorticoids promote bone loss).

3. Which of the following instructions should be given to a client who has been prescribed albuterol (Proventil) and beclomethasone dipropionate (QVAR) inhalers for the control of asthma?

A. Alternate which inhaler is used so that both are not taken the same time of day.

B. Use the albuterol inhaler 5 min before using the beclomethasone inhaler.

C. Only use beclomethasone if experiencing an acute attack.

D. Use the albuterol inhaler first and immediately follow with the beclomethasone inhaler.

When a client is prescribed an inhaled beta$_2$-agonist, such as albuterol, and an inhaled glucocorticoid, such as beclomethasone, the beta$_2$-agonist should be administered first. The beta$_2$-agonist promotes bronchodilation and enhances absorption of the glucocorticoid.

4. Albuterol (Proventil) is used in the treatment of asthma to

    A. decrease inflammation.

    B. promote bronchodilation.

    C. decrease airway mucus production.

    D. suppress the effects of leukotriene compounds.

Beta$_2$ adrenergic agonists promote bronchodilation; glucocorticoids and cromolyn decrease inflammation; montelukast (Singular), a leukotriene modifier decreases airway mucus production and suppresses the effects of leukotriene compounds.

5. Which of the following statements made by the client indicates that she has understood discharge teaching in the proper use of salmeterol (Serevent)?

    A. "I will use this medication every 6 hours."

    B. "I will take a dose of this medicine when I notice I am wheezing."

    C. "I will take this medication regularly every 12 hours."

    D. "I will use this medication when I am having an asthma attack."

Formoterol (Foradil Aerolizer) and salmeterol (Serevent) are both long-acting beta$_2$ agonist inhalers. These inhalers are used every 12 hr for long-term control and are NOT to be used to abort an asthma attack. A short-acting beta$_2$-agonist should be used if a client needs to treat an acute attack.

6. A client starting oral prednisone for treatment of chronic asthma should report signs of

    A. weight gain and fluid retention.

    B. nervousness and insomnia.

    C. chest pain and tachycardia.

    D. drowsiness and activity intolerance.

Weight gain and fluid retention can result from oral glucocorticoid use. Nervousness, insomnia, chest pain, tachycardia, drowsiness, and activity intolerance are not side effects of oral glucocorticoids.

7. Identify the two major classes of medications that are used to treat asthma.

Bronchodilators and anti-inflammatory medications.

8. A client taking triamcinolone acetonide (Azmacort) is instructed to use a spacer. What is the rationale for using a spacer with an MDI?

A spacer is used with an MDI to decrease the amount of the medication that will reach the mouth and throat, and ↑ the amount of medication that will reach its site of action (lung mucosa).

9. Match the following pharmacologic agents with the type of action they have.

Theophylline	A. Advise the client to take this short-acting beta$_2$-agonist to abort an acute asthma attack.
Albuterol	B. Advise the client to take this medication once daily at bedtime.
Salmeterol	C. Client should avoid caffeine when using this oral medication.
Montelukast	D. Client can take this inhaled beta$_2$-agonist every 12 hr.

Theophylline (C); albuterol (A); salmeterol (D); montelukast (B)

Unit 9	Medications Affecting Fluid, Electrolytes, Minerals, and/or the Renal System
	Contributor: Leona K. Pié, MPH, BSN, RN

 NCLEX® Connections:

Learning Objective: Review and apply knowledge within **"Medications Affecting Fluid, Electrolytes, Minerals, and/or the Renal System"** in readiness for performance of the following nursing activities as outlined by the NCLEX® test plans:

Δ   Assess/monitor the client for expected effects of medications.

Δ   Assess/monitor the client for side/adverse effects of medications.

Δ   Assess/monitor the client for actual/potential specific food and medication interactions.

Δ   Identify contraindications, actual/potential incompatibilities, and interactions between medications, and intervene appropriately.

Δ   Identify symptoms/evidence of an allergic reaction, and respond appropriately.

Δ   Evaluate/monitor and document the therapeutic and adverse/side effects of medications.

Δ   Provide/reinforce client teaching on actions, therapeutic effects, potential side/ adverse effects, and interactions of medications.

 General Key Points

Δ   **Homeostatic mechanisms** within the body maintain fluid and electrolyte balance.

Δ   **Homeostasis** requires maintenance of fluid volume and composition within a narrow range.

Δ   **Diuretics** are medications used to ↑ fluid loss via urine output.

Δ   Major uses of diuretics include prevention of renal failure and management of hypertension.

Δ   Diuretics are used to ↓ excess fluid seen with heart failure, cirrhosis, and renal disease.

Δ   Most diuretics work by blocking the reabsorption of sodium and chloride. The greater the amount of sodium and chloride reabsorption blocked, the greater the amount of fluid elimination.

Δ   **Diuretics** have the potential for causing hypovolemia and electrolyte/acid-base imbalances.

Δ   **Potassium** (K+) is necessary for nerve impulse conduction and regulation of acid-base balance.

Δ   **Calcium** (Ca++) is critical to normal metabolic processes of the heart, nerves, muscles, and bones. Calcium is also critical for blood coagulation.

Δ   Renal function should be monitored when administering medications that affect fluid and electrolyte balance.

Δ   It is important to carefully monitor serum levels of electrolytes to assess for the therapeutic and possible adverse effects of medications.

Δ   **Mineral supplements** tend to cause GI distress and should be administered with a full glass of water or with meals

Key Points

Medication Classification: High Ceiling Loop Diuretics

Select Prototype Medication:	**furosemide (Lasix)**
Other Medications:	ethacrynic acid (Edecrin), bumetanide (Bumex), torsemide (Demadex)

Expected Pharmacological Action

Δ   High ceiling loop diuretics work in the ascending limb of loop of Henle to:

- Block the reabsorption of sodium and chloride, and to prevent the reabsorption of water.

- Cause extensive diuresis.

Therapeutic Uses

Δ   High ceiling loop diuretics are used to treat:

- Pulmonary edema caused by heart failure

- High ceiling loop diuretics are reserved for conditions not responsive to other diuretics (e.g., edema caused by liver, cardiac, or kidney disease; hypertension).

- Works well for clients with renal impairment

- May be used to treat hypercalcemia related to kidney stone formation

Side/Adverse Effects: Nursing Interventions and Client Education

Side/Adverse Effects	Nursing Interventions/Client Education
Dehydration	• Assess/monitor the client for signs of dehydration: dry mouth, ↑ thirst, and I&O. • Report urine output < 30 mL/hr. Lasix should be stopped, and the primary care provider should be notified. • If signs of headache and/or chest, calf, or pelvic pain occur, notify the primary care provider. • Minimize the risk for dehydration by starting the client on low doses and monitoring daily weights.

Side/Adverse Effects	Nursing Interventions/Client Education
Hypotension	• Monitor the client's blood pressure. • Teach the client to get out of bed slowly.
Ototoxicity – transient with furosemide and irreversible with ethacrynic acid	• Avoid use with other ototoxic medications, such as gentamicin.
Hypokalemia (K+ < 3.0 mEq/L), potassium-wasting	• Monitor the client's cardiac status and potassium levels. • Report a ↓ in potassium level, K+ < 3.0 mEq/L. • Teach the client to consume high potassium foods (e.g., bananas, potatoes). • Teach the client signs of hypokalemia (e.g., nausea/vomiting, general weakness).
Other adverse effects – hyperglycemia, hyperuricemia, and ↓ in calcium and magnesium levels	• Monitor the client's blood glucose, uric acid, and calcium and magnesium levels. • Report elevated levels.

Contraindications/Precautions

Δ   Pregnancy Risk Category C

Δ   Avoid using these medications during pregnancy unless absolutely required.

Δ   Use cautiously in clients who have diabetes and/or gout.

Medication/Food Interactions: Nursing Interventions and Client Education

Medication/Food Interactions	Nursing Interventions/Client Education
Digoxin toxicity can occur in the presence of hypokalemia	• Monitor the client's cardiac status and potassium and digoxin levels. • Potassium-sparing diuretics are often used in conjunction with loop diuretics to reduce the risk of hypokalemia.
Antihypertensives – concurrent use can have additive hypotensive effect	• Monitor the client's blood pressure.
Lithium levels can rise due to diuresis.	• Monitor the client's lithium levels.
NSAIDs blunt diuretic effect	• Watch for a ↓ in effectiveness of diuretic, such as a ↓ in urine output.

Therapeutic Nursing Interventions and Client Education

Δ   Obtain the client's baseline data to include orthostatic blood pressure, weight, electrolytes, and location and extent of edema.

Δ   Weigh the client at the same time each day; usually upon awakening.

Δ   Monitor the client's blood pressure and I&0.

Δ   Avoid administering the medication late in the day to prevent nocturia. Usual dosing time is 0800 and 1400.

Δ   Lasix can be administered orally or as an IVP or IV infusion. Infuse IV doses slowly (20 mg/min) to avoid abrupt hypotension and hypovolemia.

Δ   If potassium level drops below 3.5 mEq/L, the client should be placed on a potassium supplement.

Δ   If the medication is used for hypertension, teach the client to self-monitor blood pressure and weight by keeping a log.

Δ   Advise the client to get up slowly to minimize postural hypotension. If faintness or dizziness occurs, instruct the client to sit or lie down.

Δ   Teach the client to report significant weight loss, lightheadedness, dizziness, GI distress, and/or general weakness to the primary care provider.

Δ   Encourage the client to consume foods high in potassium (e.g., avocados, strawberries).

Δ   Instruct clients with diabetes to monitor for elevated blood glucose levels.

Δ   Instruct the client to observe for signs of low magnesium levels (e.g., muscle twitching and tremors).

Nursing Evaluation of Medication Effectiveness

Δ   Depending on therapeutic intent, effectiveness may be evidenced by:

- ↓ in pulmonary or peripheral edema.

- Weight loss.

- ↓ in blood pressure.

- ↑ in urine output.

Key Points

Medication Classification: Thiazide Diuretics

Select Prototype Medication: **hydrochlorothiazide (HydroDIURIL)**

Other Medications: chlorothiazide (Diuril)

Expected Pharmacological Action

Δ   Thiazide diuretics work in the early distal convoluted tubule to:

- Block the reabsorption of sodium and chloride, and prevent the reabsorption of water at this site.

- Promote diuresis when renal function is not impaired.

Therapeutic Uses

Δ   Thiazide diuretics are often the medication of first choice for essential hypertension.

Δ   These medications may be used for edema of mild to-moderate heart failure, and liver and kidney disease.

Side/Adverse Effects: Nursing Interventions and Client Education

Side/Adverse Effects	Nursing Interventions/Client Education
Dehydration	• Assess/monitor the client for signs of dehydration.
Hypokalemia (K+ < 3.0 mEq/L)	• Monitor the client's cardiac status and K+ levels. • Report a ↓ in K+ level (< 3.0 mEq/L). • Teach the client to consume foods high in potassium, such as spinach and tomatoes. • Teach the client signs and symptoms of hypokalemia (e.g., nausea/vomiting, general weakness).
Hyperglycemia	• Monitor the client for an ↑ in blood glucose levels.

Contraindications/Precautions

Δ   Avoid use during pregnancy (Pregnancy Risk Category B) and lactation. If a thiazide diuretic is indicated, advise the client not to breastfeed.

Δ   Use cautiously with clients who have ↓ renal function; may not be effective.

Medication/Food Interactions: Nursing Interventions and Client Education

Medication/Food Interactions	Nursing Interventions/Client Education
Digoxin toxicity in the presence of hypokalemia	• Monitor the client's cardiac status and potassium and digoxin levels. • A potassium-sparing diuretic is used in conjunction with thiazide diuretics to reduce the risk of hypokalemia.
Antihypertensives – additive hypotensive effects	• Monitor the client's blood pressure.
Others – **lithium** levels may rise; NSAIDs blunt diuretic effect	• Monitor the client's lithium levels and observe for ↓ effectiveness of diuretic, such as ↓ urine output.

Therapeutic Nursing Interventions and Client Education

Δ   Obtain the client's baseline data to include orthostatic blood pressure, weight, electrolytes, and location and extent of edema.

Δ   There is no risk of ototoxicity when these medications are used with ototoxic medications.

Δ   Monitor the client's potassium levels.

Δ   Instruct the client to take the medication first thing in the morning; if twice-a-day dosing is prescribed, be sure the second dose is taken by 1400 to prevent nocturia.

Δ   Encourage the client to consume foods high in potassium and maintain adequate fluid intake (1,500 mL per day, unless contraindicated).

Δ   If GI upset occurs, the client should take the medication with or after meals.

Δ   Alternate day dosing can ↓ electrolyte imbalances.

Nursing Evaluation of Medication Effectiveness

Δ   Depending on therapeutic intent, effectiveness may be evidenced by:

•   ↓ in blood pressure.

•   ↓ in edema.

•   ↑ in urine output.

Key Points

Medication Classification: Potassium-Sparing Diuretics

| Select Prototype Medication: | **spironolactone (Aldactone)** |
| Other Medications: | triamterene (Dyrenium), amiloride (Midamor) |

Expected Pharmacological Action

Δ   Potassium-sparing diuretics block the action of aldosterone (sodium and water retention), which results in potassium retention and the secretion of sodium and water.

Therapeutic Uses

Δ   Potassium-sparing diuretics are combined with other diuretics for potassium-sparing effects.

Δ   Potassium-sparing diuretics are used for heart failure.

Δ   In primary hyperaldosteronism, potassium-sparing diuretics block actions of aldosterone.

Side/Adverse Effects: Nursing Interventions and Client Education

Side/Adverse Effects	Nursing Interventions/Client Education
Hyperkalemia (K+ > 5.0 mEq/L)	• Initiate cardiac monitoring for serum potassium > 5 mEq/L. • Treat hyperkalemia with the discontinuation of medication, restriction of potassium in diet, and injection of insulin to drive potassium back into the cell.
Endocrine effects (impotence in male clients; irregularities of menstrual cycle in female clients)	• Advise clients to observe for side effects. • Clients should notify the primary care provider if these responses occur.

Contraindications/Precautions

Δ   Do not administer to clients with hyperkalemia, K+ > 5.0 mEq/L.

Medication/Food Interactions: Nursing Interventions and Client Education

Medication/Food Interactions	Nursing Interventions/Client Education
ACE inhibitors, such as **lisinopril (Zestril)** – concurrent use ↑ the risk of hyperkalemia	• Monitor the client's K+ levels. Notify provider if K+ > 5.0 mEq/L.
Potassium supplements, such as **potassium chloride (K-Dur)** – concurrent use ↑ the risk of hyperkalemia	• The client should not take this medication and a potassium supplement concurrently.

Therapeutic Nursing Interventions and Client Education

Δ   Obtain the client's baseline data.

Δ   Monitor the client's potassium levels regularly.

Δ   Can only be given orally.

Δ   Teach clients to avoid potassium containing salt substitutes.

Δ   Teach the client to self-monitor blood pressure.

Δ   Instruct the client to keep a log of blood pressure and weight.

Δ   Warn the client that triamterene (Dyrenium) may turn urine a bluish color.

Nursing Evaluation of Medication Effectiveness

Δ   Depending on therapeutic intent, effectiveness may be evidenced by:

•   Maintenance of normal potassium levels: 3.5 and 5.0 mEq/L.

•   Weight loss.

•   ↓ in blood pressure and edema.

Key Points

Medication Classification: Osmotic Diuretics

Select Prototype Medication: **mannitol (Osmitrol)**

Other Medications: urea (Ureaphil), glycerin (Osmoglyn), isosorbide (Ismotic)

Expected Pharmacological Action

Δ   Osmotic diuretics create diuresis by increasing blood osmolality which attracts fluid from other compartments (e.g., third spacing, cerebral fluid, intraocular).

Therapeutic Uses

Δ   Osmotic diuretics prevent renal failure in specific situations (e.g., hypovolemic shock, severe hypotension).

Δ   These medications ↓ intracranial pressure (ICP) caused by cerebral edema.

Δ   These medications ↓ intraocular pressure (IOP).

Δ   Osmotic diuretics promote sodium retention and water excretion in clients with hyponatremia and fluid volume excess.

Side/Adverse Effects: Nursing Interventions and Client Education

Side/Adverse Effects	Nursing Interventions/Client Education
Heart failure, pulmonary edema	• If signs of heart failure (dyspnea, weakness, fatigue, distended neck veins, and/or weight gain), stop the medication immediately and instruct the client to notify the primary care provider.
Renal failure	• If signs of renal failure develop (urine output < 30 mL/hr, ↑ serum creatinine [> 1.2 mg/dL] and BUN [> 20 mg/dL]), stop the medication immediately and instruct the client to notify the primary care provider.
Fluid and electrolyte imbalances	• Monitor the client's laboratory values.

Contraindications/Precautions

Δ   Use extreme caution in clients with cardiac failure.

Δ   Lasix contributes to therapeutic effect by promoting renal excretion of fluid drawn into vasculature by osmotic diuretics.

Therapeutic Nursing Interventions and Client Education

Δ   Osmotic diuretics are most effective if given as a bolus instead of continuous infusion.

Δ   To prevent administering microscopic crystals, mannitol should be administered with a filter in the IV tubing, or use a filter needle when drawing from the vial.

Δ   Obtain the client's baseline data and continue to monitor for signs of dehydration, strict I&O, acute renal failure, and edema.

Δ   Monitor the client's serum osmolarity and electrolytes every 6 hr; urine osmolarity should be checked daily.

Δ   Use of Lasix may help prevent rebound fluid retention: contributes to therapeutic effect.

Nursing Evaluation of Medication Effectiveness

Δ   Depending on therapeutic intent, effectiveness may be evidenced by:

•   Normal renal function as demonstrated by urine output of at least 30 mL/hr, serum creatinine between 0.6 to 1.2 mg/dL for men and 0.5 to 1.1 mg/dL for women, and BUN levels between 10 to 20 mg/dL.

•   ↓ in intracranial pressure.

•   ↓ in intraocular pressure.

Key Points

Medication Classification: Phosphate Binders

Select Prototype Medication: **aluminum hydroxide gel (Amphojel)**

Other Medications: aluminum carbonate gel (Basaljel), sevelamer
                                          hydrochloride (Renagel), calcium carbonate
                                          (Tums, OsCal)

Expected Pharmacological Action

Δ   Phosphate binders bind intestinal phosphate that is eliminated in feces.

Therapeutic Uses

Δ   Phosphate binders are used in clients with end-stage kidney disease to reduce
     serum phosphorus level (hyperphosphatemia – phosphate > 4.5 mg/dL).

Δ   Phosphate binders are used as an antacid.

Side/Adverse Effects: Nursing Interventions and Client Education

Δ   These medications commonly cause constipation.

Δ   Hypophosphatemia

Contraindications/Precautions

Δ   Contraindicated in clients with hypophosphatemia, bowel obstruction, and
     women who are pregnant or breastfeeding

Δ   Use cautiously in clients who have GI motility disorders, post GI surgery, or
     vitamin deficiencies.

Medication/Food Interactions: Nursing Interventions and Client Education

Δ   These medications interfere with the absorption of many medications. Do not
     administer other medications concurrently with Amphojel. Separate by at least 1 hr.

Therapeutic Nursing Interventions and Client Education

Δ   Administer the medications with the first bite of food to bind with phosphorous contained in consumed foods.

Δ   Recommend an ↑ in dietary fiber and fluids to prevent constipation.

Δ   Advise clients to avoid foods high in phosphorous (e.g., dairy products, tuna fish, pork).

Nursing Evaluation of Medication Effectiveness

Δ   ↓ in scrum phosphorus level to within normal range: 3.0 to 4.5 mg/dL

Key Points

Medication Classification: Kayexalate

Select Prototype Medication: **sodium polystyrene sulfonate (Kayexalate)**

Other Medications: None

Expected Pharmacological Action

Δ   Kayexalate promotes potassium excretion and sodium absorption, primarily in the large intestine.

Therapeutic Uses

Δ   This medication is used to treat hyperkalemia, potassium > 5.0 mEq/L

Side/Adverse Effects: Nursing Interventions and Client Education

Side/Adverse Effects	Nursing Interventions/Client Education
Electrolyte imbalances (e.g., sodium retention, hypocalcemia, hypomagnesia, hypokalemia)	• Observe for signs of ↓ or ↑ in electrolytes. For example, hypokalemia may be manifested as a weak, thready pulse, orthostatic hypotension, and general muscle weakness. • Notify the primary provider if the client exhibits signs of electrolyte imbalance.

Contraindications/Precautions

Δ   Use cautiously in clients who are intolerant of small amounts of sodium (e.g., clients with heart failure, edema, hypertension).

Medication/Food Interactions: Nursing Interventions and Client Education

Δ   Calcium or magnesium containing antacids or laxatives may ↓ efficacy.

Δ   Clients receiving digoxin and potassium-sparing diuretics should undergo frequent potassium monitoring.

Therapeutic Nursing Interventions and Client Education

Δ   Kayexalate can be given orally or rectally.

Δ   Mix with juice when given orally.

Δ   Use warm solution for enema.

Δ   Instruct the client to retain Kayexalate solution for 30 to 60 min after administration of enema.

Δ   Irrigate the colon with non-sodium containing fluid after Kayexalate solution is expelled.

Nursing Evaluation of Medication Effectiveness

Δ   Serum potassium within normal range: 3.5 to 5.0 mEq/L

Key Points

Medication Classification: Potassium Supplements

Select Prototype Medication: **potassium chloride (K-Dur)**

Other Medications: potassium gluconate, potassium phosphate, potassium bicarbonate

Expected Pharmacological Action

Δ   Potassium is essential for conducting nerve impulses, maintaining electrical excitability of muscle, and regulation of acid/base balance.

Therapeutic Uses

Δ   Potassium supplements are used to treat hypokalemia; potassium < 3.5 mEq/L

Δ   Potassium supplements are used:

- For clients receiving potassium-sparing diuretics.

- For clients with potassium loss due to excessive or prolonged vomiting, diarrhea, abuse of laxatives, intestinal drainage, and GI fistulas.

Side/Adverse Effects: Nursing Interventions and Client Education

Side/Adverse Effects	Nursing Interventions/Client Education
GI distress – nausea, vomiting, diarrhea, and abdominal discomfort with oral administration	• Instruct the client to take the medication with meals or a full glass of water to minimize GI discomfort and prevent ulceration.
Local GI ulceration, such as esophagitis	• Instruct the client to take the medication with meals or a full glass of water to minimize GI discomfort and prevent ulceration. • Teach the client not to dissolve the tablet in the mouth because oral ulceration will develop.
Hyperkalemia, potassium > 5.0 mEq/L	• Hyperkalemia rarely occurs with oral administration • Monitor the client receiving IV potassium for signs of hyperkalemia (e.g., bradycardia, hypotension, ECG changes).

Contraindications/Precautions

Δ   Severe renal disease

Δ   Hypoaldosteronism: can place the client at risk for hyperkalemia

Medication/Food Interactions: Nursing Interventions and Client Education

Medication/Food Interactions	Nursing Interventions/Client Education
Potassium-sparing diuretics, such as **spironolactone,** or **ACE inhibitors**, such as lisinopril – concurrent use ↑ the risk of hyperkalemia	• Monitor the client's potassium levels. • Notify the primary care provider if potassium level is > 5.0 mEq/L.

Therapeutic Nursing Interventions and Client Education

Δ   Oral formulations

  • Mix powdered formulations in at least 4 oz of liquid.

  • Instruct the client not to crush extended-release tablets.

  • Instruct the client to notify the primary care provider if the client has difficulty swallowing the pills. Medication may be supplied as a powder or sustained-release tablet that is easier to tolerate.

Δ   IV administration

  • **Never give IV push**. Rapid IV infusion can result in fatal hyperkalemia.

  • Use an IV pump to control infusion rate.

  • Dilute potassium and give no more than **40 mEq/L** of IV solution to prevent vein irritation.

  • Give **no faster than 10 mEq/hr**.

  • Cardiac monitoring is indicated for serum potassium levels outside of normal parameters.

  • Assess the IV site for local irritation, phlebitis, and infiltration. Discontinue IV immediately if infiltration occurs.

  • Monitor the client's I&O to ensure an adequate urine output of at least 30 mL/hr.

Nursing Evaluation of Medication Effectiveness

Δ   Serum potassium level within normal range: 3.5 to 5.0 mEq/L

Key Points

Medication Classification: Magnesium Sulfate

Select Prototype Medication: **magnesium sulfate**

Other Medications: Magnesium gluconate, magnesium hydroxide

Expected Pharmacological Action

Δ   Magnesium activates many intracellular enzymes and plays a role in regulating skeletal muscle contractility and blood coagulation.

Therapeutic Uses

Δ   Magnesium supplements are used for clients with hypomagnesemia: magnesium level < 1.3 mEq/L.

Δ   Oral preparations are used to prevent low magnesium levels.

Δ   Parenteral magnesium is used for clients with severe hypomagnesemia.

Side/Adverse Effects: Nursing Interventions and Client Education

Side/Adverse Effects	Nursing Interventions/Client Education
Neuromuscular blockade and respiratory depression	• IV administration requires careful monitoring of the client's cardiac and neuromuscular status. • Monitor the client's serum magnesium levels.
Diarrhea	• Monitor the client's serum magnesium levels due to magnesium loss from diarrhea. • Monitor the client's I&O and observe for signs of dehydration.

Contraindications/Precautions

Δ   Use cautiously with clients with AV block, rectal bleeding, nausea/vomiting, and abdominal pain

Δ   Use cautiously with pregnant clients (Pregnancy Risk Category B).

Δ   Use cautiously with clients with renal and/or cardiac disease.

Medications/Food Interactions: Nursing Interventions and Client Education

Δ   Magnesium sulfate may ↓ the absorption of tetracyclines.

Δ   Monitor the therapeutic effect to determine if absorption has been affected.

Therapeutic Nursing Interventions and Client Education

Δ   Monitor serum magnesium, calcium, and phosphorus.

Δ   Monitor the client's blood pressure, heart rate, and respiratory rate when given intravenously.

Δ   Assess the client for depressed or absent deep tendon reflexes as a sign of toxicity.

Δ   Calcium gluconate is given for magnesium sulfate toxicity. Always have an injectable form of calcium gluconate available when administering magnesium sulfate by IV.

Δ   Teach the client about dietary sources of magnesium (e.g., whole grain cereals, nuts, legumes, green leafy vegetables, bananas).

Nursing Evaluation of Medication Effectiveness

Δ   Serum magnesium levels within normal limits: 1.3 to 2.1 mEq/L

Key Points

Medication Classification: Sodium Bicarbonate

Select Prototype Medication:	**sodium bicarbonate**
Other Medications:	None

Expected Pharmacological Action

Δ   Sodium bicarbonate is a systemic alkalinizer that is used to correct metabolic acidosis, pH < 7.45.

Therapeutic Uses

Δ   This medication is used in clients with acidosis due to diabetes mellitus, cardiac arrest, and/or vascular collapse.

Δ   Administer sodium bicarbonate orally as an antacid.

Δ   An additional use of sodium bicarbonate is to raise the urinary pH to enhance renal excretion in salicylate overdose.

Side/Adverse Effects: Nursing Interventions and Client Education

Side/Adverse Effects	Nursing Interventions/Client Education
Can cause sodium overload; sodium > 145 mEq/L	• Monitor clients with heart failure and/or hypertension for elevated blood pressure, exertional dyspnea, and activity intolerance.
Renal calculi or crystals	• Be sure the client maintains adequate fluid intake, which is at least 1,500 mL per day if not restricted.
Alkalosis; pH < 7.35	• Monitor the client for signs of alkalosis (e.g., tachycardia, irritability, and muscle twitching). • Notify the primary care provider if signs of alkalosis occur.

Contraindications/Precautions

Δ   Sodium bicarbonate is unsuitable as an antacid in peptic ulcer disease because it is short-acting, high in sodium, and can cause metabolic alkalosis

Δ   Use cautiously, or not at all in clients who have hypertension, heart failure, and/or kidney disease.

Medication/Food Interactions: Nursing Interventions and Client Education

Medication/Food Interactions	Nursing Interventions/Client Education
Corticosteroids – concurrent use can ↓ potassium levels and ↑ sodium levels	• Monitor the client's electrolyte levels. • Normal potassium range should be 3.5 to 5.0 mEq/L; normal sodium range should be 135 to 145 mEq/L.
Pseudoephedrine and quinidine – concurrent use can ↑ the effects of these medications	• Monitor the client for ↑ effects and possible side effects of these medications. • Side effects of pseudoephedrine include tachycardia, nervousness, and sleeplessness. • Side effects of quinidine include hypotension and bradycardia.
Lithium, salicylates, and benzodiazepines – concurrent use can ↓ the effects of these medications	• Monitor the client for therapeutic effects.
Numerous IV incompatibilities	• Consult with a pharmacist or other resource for IV incompatibilities.

Therapeutic Nursing Interventions and Client Education

Δ   Monitor/assess the client's fluid balance and obtain the client's baseline weight.

Δ   Obtain the client's baseline electrolyte values and blood chemistries, and monitor as indicated.

Δ   Assess the client's arterial blood gas values to confirm acidosis. Continue to monitor frequently during emergency situations.

Nursing Evaluation of Medication Effectiveness

Δ   Blood pH within normal range: 7.35 to 7.45

Δ   Absence of signs and symptoms of acidosis

Key Points

Medication Classification: Calcium Supplements

      Select Prototype Medication: **calcium citrate (Citracal)**

      Other Medications: calcium carbonate, calcium acetate

Expected Pharmacological Action

    Δ   Normal musculoskeletal, neurological, and cardiovascular function is dependent on calcium.

Therapeutic Uses

    Δ   Calcium supplements are used for clients with hypocalcemia, or deficiencies of parathyroid hormone, vitamin D, or dietary calcium.

    Δ   These medications are used in clients as a dietary supplement.

    Δ   Clients most likely to need calcium supplements include adolescents, older adults, and women who are postmenopausal, pregnant or breastfeeding.

Side/Adverse Effects: Nursing Interventions and Client Education

Side/Adverse Effects	Nursing Interventions/Client Education
Hypercalcemia – > 10.5 mg/dL	• Assess the client for signs of hypercalcemia (e.g., tachycardia, elevated blood pressure, muscle weakness, constipation, lethargy). • Monitor the client's serum calcium levels. Normal calcium range should be 9.0 to 10.5 mg/dL.

Contraindications/Precautions

    Δ   Calcium supplements are contraindicated in clients who have hypercalcemia, bone tumors, and hyperparathyroidism.

    Δ   Use cautiously in clients who are pregnant or lactating, and clients with a ↓ in GI function, kidney disease, or dehydration.

Medication/Food Interactions: Nursing Interventions and Client Education

Medication/Food Interactions	Nursing Interventions/Client Education
Glucocorticoids – absorption of calcium is reduced when taken currently with glucocorticoids	• Give medications at least 1 hr apart.
Tetracyclines and thyroid hormone – ↓ in absorption of these medications occurs when taken with calcium	• Give medications at least 1 hr apart.
Thiazide diuretics – hypercalcemia risk is ↑ when given with thiazide diuretics	• Assess the client for signs of hypercalcemia (e.g., tachycardia, elevated blood pressure, muscle weakness, constipation, lethargy).
Spinach, rhubarb, bran, and whole grains are foods that may ↓ calcium absorption.	• Do not administer calcium with foods that ↓ absorption. • Instruct the client to avoid consuming these foods at the same time as taking calcium.
Phosphates, carbonates, sulfates, and tartrates – IV calcium precipitates with these compounds	• Do not mix parenteral calcium with compounds that cause precipitation.
Digoxin and parenteral **calcium** can lead to severe bradycardia.	• IV injection of calcium must be given slowly with careful monitoring of client status.

Therapeutic Nursing Interventions and Client Education

Δ   Instruct the client to take a calcium supplement at least 1 hr apart from glucocorticoids, tetracyclines, and/or thyroid hormone.

Δ   More consistent bioavailability is obtained with chewable tablets.

Δ   Prior to administration, warm IV infusions of calcium to body temperature.

Δ   Administer IV injections at 0.5 to 2 mL/min.

Nursing Evaluation of Medication Effectiveness

Δ   Serum calcium level normal range: 9.0 to 10.5 mg/dL

Key Points

Medication Classification: Selective Estrogen Receptor Modulators/SERMs

Select Prototype Medication: **raloxifene (Evista)**

Other Medications   tamoxifen citrate (Nolvadex)

Expected Pharmacological Action

Δ   SERMs

- work as endogenous estrogen in bone, lipid metabolism, and blood coagulation.

- ↓ osteoblast activity, which thereby ↓ bone resorption. This results in slowing down of bone loss. In this way, bone mineral density is preserved.

- work as an antagonist to estrogen on breast and endometrial tissue.

- can ↓ plasma levels of cholesterol.

Therapeutic Uses

Δ   SERMS are used:

- In female clients to prevent and treat postmenopausal osteoporosis and to prevent spinal fractures.

- As protection against breast cancer.

Side/Adverse Effects: Nursing Interventions and Client Education

Side/Adverse Effects	Nursing Interventions/Client Education
↑ the risk for pulmonary embolism and deep vein thrombosis (DVT)	• Medication should be stopped prior to scheduled immobilization such as surgery. Medication can be resumed when the client is fully mobile. • Discourage long periods of sitting and inactivity.
Hot flashes	• Inform the client that hot flashes will not be reduced by medication use; instead, hot flashes may occur.

Contraindications/Precautions

Δ   SERMs should not to be used in pregnancy (Pregnancy Risk Category X).

Δ   Contraindicated in clients with a history of venous thrombosis

Medication/Food Interactions: Nursing Interventions and Client Education

Δ   No significant interactions

Therapeutic Nursing Interventions and Client Education

Δ   For maximum benefit of the medication, encourage clients to consume adequate amounts of calcium (such as dairy products) and vitamin D (such as egg yolks). Inadequate amounts of dietary calcium and vitamin D cause release of parathyroid hormone. The parathyroid hormone stimulates calcium release from the bone.

Δ   Monitor the client's serum calcium: normal range 9.0 to 10.5 mg/dL.

Δ   Medication may be taken with or without food once a day.

Nursing Evaluation of Medication Effectiveness

Δ   ↑ in bone density

Δ   No fractures

Key Points

Medication Classification: Bisphosphonates

Select Prototype Medication:	**alendronate sodium (Fosamax)**
Other Medications:	ibandronate sodium (Boniva), risedronate (Actonel)

Expected Pharmacological Action

Δ   Bisphosphonates ↓ the number and action of osteoclasts, which thereby inhibits bone resorption.

Therapeutic Uses

Δ   Use bisphosphonates:

- In women to treat and prevent postmenopausal osteoporosis.

- In male clients who have osteoporosis.

- For clients with osteoporosis produced by the use of glucocorticoid-induced osteoporosis.

- For clients who have Paget's disease of the bone and hypercalcemia of malignancy.

Side/Adverse Effects: Nursing Interventions and Client Education

Side/Adverse Effects	Nursing Interventions/Client Education
Esophagitis	• To facilitate passage through the esophagus, administer with a full glass of water and instruct the client to sit up or stand for 30 min after taking the medication.
Risk for hyperparathyroidism at higher dose – used for Paget's disease	• Monitor the client's parathyroid hormone (PTH) levels.

Contraindications/Precautions

Δ   Use cautiously with women who are lactating (Pregnancy Risk Category C).

Δ   Clients who have prior esophageal disorders, such as gastroesophageal reflux disease should not use bisphosphonates.

Medication/Food Interactions: Nursing Interventions and Client Education

Medication/Food Interactions	Nursing Interventions/Client Education
Calcium supplements, antacids, orange juice, and caffeine – alendronate sodium absorption ↓ when taken concurrently	• Advise the client to take the medication on an empty stomach with at least 8 oz of water.

Therapeutic Nursing Interventions and Client Education

Δ Instructions for the client should include:

• Taking the medication first thing in the morning after getting out of bed.

• Taking medication on an empty stomach with a full glass (8 oz) of water.

• Sitting or standing for 30 min after taking the medication.

• Not taking any other medication within 30 min of taking Fosamax.

Δ Advise the client to avoid chewing or sucking on the tablet.

Δ Medication is available in liquid form; advise the client to drink at least 2 oz, and preferable 8 oz of liquid after taking the medication.

Δ Tablets are prescribed once daily or once a week; liquid form is prescribed for once a week.

Δ If dose is skipped, advise the client to wait until the next day to take the next dose. The client should not take the skipped dose.

Δ For maximum benefit of the medication, encourage clients to consume adequate amounts of calcium (such as dairy products) and vitamin D (such as egg yolks). Inadequate amounts of dietary calcium and vitamin D cause release of parathyroid hormone. Parathyroid hormone stimulates calcium release from the bone.

Δ Monitor the client's bone density; perform a bone density scan every 12 to 18 months.

Δ Monitor the client's serum calcium. Normal range is between 9.0 to 10.5 mg/dL.

Δ Teach the client about signs of hypercalcemia (e.g., numbness, tingling, twitching).

Δ Encourage the client to perform weight-bearing exercises daily such as walking 30 to 40 min each day.

Δ Teach the client to notify the primary care provider if the client experiences difficulty swallowing, painful swallowing, and/or new or worsening heartburn.

Nursing Evaluation of Medication Effectiveness

Δ ↑ in bone density

Δ No fractures

Key Points

Medication Classification: Calcitonin-Salmon

Select Prototype Medication: **calcitonin salmon (Fortical, Miacalcin)**

Other Medications: None

Expected Pharmacological Action

Δ   Calcitonin-salmon ↓ bone resorption by inhibiting activity of osteoclasts in osteoporosis.

Δ   This medication ↑ calcium excretion by inhibiting tubular resorption of calcium for conditions that cause hypercalcemia.

Therapeutic Uses

Δ   Calcitonin-salmon is used for clients with postmenopausal osteoporosis and moderate to severe Paget's disease.

Δ   Calcitonin-salmon is used for clients with hypercalcemia due to hyperparathyroidism and cancer.

Side/Adverse Effects: Nursing Interventions and Client Education

Δ   With intranasal route, nasal dryness and irritation can occur.

Δ   With IM or SC injection, an inflammatory reaction can occur at the injection site.

Δ   Nausea may occur, but it is usually self-limiting.

Contraindications/Precautions

Δ   Hypersensitivity to the medication and fish protein: Perform an allergy skin test prior to administration.

Δ   Pregnancy Risk Category C

Δ   Use cautiously with women who are lactating, children, and clients diagnosed with kidney disease.

Medication/Food Interactions: Nursing Interventions and Client Education

Δ   May ↓ serum lithium levels: Monitor lithium levels closely.

Therapeutic Nursing Interventions and Client Education

Δ   Calcitonin-salmon is most commonly given by nasal spray. It can also be given IM or SC.

Δ   Keep container in an upright position.

Δ   Teach the client to alternate nostrils daily.

Δ   Check for Chvostek's or Trousseau's signs to monitor for hypocalcemia.

Δ   Monitor serum calcium in clients with hypercalcemia or Paget's disease.

Δ   Monitor the client's bone density scans periodically.

Δ   Encourage the client to engage in a diet high in calcium (such as dairy products) vitamin D (egg yolks) and leafy green vegetables. Inadequate amounts of dietary calcium and vitamin D cause release of parathyroid hormone. Parathyroid hormone stimulates calcium release from the bone.

Nursing Evaluation of Medication Effectiveness

Δ   ↑ in bone density

Δ   Serum calcium: normal range between 9.0 to 10.5 mg/dL

Primary Reference:

Lehne, R. A. (2007). *Pharmacology for nursing care.* (6th ed.). St. Louis, MO: Saunders.

Additional Resources:

Grodner, M., Long, S., & DeYoung, S. (2004). *Foundations and clinical applications of nutrition.* St. Louis, MO: Mosby.

Medline Plus. (2006). *Alendronate.* Retrieved July 20, 2006 from www.nlm.nih.gov/medlineplus/druginfo/medmaster/a601011.html#side-effects.

Skidmore-Roth, L. (2006). *Mosby's nursing drug reference.* St. Louis, MO: Elsevier.

Wilson, B. A., Shannon, M. T., & C. L., Stang. (2006). *Nurse's drug guide.* Upper Saddle River, NJ: Prentice Hall.

Unit 9 Medications Affecting Fluid, Electrolytes, Minerals, and/or the Renal System

Application Exercises

1. Hydrochlorothiazide has just been prescribed for a client with hypertension. Which of the following instructions should the nurse include in the client's teaching?

    A. "Your diet should include foods high in potassium."

    B. "Take the medication right before bedtime."

    C. "You may notice some swelling in your feet."

    D. "Avoid drinking liquids early in the morning."

2. Which of the following side effects should a client taking furosemide (Lasix) for hypertension be assessed for?

    A. Visual disturbances

    B. Hearing loss

    C. Tremors

    D. Restlessness

3. A client who is taking spironolactone (Aldactone) and lisinopril (Zestril) should be observed for which of the following additive effects? (Select all that apply.)

    _____   Hyperglycemia

    _____   Hyperkalemia

    _____   Hypotension

    _____   Hyponatremia

    _____   Hypercalcemia

4. A client who has a serum potassium of 3.6 mEq/L is receiving an oral potassium supplementation. The client is having difficulty swallowing the large tablet. Which of the following is the most appropriate nursing intervention?

    A. Instruct the client to allow the tablet to dissolve in the mouth.

    B. Contact the pharmacist to provide a powdered formulation that can be mixed with fluid.

    C. Contact the primary care provider to change the dose to an IV route.

    D. Notify the primary care provider that the dose will be withheld until swallowing improves.

5. A client with hyperkalemia has been prescribed Kayexalate rectally. Which of the following is an appropriate nursing intervention related to this route of administration?

        A. Refrigerate the Kayexalate prior to administration.

        B. Instruct the client to retain the enema for 10 min, then expel it.

        C. Irrigate the colon after the Kayexalate solution has been expelled.

        D. Provide for a sodium increase in the diet for 1 to 2 days after Kayexalate enema.

6. A client receiving IV magnesium sulfate is being evaluated for toxicity. Which of the following medications should the nurse anticipate administering?

        A. Calcium gluconate

        B. Potassium chloride

        C. Sodium bicarbonate

        D. Sodium polystyrene sulfonate

7. Which of the following signs of toxicity should a client be monitored for when receiving magnesium sulfate by the intravenous route?

        A. Constipation

        B. Increased respiratory rate

        C. Depressed deep tendon reflexes

        D. Peripheral edema

8. For which of the following clients is raloxifene (Evista) contraindicated? (Select all that apply.)

        _____ Menopausal woman experiencing hot flashes

        _____ Postmenopausal woman with low bone density

        _____ Woman who is pregnant

        _____ Woman who has had DVT in the past

        _____ Woman at high risk for breast cancer

9. Which of the following should be included in the teaching plan for a client who is starting alendronate sodium (Fosamax) to prevent osteoporosis? (Select all that apply.)

        _____ Take the medication with breakfast.

        _____ Do not chew or suck on the tablet.

        _____ Remain standing or sitting for 30 min after taking medication.

        _____ Notify the primary care provider if difficulty swallowing develops.

        _____ Take an extra dose if the prior dose was missed.

Unit 9 Medications Affecting Fluid, Electrolytes, Minerals, and/or the Renal System

Application Exercises Answer Key

1. Hydrochlorothiazide has just been prescribed for a client with hypertension. Which of the following instructions should the nurse include in the client's teaching?

    A. "Your diet should include foods high in potassium."
    B. "Take the medication right before bedtime."
    C. "You may notice some swelling in your feet."
    D. "Avoid drinking liquids early in the morning."

    Clients who take hydrochlorothiazide are at risk for potassium loss. Eating foods high in potassium (e.g., bananas, cantaloupe, white potatoes) can help prevent this. Diuretics should be taken early in the morning and usually no later than 1400. Clients should notice decreased swelling. Clients need adequate fluid intake to promote urine output. Fluids are best taken in the morning.

2. Which of the following side effects should a client taking furosemide (Lasix) for hypertension be assessed for?

    A. Visual disturbances
    B. Hearing loss
    C. Tremors
    D. Restlessness

    Lasix is ototoxic and may cause hearing loss. Visual disturbances, tremors, and restlessness are not side effects of Lasix.

3. A client who is taking spironolactone (Aldactone) and lisinopril (Zestril) should be observed for which of the following additive effects? (Select all that apply.)

_____ Hyperglycemia

__X__ **Hyperkalemia**

__X__ **Hypotension**

_____ Hyponatremia

_____ Hypercalcemia

Both medications have a potassium-sparing effect; both medications contribute to antihypertension effects. Hyperglycemia, hyponatremia, and hypercalcemia are not effects of either medication.

4. A client who has a serum potassium of 3.6 mEq/L is receiving an oral potassium supplementation. The client is having difficulty swallowing the large tablet. Which of the following is the most appropriate nursing intervention?

A. Instruct the client to allow the tablet to dissolve in the mouth.

B. Contact the pharmacist to provide a powdered formulation that can be mixed with fluid.

C. Contact the primary care provider to change the dose to an IV route.

D. Notify the primary care provider that the dose will be withheld until swallowing improves.

Potassium is available in powdered form, and the pharmacist can provide an equivalent dose without changing the route. Potassium should not be dissolved in the mouth because it can cause mouth ulceration, and there is more risk with IV administration. Swallowing may not improve, and the client needs the potassium supplement.

5. A client with hyperkalemia has been prescribed Kayexalate rectally. Which of the following is an appropriate nursing intervention related to this route of administration?

A. Refrigerate the Kayexalate prior to administration.

B. Instruct the client to retain the enema for 10 min, then expel it.

C. Irrigate the colon after the Kayexalate solution has been expelled.

D. Provide for a sodium increase in the diet for 1 to 2 days after Kayexalate enema.

Irrigation prevents impaction and avoids complication of resulting hypokalemia; cool fluid will cause cramping. The enema should be retained for 30 to 60 min; Kayexalate is high in sodium and clients need to be monitored for hypernatremia.

6. A client receiving IV magnesium sulfate is being evaluated for toxicity. Which of the following medications should the nurse anticipate administering?

> **A. Calcium gluconate**
>
> B. Potassium chloride
>
> C. Sodium bicarbonate
>
> D. Sodium polystyrene sulfonate

Calcium gluconate is given for magnesium sulfate toxicity. Potassium chloride is given for hypokalemia. Sodium bicarbonate is given to reverse metabolic acidosis. Sodium polystyrene sulfate (Kayexalate) is given for hyperkalemia.

7. Which of the following signs of toxicity should a client be monitored for when receiving magnesium sulfate by the intravenous route?

> A. Constipation
>
> B. Increased respiratory rate
>
> **C. Depressed deep tendon reflexes**
>
> D. Peripheral edema

Magnesium sulfate depresses the neuromuscular system and can depress deep tendon reflexes. Diarrhea and respiratory depression may be a side effect, and edema is not a side effect of magnesium sulfate toxicity.

8. For which of the following clients is raloxifene (Evista) contraindicated? (Select all that apply.)

> _____ Menopausal woman experiencing hot flashes
>
> _____ Postmenopausal woman with low bone density
>
> __X__ **Woman who is pregnant**
>
> __X__ **Woman who has had DVT in the past**
>
> _____ Woman at high risk for breast cancer

Evista causes fetal harm and can contribute to thrombotic events. Hot flashes may also occur with Evista but they are not a contraindication for use. Evista is indicated for menopausal women with hot flashes and postmenopausal women with low bone density. Evista may protect against breast cancer.

9. Which of the following should be included in the teaching plan for a client who is starting alendronate sodium (Fosamax) to prevent osteoporosis? (Select all that apply.)

_____	Take the medication with breakfast.
__X__	**Do not chew or suck on the tablet.**
__X__	**Remain standing or sitting for 30 min after taking medication.**
__X__	**Notify the primary care provider if difficulty swallowing develops.**
_____	Take an extra dose if the prior dose was missed.

Alendronate sodium should be swallowed whole, and the client should remain in an upright position for 30 min after taking it. Difficulty swallowing may be a sign of esophagitis. The medication should be taken on an empty stomach. If one dose is missed, the client should not take two doses at one time.

| Unit 10 | Medications Affecting the Digestive System and Nutrition |

Contributor: Leona K. Pié, MPH, BSN, RN

 NCLEX® Connections:

Learning Objective: Review and apply knowledge within **"Medications Affecting the Digestive System and Nutrition"** in readiness for performance of the following nursing activities as outlined by the NCLEX® test plans:

Δ   Assess/monitor the client for expected effects of medications.

Δ   Assess/monitor the client for side/adverse effects of medications.

Δ   Assess/monitor the client for actual/potential specific food and medication interactions.

Δ   Identify contraindications, actual/potential incompatibilities, and interactions between medications, and intervene appropriately.

Δ   Identify symptoms/evidence of an allergic reaction, and respond appropriately.

Δ   Evaluate/monitor and document the therapeutic and adverse/side effects of medications.

Δ   Provide/reinforce client teaching on actions, therapeutic effects, potential side/adverse effects and interactions of medications.

 General Key Points

Δ   The **GI tract** is used as a route of medication administration and as a target for pharmacological treatment of GI disorders.

Δ   **GI side effects** and adverse effects (e.g., abdominal pain, nausea/vomiting, diarrhea, constipation) are common with the administration of many medications.

Δ   Systemic conditions and surgery can also lead to **GI symptoms** (e.g., postoperative clients often experience nausea and vomiting).

Δ   **GI complaints** may actually be signs of more serious health conditions (e.g., heartburn may be a manifestation of peptic ulcer disease).

Δ   When **peptic ulcer disease** is caused by *H. pylori*, non-antibiotic medications promote healing, but do not cure the disease.

Δ   Medication therapy for **peptic ulcer disease** is directed at controlling symptoms, facilitating healing, decreasing the risk of complications, and preventing relapse.

Δ   Many medications for the GI system are available over-the-counter (OTC). Obtain a complete health history on clients to determine dosage and frequency of use of OTC medications.

Δ   Many medications can be used to treat **nausea and vomiting**. Prevention of emesis is more effective than treatment (e.g., prevention of vomiting caused by chemotherapy should be managed by administering antiemetics **prior** to chemotherapy).

Δ   **Diarrhea** is not a specific disease, but rather a symptom of some underlying condition (e.g., infection and inflammatory bowel disease).

Δ   Client reports of constipation should be carefully assessed to determine appropriate use of **laxatives.**

Key Points

Medication Classification: Histamine$_2$-Receptor Antagonists

Select Prototype Medication: **ranitidine hydrochloride (Zantac)**

Other Medications: cimetidine (Tagamet), nizatidine (Axid), famotidine (Pepcid)

Expected Pharmacological Action

Δ Histamine$_2$-receptor antagonists suppress the secretion of gastric acid by selectively blocking H$_2$ receptors in parietal cells lining the stomach.

Therapeutic Uses

Δ Histamine$_2$-receptor antagonists are prescribed for gastric and peptic ulcers, gastroesophageal reflux disease (GERD), and hypersecretory conditions, such as Zollinger-Ellison syndrome.

Δ Histamine$_2$-receptor antagonists are used in conjunction with antibiotics to treat ulcers caused by *H. pylori*.

Δ Clients can now purchase OTC agents to self treat heartburn, sour stomach, and acid indigestion.

Side/Adverse Effects: Nursing Interventions and Client Education

Side/Adverse Effects	Nursing Interventions/Client Education
↓ libido and impotence	• Cimetidine may block androgen receptors resulting in ↓ libido and impotence. • Inform the client of these possible effects.
CNS effects (e.g., lethargy, depression, confusion)	• These effects are seen more often in an older adult with kidney or liver dysfunction. • Avoid the use of cimetidine in older adults.

Δ Ranitidine, nizatidine, and famotidine have few adverse effects and interactions.

Contraindications/Precautions

Δ   Pregnancy Risk Category B

Δ   Use cimetidine cautiously in older adults. Use in older adults can cause antiadrenergic effects (e.g., impotence) and CNS effects (e.g., confusion).

Δ   Ranitidine ↓ gastric acid pH, which promotes bacterial colonization of the stomach and the respiratory tract. Use cautiously in clients who at a high risk for pneumonia, such as clients with chronic obstructive pulmonary disease (COPD).

Medication/Food Interactions: Nursing Interventions and Client Education

Medication/Food Interactions	Nursing Interventions/Client Education
Warfarin, phenytoin – drug-metabolizing enzymes can be inhibited by cimetidine, and thus ↑ the levels of these medications.	• In clients taking warfarin, monitor for signs of bleeding. • Monitor international normalized ratio (INR) and prothrombin time (PT) levels, and adjust warfarin dosages accordingly. • In clients taking phenytoin, monitor serum levels and adjust phenytoin dosages accordingly.
Antacids – concurrent use can ↓ absorption of histamine₂-receptor antagonists	• Advise the client not to take an antacid 1 hr before or after taking a Histamine₂-receptor antagonist.

Therapeutic Nursing Interventions and Client Education

Δ   Cimetidine, ranitidine, and famotidine can be administered IV for acute situations.

Δ   Advise the client to practice good nutrition. Suggest eating six small meals rather than three large meals a day.

Δ   Inform the client that adequate rest and reduction of stress may promote healing.

Δ   Clients should avoid smoking, because smoking can delay healing.

Δ   Encourage the client to avoid aspirin and other nonsteroidal anti-inflammatory drugs (NSAIDs) unless taking low-dose aspirin therapy for prevention of cardiovascular disease.

Δ   If alcohol exacerbates symptoms, advise the client to stop drinking.

Δ   Availability of these medications OTC may discourage clients from seeking appropriate healthcare. Encourage clients to see the primary care provider if symptoms persist.

Δ   The medication regimen can be complex, often requiring clients to take two to three different medications for an extended period of time. Encourage the client to be compliant with the medication regimen and provide support.

Δ   Ranitidine can be taken with or without food.

Δ   Treatment of peptic ulcer disease is usually started as an oral dose twice a day until the ulcer is healed, followed by a maintenance dose, which is usually taken once a day at bedtime.

Δ   Teach clients to notify the primary care provider for any sign of obvious or occult GI bleeding (e.g., coffee ground emesis).

Nursing Evaluation of Medication Effectiveness

Δ   Depending on therapeutic intent, effectiveness may be evidenced by:

- Reduced frequency or absence of GERD symptoms (e.g., heartburn, bloating, belching).

- No signs or symptoms of GI bleeding.

- Healing of gastric and duodenal ulcers.

Key Points

Medication Classification: Proton Pump Inhibitor

Select Prototype Medication: **omeprazole (Prilosec)**

Other Medications: pantoprazole (Protonix), lansoprazole (Prevacid), rabeprazole sodium (Aciphex), esomeprazole (Nexium)

Expected Pharmacological Action

Δ   Proton pump inhibitors reduce gastric acid secretion by **irreversibly** inhibiting the enzyme that produces gastric acid.

Δ   Proton pump inhibitors reduce basal and stimulated acid production.

Therapeutic Uses

Δ   Proton pump inhibitors are prescribed for gastric and peptic ulcers, GERD, and hypersecretory conditions (e.g., Zollinger-Ellison syndrome).

Side/Adverse Effects: Nursing Interventions and Client Education

Δ   Insignificant side effects and adverse effects with short-term treatment

Δ   Low incidence of headache, diarrhea, and nausea/vomiting

Contraindications/Precautions

Δ   Pregnancy Risk Category C

Δ   Use cautiously with children and women who are breastfeeding.

Δ   Contraindicated for clients hypersensitive to medication

Δ   These medications ↑ the risk for pneumonia. Omeprazole ↓ gastric acid pH, which promotes bacterial colonization of the stomach and the respiratory tract. Use cautiously in clients at high risk for pneumonia (e.g., clients with COPD).

Medication/Food Interactions: Nursing Interventions and Client Education

Medication/Food Interactions	Nursing Interventions/Client Education
Ampicillin, digoxin, iron, and ketoconazole – delayed absorption of these medications may occur if taken concurrently with omeprazole	• Allow at a least 2 hr interval between these medications and omeprazole.

Therapeutic Nursing Interventions and Client Education

Δ   Do not crush, chew, or break sustained-release capsules.

Δ   The client may sprinkle the contents of the capsule over food to facilitate swallowing.

Δ   The client should take omeprazole once a day prior to eating.

Δ   Encourage the client to avoid irritating medications (e.g., ibuprofen and alcohol).

Δ   Active ulcers should be treated for 4 to 6 weeks.

Δ   Pantoprazole (Protonix) can be administered to the client intravenously. In addition to low incidence of headache and diarrhea, there may be irritation at the injection site leading to thrombophlebitis. Monitor the client's IV site for signs of inflammation (e.g., redness, swelling, local pain) and change the IV site if indicated.

Δ   Teach clients to notify the primary care provider for any sign of obvious or occult GI bleeding (e.g., coffee ground emesis).

Nursing Evaluation of Medication Effectiveness

Δ   Depending on therapeutic intent, effectiveness may be evidenced by:

• Healing of gastric and duodenal ulcers.

• Reduced frequency or absence of GERD symptoms (e.g., heartburn, sour stomach).

• No signs or symptoms of GI bleeding.

Key Points

Medication Classification: Sucralfate

Select Prototype Medication:	**sucralfate (Carafate)**
Other Medications:	None

Expected Pharmacological Action

- Δ The acidic environment of the stomach and duodenum changes sucralfate into a viscous substance that adheres to an ulcer. This protects the ulcer from further injury that may be caused by acid and pepsin.

- Δ This viscous substance can stick to the ulcer for up to 6 hr.

- Δ Sucralfate has no systemic effects.

Therapeutic Uses

- Δ Sucralfate is used for clients with acute duodenal ulcers and those requiring maintenance therapy.

- Δ Investigational use of sucralfate includes gastric ulcers and gastroesophageal reflux disease.

Side/Adverse Effects: Nursing Interventions and Client Education

- Δ To prevent constipation, encourage the client to ↑ dietary fiber and drink at least 1,500 mL/day if fluids are not restricted.

- Δ No systemic effects

Contraindications/Precautions

- Δ Pregnancy Risk Category B

- Δ Contraindicated in clients who are hypersensitive to the medication

Medication/Food Interactions: Nursing Interventions and Client Education

Medication/Food Interactions	Nursing Interventions/Client Education
Phenytoin, digoxin, warfarin, and ciprofloxacin – sucralfate may interfere with the absorption of these medications	• Maintain a 2 hr interval between these medications and sucralfate to minimize this interaction.
Antacids interfere with the absorption of sucralfate.	• Antacids should not be administered within 30 min of sucralfate.

Therapeutic Nursing Interventions and Client Education

Δ   Assist the client with the medication regimen.

Δ   Instruct the client that the medication should be taken on an empty stomach.

Δ   Instruct the client that sucralfate should be taken four times a day, 1 hr before meals, and again at bedtime.

Δ   The client can break or dissolve the medication in water, but should not crush or chew the tablet.

Δ   Encourage the client to complete the course of treatment.

Nursing Evaluation of Medication Effectiveness

Δ   Depending on therapeutic intent, effectiveness may be evidenced by:

•   Healing of gastric and duodenal ulcers.

•   No signs or symptoms of GI bleeding.

Key Points

Medication Classification: Antacids

Select Prototype Medication: **aluminum hydroxide gel (Amphojel)**

Other Medications: aluminum carbonate, magnesium hydroxide
(Milk of Magnesia), sodium bicarbonate

Expected Pharmacological Action

Δ   Antacids neutralize gastric acid and inactivate pepsin.

Δ   Mucosal protection may occur by the antacid's ability to stimulate the production
of prostaglandins.

Therapeutic Uses

Δ   Antacids are used in clients to treat peptic ulcer disease (PUD) by promoting
healing and relieving pain.

Δ   Antacids provide symptomatic relief for clients with GERD.

Side/Adverse Effects: Nursing Interventions and Client Education

Side/Adverse Effects	Nursing Interventions/Client Education
Aluminum and calcium compounds cause constipation, whereas magnesium compounds cause diarrhea.	• Advise clients that alternate use of these compounds can be used to offset intestinal effects and to normalize bowel function. • If the client has difficulty managing bowel function, recommend the use of a combination product, such as Mylanta DS liquid. This product contains aluminum hydroxide, magnesium hydroxide, and simethicone.
Sodium containing antacids may result in fluid retention.	• Teach the client with hypertension or heart failure to avoid sodium containing antacids.
Aluminum hydroxide can lead to hypophosphatemia.	• Monitor the client's phosphate level.
Magnesium compounds can lead to toxicity in clients with renal impairment.	• Teach the client with renal impairment to avoid antacids that contain magnesium.

Contraindications/Precautions

- Δ   Pregnancy Risk Category C

- Δ   Antacids should be not administered to clients with GI perforation or obstruction.

- Δ   Use cautiously in clients with abdominal pain.

Medication/Food Interactions: Nursing Interventions and Client Education

Medication/Food Interactions	Nursing Interventions/Client Education
Warfarin, tetracycline – aluminum compounds bind to these medications and interfere with absorption.	• Teach the client to take these medications 1 hr apart.

Therapeutic Nursing Interventions and Client Education

- Δ   Clients taking tablets should be instructed to chew the tablets thoroughly and then drink at least 8 oz of water or milk.

- Δ   Teach the client to shake liquid formulations to ensure even dispersion of the medication.

- Δ   Compliance is difficult for clients because of the frequency of administration. Medication is administered seven times a day: 1 hr before and 3 hr after meals, and again at bedtime. Encourage compliance by reinforcing the intended effect of the antacid (e.g., relief of pain, healing of ulcer).

- Δ   Teach clients to take all medications at least 1 hr before or after taking an antacid.

Nursing Evaluation of Medication Effectiveness

- Δ   Depending on therapeutic intent, effectiveness may be evidenced by:

  - •   Healing of gastric and duodenal ulcers.

  - •   Reduced frequency or absence of GERD symptoms.

  - •   No signs or symptoms of GI bleeding.

Key Points

Medication Classification: Prostaglandin E Analog

Select Prototype Medication: **misoprostol (Cytotec)**

Other Medications: None

Expected Pharmacological Action

Δ   Prostaglandin E analog acts as an endogenous prostaglandin in the GI tract to ↓ acid secretion, ↑ the secretion of bicarbonate and protective mucus, and promote vasodilation to maintain submucosal blood flow. These actions all serve to prevent gastric ulcers.

Therapeutic Uses

Δ   Prostaglandin E analog is used in clients taking long-term NSAIDs to prevent gastric ulcers.

Δ   Prostaglandin E analog is used in clients who are pregnant to induce labor by causing cervical ripening.

Side/Adverse Effects: Nursing Interventions and Client Education

Side/Adverse Effects	Nursing Interventions/Client Education
Diarrhea and abdominal pain	• Instruct the client to notify the primary care provider of symptoms of diarrhea or abdominal pain. • Dosage may need to be reduced.
Women may experience dysmenorrhea and spotting	• Instruct the client to notify the primary care provider if dysmenorrhea and spotting occur. • The provider may discontinue the medication.

Contraindications/Precautions

Δ   Pregnancy Risk Category X

Medication/Food Interactions: Nursing Interventions and Client Education

Δ   None

Therapeutic Nursing Interventions and Client Education

Δ   For women of childbearing capacity, specific guidelines must be followed regarding contraception and notification of warnings (e.g., woman must be able to use birth control effectively).

Δ   Teach the client to take misoprostol with meals and at bedtime.

Nursing Evaluation of Medication Effectiveness

Δ   Depending on therapeutic intent, effectiveness may be evidenced by:

- Healing of gastric and duodenal ulcers.

- No signs or symptoms of GI bleeding.

Key Points

Medication Classification: Antiemetics

Select Prototype Medication:	Serotonin antagonists: **ondansetron (Zofran)** Dopamine antagonists: **prochlorperazine (Compazine)** Glucocorticoids: **dexamethasone (Decadron)** Cannabinoids: **dronabinol (Marinol)** Anticholinergics: **scopolamine (Transderm Scop)** Antihistamine: **dimenhydrinate (Dramamine)**
Other Medications:	granisetron (Kytril), promethazine (Phenergan), metoclopramide (Reglan), hydroxyzine (Vistaril), aprepitant (Emend)

Expected Pharmacological Action and Therapeutic Uses

Medication	Expected Pharmacological Action	Therapeutic Uses
Serotonin antagonist – ondansetron (Zofran)	• Ondansetron prevents emesis by blocking the serotonin receptors in the chemoreceptor trigger zone (CTZ), and antagonizing the serotonin receptors on the afferent vagal neurons that travel from the upper GI tract to the CTZ.	• Ondansetron prevents emesis related to chemotherapy, radiation therapy, and postoperative recovery.
Dopamine antagonists – prochlorperazine (Compazine) in the subset phenothiazine	• Antiemetic effects of prochlorperazine result from blockade of dopamine receptors in the CTZ.	• Prochlorperazine prevents emesis related to chemotherapy, opioids, and postoperative recovery.
Glucocorticoids – dexamethasone (Decadron)	• The antiemetic mechanism of dexamethasone is unknown.	• Dexamethasone is usually used in combination with other antiemetics to treat emesis related to cancer chemotherapy.

Medication	Expected Pharmacological Action	Therapeutic Uses
Cannabinoids – dronabinol (Marinol)	• Antiemetic mechanism of dronabinol is unknown.	• Dronabinol is used to control chemotherapy-induced nausea and vomiting (CINV).
Anticholinergics – scopolamine (Transderm Scop)	• Scopolamine interferes with the transmission of nerve impulses traveling from the vestibular apparatus of the inner ear to the vomiting center (VC) in the brain.	• Scopolamine treats motion sickness.
Antihistamine (subset of anticholinergics) – dimenhydrinate (Dramamine)	• Dimenhydrinate blocks muscarinic and histaminergic receptors in nerve pathways between inner ear and VC.	• Dimenhydrinate treats motion sickness.

Side/Adverse Effects: Nursing Interventions and Client Education

Side/Adverse Effects	Nursing Interventions/Client Education
Serotonin antagonist: ondansetron (Zofran)	
Headache, diarrhea, dizziness	• Treat headache with non-opioid analgesics. • Monitor stool pattern.
Dopamine antagonists: prochlorperazine (Compazine)	
Extrapyramidal symptoms (EPS)	• Inform the client of possible side effects (e.g., restlessness, anxiety, spasms of face and neck). • Administer an anticholinergic medication, such as diphenhydramine (Benadryl), or a benzodiazepine, such as lorazepam (Ativan), to control EPS.
Hypotension	• Monitor clients receiving antihypertensive medications for ↓ blood pressure.
Sedation	• Inform the client of the potential for sedation. • Advise the client to avoid activities that require alertness, such as driving.

Side/Adverse Effects	Nursing Interventions/Client Education
Anticholinergic effects (e.g., dry mouth, urinary retention, constipation)	• Instruct the client to ↑ fluid intake. • Instruct the client to ↑ physical activity by engaging in regular exercise. • Tell the client to suck on hard candy or chew gum to help relieve dry mouth. • Administer a stimulant laxative, such as senna (Senokot) to counteract a ↓ in bowel motility, or stool softeners, such as docusate sodium (Colace), to prevent constipation. • Advise the client to void every 4 hr, monitor I&O, and palpate the client's lower abdomen area every 4 to 6 hr to assess the client's bladder.
Cannabinoids: dronabinol (Marinol)	
Potential for dissociation, dysphoria	• Avoid using in clients with mental health disorders.
Hypotension, tachycardia	• Use cautiously in clients with cardiovascular disorders.
Anticholinergics: scopolamine (Transderm Scop) and Antihistamine: dimenhydrinate (Dramamine)	
Sedation	• Inform the client of the potential for sedation. • Advise the client to avoid activities that require alertness, such as driving.
Anticholinergic effects (e.g., dry mouth, urinary retention, constipation)	• Instruct the client to ↑ fluid intake. • Instruct the client to ↑ physical activity by engaging in regular exercise. • Tell the client to suck on hard candy or chew gum to help relieve dry mouth. • Administer a stimulant laxative, such as senna (Senokot), to counteract a ↓ in bowel motility or stool softeners, such as docusate sodium (Colace), to prevent constipation. • Advise the client to void every 4 hr, monitor I&O, and palpate the client's lower abdomen area every 4 to 6 hr to assess the client's bladder.

Contraindications/Precautions

Δ   Use dopamine antagonists cautiously, if at all, with children and older adults due to the ↑ risk of extrapyramidal side effects.

Δ   Dopamine antagonists, antihistamine, and anticholinergic antiemetics should be used cautiously in clients with urinary retention or obstruction, asthma, and narrow angle glaucoma.

Medication/Food Interactions: Nursing Interventions and Client Education

Medication/Food Interactions	Nursing Interventions/Client Education
CNS depressants, such as **opioids** – medications can intensify CNS depression of antiemetics	• Advise the client that CNS depression is more likely and to avoid activities that require mental alertness.
Antihypertensives – concurrent use can intensify hypotensive effects of antiemetics	• Advise the client to sit or lie down if symptoms of lightheadedness or dizziness occur. The client should avoid sudden changes in position by moving slowly from a lying to a sitting or standing position. • Provide assistance with ambulation as needed.
Anticholinergic medications (e.g., antihistamines) – concurrent use can intensify anticholinergic effects of antiemetics	• Provide teaching to reduce anticholinergic effects (e.g., sipping on fluids, use of laxatives, voiding on a regular basis).

Therapeutic Nursing Interventions and Client Education

Δ   Antiemetics prevent or treat nausea and vomiting from various causes. Match medication with the cause.

Δ   Combining more than one antiemetic allows for lower doses of each therapy, thereby ↓ the risk of side effects. For example, use of lorazepam (Ativan) can ↓ the risk of EPS caused by phenothiazine antiemetics).

Δ   Antiemetic medications are more effective when used to **prevent** nausea and vomiting than to treat nausea and vomiting that has already occurred.

Nursing Evaluation of Medication Effectiveness

Δ   Depending on therapeutic intent, effectiveness may be evidenced by:

•   Control of emesis.

•   Absence of nausea and vomiting.

Key Points

Medication Classification: Laxatives

Select Prototype Medications: **psyllium (Metamucil)**
docusate sodium (Colace)
bisacodyl (Dulcolax)
magnesium hydroxide

Other Medications: senna (Ex-Lax), lactulose

Expected Pharmacological Action and Therapeutic Uses

Medication	Expected Pharmacological Action	Therapeutic Uses
Bulk-forming laxatives (e.g., psyllium [Metamucil])	• Bulk-forming laxatives soften fecal mass and ↑ bulk which is identical to the action of dietary fiber.	• Bulk-forming laxatives ↓ diarrhea in clients with diverticulosis and irritable bowel syndrome (IBS). • Bulk-forming laxatives control stool for clients with an ileostomy or colostomy. • Bulk-forming laxatives promote defecation in older adults with ↓ in peristalsis due to age-related changes in the GI tract.
Surfactant laxatives (e.g., docusate sodium [Colace])	• Surfactant laxatives lower surface tension of the stool to allow penetration of water.	• Surfactant laxatives are used short-term in clients with constipation related to pregnancy or opioid use. • Surfactant laxatives are used in clients to prevent painful elimination (e.g., clients with episiotomy or hemorrhoids). • Surfactant laxatives are used in clients to prevent straining (e.g., clients with cerebral aneurysm or post MI). • Surfactant laxatives ↓ the risk of fecal impaction in immobile clients. • Surfactant laxatives promote defecation in older adults with ↓ in peristalsis due to age-related changes in the GI tract.

Medication	Expected Pharmacological Action	Therapeutic Uses
Stimulant laxatives (e.g., bisacodyl [Dulcolax])	• Stimulant laxatives stimulate intestinal peristalsis. They act on the colon by reducing water and electrolyte absorption and increasing the secretion of water and ions into the intestine.	• Stimulant laxatives are used for client preparation prior to surgery or diagnostic tests such as a colonoscopy. • Stimulant laxatives are used for short-term treatment of constipation caused by high-dose opioid use.
Osmotic laxatives (e.g., magnesium hydroxide [Milk of Magnesia])	• Osmotic laxatives draw water into the intestine to ↑ the mass of stool, stretching musculature, thereby stimulating peristalsis.	• Low dose – Osmotic laxatives are used in clients to prevent painful elimination (e.g., clients with episiotomy or hemorrhoids). • High dose – Osmotic laxatives are used for client preparation prior to surgery or diagnostic tests such as a colonoscopy. • Osmotic laxatives rapidly evacuate the bowel after ingestion of poisons or following antihelminthic therapy to rid the body of dead parasites.

Side/Adverse Effects: Nursing Interventions and Client Education

Side/Adverse Effects	Nursing Interventions/Client Education
GI irritation	• Instruct the client not to crush or chew enteric-coated tablets.
Rectal burning sensation leading to proctitis	• Discourage clients from using bisacodyl suppositories on a regular basis.
Laxatives with magnesium salts, such as magnesium hydroxide can lead to accumulation of toxic levels of magnesium.	• Advise clients with renal dysfunction to read labels carefully and to avoid laxatives that contain magnesium.
Laxatives with sodium salts, such as sodium phosphate place clients at risk for sodium absorption and fluid retention.	• Advise clients with heart disease to read labels carefully and to avoid laxatives that contain sodium.
Osmotic diuretics may cause dehydration	• Monitor I&O. • Monitor/assess for signs of dehydration, such as poor skin turgor. • Encourage adequate fluid intake, 1,500 mL/day, unless on fluid restriction.

Contraindications/Precautions

Δ   Contraindicated in clients with fecal impaction, bowel obstruction, and acute surgical abdomen to prevent perforation

Δ   Contraindicated in clients with nausea, cramping, and abdominal pain

Δ   Contraindicated in clients with ulcerative colitis and diverticulitis with the exception of bulk-forming laxatives

Δ   Use cautiously during pregnancy and lactation.

Medication/Food Interactions: Nursing Interventions and Client Education

Medication/Food Interactions	Nursing Interventions/Client Education
Milk and antacids – can destroy enteric coating of bisacodyl	• Instruct the client to take bisacodyl at least 1 hr apart from these medications.

Therapeutic Nursing Interventions and Client Education

Δ   Obtain a complete history of laxative use and provide teaching as appropriate.

Δ   Teach clients that chronic laxative use can lead to fluid and electrolyte imbalances.

Δ   To promote defecation and resumption of normal bowel function, instruct clients to ↑ daily high-fiber foods in daily diet (e.g., bran, fresh fruit, vegetables) and amount of fluids. Recommend at least 1,500 mL of fluid, unless restricted.

Δ   Encourage clients to exercise to improve bowel function.

Δ   Instruct clients to take bulk-forming and surfactant laxatives with a glass of water.

Nursing Evaluation of Medication Effectiveness

Δ   Depending on therapeutic intent, effectiveness may be evidenced by:

• Regulation of bowel function.

• Evacuation of bowel in preparation for surgery or diagnostic tests.

• Facilitation of defecation for clients with ↓ bowel function.

Key Points

Medication Classification: Antidiarrheals

Select Prototype Medication: **diphenoxylate (Lomotil)**

Other Medications: loperamide (Imodium), difenoxin (Motofen)

Expected Pharmacological Action

Δ   Antidiarrheals activate opioid receptors in the GI tract to ↓ intestinal motility and to ↑ the absorption of fluid and sodium in the intestine.

Therapeutic Uses

Δ   Specific antidiarrheal agents may be used to treat the underlying cause of diarrhea. For example, antibiotics may be used to treat diarrhea caused by a bacterial infection).

Δ   Nonspecific antidiarrheal agents provide symptomatic treatment of diarrhea (e.g., ↓ in frequency of stool and ↓ in fluid content of stool).

Side/Adverse Effects: Nursing Interventions and Client Education

Δ   At recommended doses for diarrhea, diphenoxylate does not affect the CNS system.

Δ   At high doses, the client may experience **typical opioid effects** (e.g., euphoria, CNS depression).

Contraindications/Precautions

Δ   There is an ↑ risk of megacolon in clients with inflammatory bowel disorders. This could lead to a serious complication such as perforation of the bowel.

Medication/Food Interactions: Nursing Interventions and Client Education

Δ   Alcohol or other CNS depressants may enhance CNS depression.

Therapeutic Nursing Interventions and Client Education

Δ   Administer initial dose of diphenoxylate, 4 mg; follow each loose stool with additional dose of 2 mg, but do not exceed 16 mg/day.

Δ   Loperamide (Imodium) is an analog of the opioid meperidine. This medication is not a controlled substance, and at high doses loperamide **does not** mimic morphine-like symptoms.

Δ   Advise clients with diarrhea to drink small amounts of clear liquids or a commercial oral electrolyte solution to maintain electrolyte balance for the first 24 hr.

Δ   Advise the client to avoid drinking plain water. Water does not contain necessary electrolytes that have been lost in the stool.

Δ   Advise the client to avoid caffeine. Caffeine exacerbates diarrhea by increasing GI motility.

Δ   Clients with severe cases of diarrhea may be hospitalized for management of dehydration.

Δ   Management of dehydration should include monitoring of weight, I&O, and vital signs. A hypotonic solution such as 0.45% NS may be prescribed.

Nursing Evaluation of Medication Effectiveness

Δ   Return to normal bowel pattern as evidenced by ↓ in frequency and fluid volume of stool

Key Points

Medication Classification: Prokinetic Agents

Select Prototype Medication: **metoclopramide (Reglan)**

Other Medications: None

Expected Pharmacological Action

Δ   Prokinetic agents block dopamine and serotonin receptors in the CTZ, and thereby suppress emesis.

Δ   Prokinetic agents augment action of acetylcholine which causes an ↑ in upper GI motility.

Therapeutic Uses

Δ   Prokinetic agents control postoperative and chemotherapy-induced nausea and vomiting.

Δ   Prokinetic agents are used to treat GERD.

Δ   Prokinetic agents are used to treat diabetic gastroparesis.

Side/Adverse Effects: Nursing Interventions and Client Education

Side/Adverse Effects	Nursing Interventions/Client Education
Extrapyramidal symptoms (EPS)	• Inform the client of the possible side effects (e.g., restlessness, anxiety, spasms of face and neck). • Administer a benzodiazepine, such as lorazepam (Ativan), to minimize EPS.
Sedation	• Inform the client of the potential for sedation. • Advise the client to avoid activities that require alertness, such as driving.
Diarrhea	• Monitor the client's bowel function and for signs of dehydration.

Contraindications/Precautions

△ Contraindicated in clients with GI perforation, GI bleeding, bowel obstruction, and hemorrhage

△ Contraindicated in clients with a seizure disorder due to ↑ risk of seizures

△ Use cautiously in children and older adults due to the ↑ risk for EPS.

Medication/Food Interactions: Nursing Interventions and Client Education

Medication/Food Interactions	Nursing Interventions/Client Education
↑ risk of seizures the risk of sedation with concurrent use of alcohol and other CNS depressants	• Advise the client to avoid the use of alcohol. • Use cautiously with other CNS depressants.
Opioids and anticholinergics will ↓ effects metoclopramide.	• Advise the client to avoid using opioids and medications with anticholinergic effects.

Therapeutic Nursing Interventions and Client Education

△ Monitor clients for CNS depression and EPS.

△ The medication can be given orally or intravenously. If dose is ≤ 10 mg, it may be administered undiluted over 2 min. If the dose is ≥ 10 mg, it should be diluted and infused over 15 min. Dilute medication in at least 50 mL of D_5W or lactated Ringer's solution.

Nursing Evaluation of Medication Effectiveness

△ Control of nausea and vomiting

Primary Reference:

Lehne, R. A. (2007). *Pharmacology for nursing care.* (6th ed.). St. Louis, MO: Saunders.

Additional Resources:

Ignatavicius, D. D., & Workman, M. L. (2006). *Medical-surgical nursing.* (5th ed.). St. Louis, MO: Saunders.

Skidmore-Roth, L. (2006). *Mosby's Nursing drug reference.* St. Louis, MO: Elsevier.

Wilson, B. A., Shannon, M. T., & Stang, C. L. (2006). *Nurse's drug guide.* Upper Saddle River, NJ: Prentice Hall.

Unit 10 Medications Affecting the Digestive System and Nutrition

Application Exercises

1. A client is receiving ranitidine (Zantac) and an antacid for treatment of PUD. The nurse should instruct the client to take these medications

   A. at the same time.

   B. at least 1 hr apart.

   C. on an empty stomach.

   D. only when the client is feeling pain.

2. A nurse is teaching a client with PUD how to properly self-administer ranitidine (Zantac). Which of the following client statements indicates effective teaching by the nurse?

   A. "I will call my doctor if my stools look black and sticky."

   B. "I will take Zantac regularly until my burning symptoms disappear."

   C. "I need to take Zantac on an empty stomach."

   D. "I can take ibuprofen if I have minor aches and pains."

3. For which of the following clients is a laxative indicated? (Select all that apply.)

   _____   An adult female who is postpartum from a vaginal delivery with an episiotomy

   _____   A young adult male with constipation and periumbilical pain

   _____   A client affected by IBS

   _____   An older adult client with limited mobility and minor incontinence

   _____   A client preparing for a colonoscopy

4. A client is receiving scopolamine (Transderm Scop). Which of the following client statements should alert the nurse that the client is experiencing side effects of this medication?

   A. "I'm having frequent loose stools."

   B. "I'm urinating little and my abdomen feels full."

   C. "My bowel movements are black and very sticky."

   D. "I have a headache and feel dizzy."

5. Children and older adults are usually not administered prochlorperazine (Compazine) for nausea and vomiting due to the ↑ risk for _____.

6. A nurse is providing teaching to a client starting omeprazole (Prilosec) for management of GERD. The nurse knows teaching has been effective when the client states that this medication works by

    A. improving gastric motility.

    B. decreasing the production of gastric acid.

    C. neutralizing gastric acid.

    D. antagonizing serotonin receptors.

7. Laxatives containing sodium are contraindicated for which of the following client conditions?

    A. Hypertension

    B. Arthritis

    C. Depression

    D. Seizure disorder

8. A client taking sucralfate (Carafate) for peptic ulcer disease has been started on phenytoin (Dilantin) to control seizures. Which of the following should be included in the client's teaching?

    A. Take both of these medications at the same time.

    B. Take sucralfate with a glass of milk.

    C. Allow a 2-hr interval between these medications.

    D. Chew the sucralfate thoroughly before swallowing.

9. For which of the following clients with peptic ulcer disease is misoprostol (Cytotec) contraindicated?

    A. 27-year-old pregnant woman

    B. 75-year-old client with osteoarthritis

    C. 37-year-old client with a kidney stone

    D. 46-year-old client with a urinary tract infection

Unit 10 Medications Affecting the Digestive System and Nutrition

Application Exercises Key

1. A client is receiving ranitidine (Zantac) and an antacid for treatment of PUD. The nurse should instruct the client to take these medications

       A. at the same time.

       B. at least 1 hr apart.

       C. on an empty stomach.

       D. only when the client is feeling pain.

Antacids can interfere with absorption of ranitidine, so they should be taken at least 1 hr apart. Ranitidine can be taken without regard to food, and both medications should be taken on a regular schedule (not only when the client is feeling pain).

2. A nurse is teaching a client with PUD how to properly self-administer ranitidine (Zantac). Which of the following client statements indicates effective teaching by the nurse?

       A. "I will call my doctor if my stools look black and sticky."

       B. "I will take Zantac regularly until my burning symptoms disappear."

       C. "I need to take Zantac on an empty stomach."

       D. "I can take ibuprofen if I have minor aches and pains."

Clients need to notify the primary care provider if signs of GI bleeding develop. Symptom relief is not indicative of ulcer healing. Ranitidine can be taken without regard to food and NSAIDs, such as ibuprofen, should be avoided for clients with PUD due to the risk of bleeding.

3. For which of the following clients is a laxative indicated? (Select all that apply.)

    __X__   **An adult female who is postpartum from a vaginal delivery with an episiotomy**

    _____   A young adult male with constipation and periumbilical pain

    __X__   **A client affected by IBS**

    _____   An older adult client with limited mobility and minor incontinence

    __X__   **A client preparing for a colonoscopy**

Laxatives will prevent straining until the episiotomy heals. Bulk-forming laxatives can provide relief of diarrhea for clients with IBS. Laxatives are used for bowel cleansing prior to diagnostic procedures of the GI tract. Appendicitis can begin in the periumbilical area before progressing to the right lower quadrant. The older adult may be experiencing fecal impaction and a laxative could cause perforation.

4. A client is receiving scopolamine (Transderm Scop). Which of the following client statements should alert the nurse that the client is experiencing side effects of this medication?

    A. "I'm having frequent loose stools."

    B. "I'm urinating little and my abdomen feels full."

    C. "My bowel movements are black and very sticky."

    D. "I have a headache and feel dizzy."

Urinary retention is a side effect from this medication. Constipation is a side effect of anticholinergic medications. Black, tarry stools are a sign of GI bleeding, but are not a side effect from an anticholinergic medication. Headache and dizziness are side effects of ondansetron (Zofran), a serotonin antagonist.

5. Children and older adults are usually not administered prochlorperazine (Compazine) for nausea and vomiting due to the ↑ risk for _____.

Extrapyramidal symptoms. EPS such as restlessness, anxiety, and spasms of the face and neck are more common in children and older adults.

6. A nurse is providing teaching to a client starting omeprazole (Prilosec) for management of GERD. The nurse knows teaching has been effective when the client states that this medication works by

    A. improving gastric motility.

    B. decreasing the production of gastric acid.

    C. neutralizing gastric acid.

    D. antagonizing serotonin receptors.

Omeprazole reduces gastric acid secretion by irreversibly inhibiting the enzyme that produces gastric acid. Metoclopramide (Reglan) improves gastric motility. Antacids neutralize gastric acid. Ondansetron (Zofran) antagonizes serotonin receptors, decreasing nausea and vomiting.

7. Laxatives containing sodium are contraindicated for which of the following client conditions?

    A. Hypertension

    B. Arthritis

    C. Depression

    D. Seizure disorder

Laxatives containing sodium can lead to sodium and water retention, which could exacerbate hypertension. Laxatives with sodium are not contraindicated for arthritis, depression, or seizure disorders.

8. A client taking sucralfate (Carafate) for peptic ulcer disease has been started on phenytoin (Dilantin) to control seizures. Which of the following should be included in the client's teaching?

    A. Take both of these medications at the same time.

    B. Take sucralfate with a glass of milk.

    C. Allow a 2-hr interval between these medications.

    D. Chew the sucralfate thoroughly before swallowing.

Sucralfate can interfere with the absorption of phenytoin, so the client should allow a 2-hr interval between the sucralfate and phenytoin. Sucralfate should be taken on an empty stomach and it should be swallowed whole.

9. For which of the following clients with peptic ulcer disease is misoprostol (Cytotec) contraindicated?

    A. 27-year-old pregnant woman
    B. 75-year-old client with osteoarthritis
    C. 37-year-old client with a kidney stone
    D. 46-year-old client with a urinary tract infection

Misoprostol can induce labor, and therefore is contraindicated in pregnancy. There are no contraindications for use in clients with osteoarthritis, kidney stones, or urinary tract infections.

Unit 11   Medications Affecting the Endocrine System

Contributor: Judith A. Harris, MSN, RNC

 NCLEX® Connections:

Learning Objective: Review and apply knowledge within **"Medications Affecting the Endocrine System"** in readiness for performance of the following nursing activities as outlined by the NCLEX® test plans:

Δ   Assess/monitor the client for expected effects of medications.

Δ   Assess/monitor the client for side/adverse effects of medications.

Δ   Assess/monitor the client for actual/potential specific food and medication interactions.

Λ   Identify contraindications, actual/potential incompatibilities, and interactions between medications, and intervene appropriately.

Δ   Identify symptoms/evidence of an allergic reaction, and respond appropriately.

Δ   Evaluate/monitor and document the therapeutic and adverse/side effects of medications.

Δ   Provide/reinforce client teaching on actions, therapeutic effects, potential side/adverse effects, and interactions of medications.

 General Key Points

Δ   Diabetes mellitus is classified as an endocrine disorder. Diabetes is not a single disease but a group of chronic disorders resulting from pancreatic dysfunction.

Δ   Carbohydrate, fat, and protein metabolism are all affected by an **absolute** or **relative** lack of insulin secretion by the beta cells in the islets of Langerhans of the pancreas. The body is unable to **produce** or **use** insulin.

Δ   All clients with type 1 diabetes mellitus require insulin for the management of blood glucose.

Δ   Clients with type 2 diabetes mellitus require insulin when undergoing surgery, experiencing high levels of physiologic stress, such as infection, and during pregnancy.

Δ   Insulin can be classified in two ways:

- **Type** – how the insulin is made.

  ◊   Natural or regular

  ◊   Addition of protein to prolong duration

      °   NPH

  ◊   Insulin analogs

      °   Lispro insulin and aspart insulin have shorter durations than Regular insulin

      °   Glargine insulin has a longer duration than Regular insulin

- **Group** – time course of action. The time course of action identifies how fast a specific insulin will work, when it will peak, and how long its action will last.

Δ   **Oral hypoglycemic** agents are indicated for clients who have type 2 diabetes mellitus and cannot achieve glycemic control with diet and exercise modification alone.

Δ   There are five classes of **oral hypoglycemic** medications. These classes have different mechanisms of actions, are beneficial to different clients, and may cause different side effects.

Oral Hypoglycemic Medications	Comments
Sulfonylureas – 1st generation: • tolbutamide (Orinase) • chlorpropamide (Diabinese) 2nd generation: • glipizide (Glucotrol, Glucotrol XL) – 30 min before first meal of day • glyburide (DiaBeta, Micronase) – daily with first main meal • glimepiride (Amaryl) – daily with first main meal	• Second generation agents are more likely seen in clinical practice. These medications have a longer duration of action than 1st generation, and therefore can be given once/day. • Begin client at low doses and increase gradually.
Meglitinides – • repaglinide (Prandin)	• Fast, but short-lived release of insulin; act fast and last a short time. • Meglitinides ↓ the risk of hypoglycemia, as action only lasts during digestion. • Take the dose within 30 min before each meal.
Biguanides – • metformin (Glucophage)	• Biguanides do not promote insulin release from pancreas, and therefore do not cause hypoglycemia. • Take biguanides with food during the morning and evening meal. Medication may be taken 3 times/day.

Oral Hypoglycemic Medications	Comments
Thiazolidinediones – • rosiglitazone (Avandia)	• Thiazolidinediones may be given without regard to food. • Dosing is usually once daily or bid in divided doses.
Alpha-glucosidase inhibitors – • acarbose (Precose)	• Alpha-glucosidase inhibitors should be taken with the first bite of food at three daily meals.

Δ   Teach clients receiving thyroid replacement therapy for **hypothyroidism** that therapy is **life-long.** Medication should not be discontinued when symptoms are resolved.

• Clients with chronic hypothyroidism will be very sensitive to thyroid replacement medications. Therapy needs to begin with **low** doses and ↑ gradually.

• Encourage clients not to be discouraged at the start of treatment. Advise clients that effects may take several weeks to months to be noticed. Doses will be changed gradually based on clinical signs and blood levels.

Δ   Therapy for **hyperthyroidism** includes: antithyroid medications (e.g., propylthiouracil [PTU] and strong iodine solution [Lugol's Solution]); radioactive iodine (^{131}I) to destroy thyroid tissue; and surgical removal of part or all of the thyroid gland.

Key Points

Medication Classification: Insulin

Select Prototype Medication: Regular insulin (Humulin R, Novolin R)

Insulin	Duration	Routes of administration	For meal time doses, administer	Onset	Peak
Lispro insulin (Humalog)	Short, rapid-acting (3 to 6.5 hr)	SC SC infusion pump	15 min ac	Rapid 15 to 30 min	½ to 2½ hr
Aspart insulin (NovoLog)	Short, rapid-acting (3 to 5 hr)	SC SC infusion pump	5 to 10 min ac	Rapid 10 to 20 min	1 to 3 hr
Regular insulin (Humulin R, Novolin R)	Short, slower-acting (6 to 10 hr)	SC SC infusion pump IH IM IV	30 min ac Bolus 30 min ac 20 min ac	30 to 60 min	1 to 5 hr
NPH insulin (Humulin-N, Novolin-N)	Intermediate (16 to 24 hr)	SC inj	Administer 2 times/day (same time)	1 to 2 hr	6 to 14 hr
Glargine insulin (Lantus)	Long (24 hr)	SC inj	Administer 1 time/day (same time)	70 min	None

Expected Pharmacological Action

Δ   Insulin promotes cellular uptake of glucose (↓ glucose levels)

Δ   Insulin converts glucose into glycogen

Δ   Insulin moves potassium into cells (along with glucose)

Therapeutic Uses

Δ   Insulin is used for glycemic control of diabetes mellitus (type 1, type 2, gestational) to prevent complications.

Δ   Clients with type 2 diabetes mellitus may require insulin when:

•   Oral hypoglycemics, diet, and exercise are unable to control BG levels.

•   Severe renal or liver disease is present.

- Painful neuropathy is present.

- Undergoing surgery or diagnostic tests.

- Experiencing severe stress such as infection and trauma.

Δ Emergency treatment of diabetes ketoacidosis (DKA) and hyperosmolar hyperglycemic nonketotic syndrome (HHNS)

Δ Treatment of hyperkalemia

Side/Adverse Effects: Nursing Interventions and Client Education

Side/Adverse Effects	Nursing Interventions/Client Education
Risk for hypoglycemia (too much insulin)	• Monitor the client for signs of hypoglycemia. If abrupt onset, client will experience sympathetic nervous system (SNS) symptoms (e.g., tachycardia, palpitations, diaphoresis, shakiness). If gradual onset, client will experience CNS symptoms (e.g., headache, tremors, weakness, diaphoresis). • Administer glucose. For conscious clients, administer a fast-acting source (e.g., glucose tablet, orange juice, non-diet soda, candy). If the client is not fully conscious, do not risk aspiration and instead administer glucose parenterally (e.g., IV glucose, SC/IM glucagon). • Encourage the client to wear a medical alert bracelet.
Lipohypertrophy	• Instruct the client to systematically rotate injection sites and to allow 1 in between injection sites.

Contraindications/Precautions

Δ **Only regular insulin** may be administered **intravenously**.

Side/Adverse Effects: Nursing Interventions and Client Education

Medication/Food Interactions	Nursing Interventions/Client Education
Sulfonylureas, meglitinides, beta-blockers, and alcohol – additive glucose reducing effects with concurrent use	• Monitor the client's serum glucose levels for hypoglycemia (< 50 mg/dL) and adjust insulin or oral hypoglycemic dosages accordingly.
Thiazide diuretics and glucocorticoids – concurrent use will ↓ glucose-reducing effects of insulin.	• Monitor the client's serum glucose levels for hyperglycemia and adjust insulin doses accordingly. Higher insulin doses may be indicated.

Therapeutic Nursing Interventions and Client Education

Δ   Adjust the client's insulin dosage to meet insulin needs.

   • ↑ the client's dosage in response to the client's ↑ in caloric intake, infection, stress, growth spurts, and in the second and third trimesters of pregnancy.

   • ↓ the client's dosage in response to the client's exercise and first trimester of pregnancy.

Δ   When mixing short-acting insulin with longer-acting insulin, draw the short-acting insulin up into the syringe first then the longer-acting insulin. This prevents the possibility of accidentally injecting some of the longer-acting insulin into the shorter-acting insulin vial (this would pose a risk for unexpected insulin effects with subsequent uses of the vial).

Δ   For insulin suspensions, the nurse should gently rotate the vial between palms to disperse the particles throughout the vial prior to withdrawing insulin.

Δ   Do not administer short-acting insulins if they appear cloudy or discolored.

Δ   Insulin glargine is not administered IV and should not to be mixed in a syringe with any other insulin.

Δ   Instruct the client to administer SC insulin in one general locale to have consistent rates of absorption. Absorption rates from subcutaneous tissue ↑ from thigh to upper arm to abdomen.

Δ   Select an appropriate needle length to ensure insulin is injected into subcutaneous tissue versus intradermal (too short) or intramuscular (too long).

Δ   Encourage clients to enhance their diabetes medication therapy with a proper diet and consistent exercise.

Nursing Evaluation of Medication Effectiveness

Δ   Glucose levels of 90 to 130 mg/dL preprandial and < 180 mg/dL postprandial

Δ   HgA1c < 7%

Δ   Normotensive (< 130/80 mm Hg)

Δ   Cholesterol levels within normal ranges

Key Points

Medication Classification: Oral Hypoglycemics-Sulfonylureas

Select Prototype Medication:	1ˢᵗ generation – **tolbutamide (Orinase)**

Select Prototype Medication: 1ˢᵗ generation – **tolbutamide (Orinase)**
2ⁿᵈ generation – **glipizide (Glucotrol, Glucotrol XL)**

Other Medications: 1ˢᵗ generation – chlorpropamide (Diabinese)
2ⁿᵈ generation – glyburide (DiaBeta, Micronase)
glimepiride (Amaryl)

Expected Pharmacological Action

Δ   Oral hypoglycemics-sulfonylureas promote insulin release from the pancreas.

Therapeutic Uses

Δ   Oral hypoglycemics-sulfonylureas control blood glucose levels in clients with type 2 diabetes mellitus.

Δ   Oral hypoglycemics-sulfonylureas are used in conjunction with diet and exercise life-style changes.

Side/Adverse Effects: Nursing Interventions and Client Education

Side/Adverse Effects	Nursing Interventions/Client Education
Hypoglycemia	• Monitor the client for signs of hypoglycemia. If abrupt onset, the client will experience SNS symptoms (e.g., tachycardia, palpitations, diaphoresis, shakiness). If gradual onset, the client will experience CNS symptoms (e.g., headache, tremors, weakness, diaphoresis). • Instruct the client to self-administer a fast-acting source (e.g., glucose tablet, orange juice, non-diet soda, candy). • Instruct the client to notify the primary care provider if there is a recurrent problem. • If severe hypoglycemia occurs, IV glucose may be needed. • Encourage the client to wear a medical alert bracelet.

Contraindications/Precautions

△   Pregnancy Risk Category C

△   Avoid use in pregnancy and lactation (risk for fetal/infant hypoglycemia).

△   Use is ineffective in clients with type 1 diabetes mellitus, since the pancreatic islets are not capable of producing insulin

△   Contraindicated in the treatment of diabetic ketoacidosis (DKA)

△   Use cautiously in clients with renal or hepatic dysfunction due to the risk of medication accumulation and resulting hypoglycemia.

Medication/Food Interactions, Nursing Interventions, and Client Education

Medication/Food Interactions	Nursing Interventions/Client Education
Alcohol – use of alcohol can result in disulfiram-like reaction (intense nausea and vomiting, flushing, palpitations)	• Inform the client about the risk and encourage the client to avoid alcohol.
Alcohol, NSAIDs, sulfonamide antibiotics, ranitidine (Zantac), and cimetidine (Tagamet) – additive hypoglycemia effect	• Inform the client of risk of additive hypoglycemic effect. Encourage the client to avoid alcohol. • Instruct the client to closely monitor glucose levels when these other agents are concurrently used. • If the client is taking a medication with an additive hypoglycemic effect, dosage adjustment of the oral hypoglycemic medication may be indicated.
Concurrent use of **beta-blockers** may mask the "typical awareness symptoms" of hypoglycemia, specifically the SNS symptoms of tachycardia, palpitations, and diaphoresis	• Advise the client of the importance of monitoring glucose levels and not relying on SNS symptoms as an alert to developing hypoglycemia.

Therapeutic Nursing Interventions and Client Education

△   Encourage clients to consistently exercise and to follow appropriate dietary guidelines.

△   Encourage clients to maintain a log of glucose levels and to note patterns that impact glucose levels (e.g., ↑ dietary intake, infection).

△   Consider referring the client to a dietician and/or diabetes educator.

Nursing Evaluation of Medication Effectiveness

Δ   Glucose levels of 90 to 130 mg/dL preprandial and < 180 mg/dL postprandial

Δ   HgA1c < 7%

Δ   Normotensive (< 130/80 mm Hg)

Δ   Cholesterol levels within normal ranges

Key Points

Medication Classification: Oral Hypoglycemics-Meglitinides

Select Prototype Medication: **repaglinide (Prandin)**

Other Medications: nateglinide (Starlix)

Expected Pharmacological Action

Δ   Oral hypoglycemics-meglitinides promote insulin release from the pancreas.

Therapeutic Uses

Δ   Oral hypoglycemics-meglitinides control blood glucose levels in clients with type 2 diabetes mellitus.

Δ   Oral hypoglycemics-meglitinides are used in conjunction with diet and exercise life-style changes.

Δ   Oral hypoglycemics-meglitinides are used in combination with metformin.

Side/Adverse Effects: Nursing Interventions and Client Education

Side/Adverse Effects	Nursing Interventions/Client Education
Hypoglycemia	• Monitor for signs of hypoglycemia. If gradual onset, the client will experience CNS symptoms (e.g., headache, tremors, weakness, diaphoresis). If abrupt onset, the client will experience SNS symptoms (e.g., tachycardia, palpitations, diaphoresis, shakiness). • Instruct the client to self-administer a fast-acting source (e.g., glucose tablet, orange juice, non-diet soda, candy). • Instruct the client to notify the primary care provider if there is a recurrent problem. • If severe hypoglycemia occurs, IV glucose may be needed. • Encourage the client to wear a medical alert bracelet.

Contraindications/Precautions

Δ   Pregnancy Risk Category C

Δ   Use is ineffective in clients with type 1 diabetes mellitus, since the pancreatic islets are not capable of producing insulin.

Δ   Contraindicated in the treatment of diabetic ketoacidosis (DKA)

Δ   Use cautiously in clients with hepatic dysfunction due to the risk of medication accumulation and resulting hypoglycemia.

Medication/Food Interactions, Nursing Interventions, and Client Education

Medication/Food Interactions	Nursing Interventions/Client Education
Gemfibrozil (Lopid) – concurrent use results in inhibition of repaglinide metabolism, leading to an ↑ risk for hypoglycemia	• Avoid concurrent use of repaglinide and gemfibrozil. • If used, closely monitor the client for signs of hypoglycemia.

Therapeutic Nursing Interventions and Client Education

Δ   Instruct the client to eat within 30 min of taking a dose of the medication.

Δ   Encourage the client to consistently exercise and to follow appropriate dietary guidelines.

Δ   Encourage the client to maintain a log of glucose levels and to note patterns that impact glucose levels (e.g., ↑ dietary intake, infection).

Δ   Consider referring the client to a dietician and/or diabetes educator.

Nursing Evaluation of Medication Effectiveness

Δ   Glucose levels of 90 to 130 mg/dL preprandial and < 180 mg/dL postprandial

Δ   HgA1c < 7%

Δ   Normotensive (< 130/80 mm Hg)

Δ   Cholesterol levels within normal ranges

Key Points

Medication Classification: Oral Hypoglycemics-Biguanides

Select Prototype Medication: **metformin HCl (Glucophage)**

Other Medications: None

Expected Pharmacological Action

Δ   Oral hypoglycemics-biguanides reduce the production of glucose within the liver through suppression of gluconeogenesis.

Δ   Oral hypoglycemics-biguanides ↑ muscles' glucose uptake and use.

Therapeutic Uses

Δ   Oral hypoglycemics-biguanides control blood glucose levels in clients with type 2 diabetes mellitus.

Δ   Oral hypoglycemics-biguanides are used in conjunction with diet and exercise life-style changes.

Δ   Oral hypoglycemics-biguanides are used to treat polycystic ovary syndrome (PCOS).

Side/Adverse Effects: Nursing Interventions and Client Education

Side/Adverse Effects	Nursing Interventions/Client Education
Gastrointestinal effects (e.g., anorexia, nausea, vomiting, which frequently results in weight loss of 3 to 4 kg [6 to 8 lb])	• Monitor the client for severity of these effects. • Discontinue the client's medication if necessary.
Vitamin B$_{12}$ and folic acid deficiency due to altered absorption	• Provide the client supplements as needed.
Lactic acidosis (hyperventilation, myalgia, sluggishness) – 50% mortality rate	• Instruct the client to discontinue use of metformin if these symptoms occur, and to inform the primary care provider immediately. Severe lactic acidosis can be treated with hemodialysis.

Contraindications/Precautions

Δ   Pregnancy Risk Category B

Δ   Contraindicated in the treatment of diabetic ketoacidosis (DKA)

Δ   Clients with renal, hepatic, and/or cardiac failure are at greater risk for medication accumulation and resulting lactic acidosis, therefore use is generally contraindicated.

Δ   Clients with severe infection, shock, and any hypoxic condition

Medication/Food Interactions, Nursing Interventions, and Client Education

Medication/Food Interactions	Nursing Interventions/Client Education
Alcohol – ↑ the risk of lactic acidosis with concurrent use	• Encourage the client to avoid consuming alcohol. Warn client of the risks.

Therapeutic Nursing Interventions and Client Education

Δ   Instruct the client to take immediate release tablets twice a day with breakfast and dinner and to take sustained release tablets once a day with dinner.

Nursing Evaluation of Medication Effectiveness

Δ   Glucose levels of 90 to 130 mg/dL preprandial and < 180 mg/dL postprandial

Δ   HgA1c < 7%

Δ   Normotensive (< 130/80 mm Hg)

Δ   Cholesterol levels within normal ranges

Key Points

Medication Classification: Oral Hypoglycemics-Thiazolidinediones "Glitazones"

Select Prototype Medication:	**rosiglitazone (Avandia)**
Other Medications:	pioglitazone (Actos)

Expected Pharmacological Action

Δ   Oral hypoglycemics-thiazolidinediones ↑ cellular response to insulin by decreasing insulin resistance.

Therapeutic Uses

Δ   Oral hypoglycemics-thiazolidinediones control blood glucose levels in clients with type 2 diabetes mellitus.

Δ   Oral hypoglycemics-thiazolidinediones are used in conjunction with diet and exercise life-style changes.

Side/Adverse Effects: Nursing Interventions and Client Education

Side/Adverse Effects	Nursing Interventions/Client Education
Fluid retention	• Monitor the client for edema, weight gain, and/or signs of congestive heart failure.
Elevations in low density lipoproteins (LDL) cholesterol	• Monitor the client's cholesterol levels.
Hepatotoxicity	• Baseline and periodic liver function tests should be performed, and the client should be instructed to report any hepatotoxicity symptoms (e.g., jaundice, dark urine).

Contraindications/Precautions

Δ   Pregnancy Risk Category C

Δ   Use is ineffective in clients with type 1 diabetes mellitus, since in type 1 diabetes mellitus the pancreatic islets are not capable of producing insulin

Δ   Contraindicated in the treatment of diabetic ketoacidosis (DKA)

Δ   Contraindicated in clients with severe heart failure

Δ   Use cautiously in clients with mild heart failure due to fluid retention effects.

Medication/Food Interactions, Nursing Interventions, and Client Education

Medication/Food Interactions	Nursing Interventions/Client Education
Gemfibrozil (Lopid) – concurrent use results in inhibition of rosiglitazone metabolism, which leads to an ↑ risk for hypoglycemia	• The client should avoid concurrent use. • If used, closely monitor the client for signs of hypoglycemia.
Insulin – ↑ risk for hypoglycemia with concurrent use	• If used, closely monitor the client for signs of hypoglycemia.

Therapeutic Nursing Interventions and Client Education

Δ   Encourage the client to consistently exercise and to follow appropriate dietary guidelines.

Δ   Encourage the client to maintain a log of glucose levels and to note patterns that impact glucose levels (e.g., ↑ dietary intake, infection).

Δ   Consider referring the client to a dietician and/or diabetes educator.

Nursing Evaluation of Medication Effectiveness

Δ   Glucose levels of 90 to 130 mg/dL preprandial < 180 mg/dL postprandial

Δ   HgA1c < 7%

Δ   Normotensive (< 130/80 mm Hg)

Δ   Cholesterol levels within normal ranges

Key Points

Medication Classification: Oral Hypoglycemics-Alpha Glucosidase Inhibitors

    Select Prototype Medication: **acarbose (Precose)**

    Other Medications: miglitol (Glyset)

Expected Pharmacological Action

    Δ   Oral hypoglycemics-alpha glucosidase inhibitors slow carbohydrate absorption and digestion.

Therapeutic Uses

    Δ   Oral hypoglycemics-alpha glucosidase inhibitors control postprandial blood glucose levels in clients with type 2 diabetes mellitus.

    Δ   Oral hypoglycemics-alpha glucosidase inhibitors are used in conjunction with diet and exercise lifestyle changes.

Side/Adverse Effects: Nursing Interventions and Client Education

Side/Adverse Effects	Nursing Interventions/Client Education
Intestinal effects (e.g., abdominal distention and cramping, hyperactive bowel sounds, diarrhea, flatulence)	• Monitor impact of these symptoms on the client. • Discontinue the medication if necessary.
Risk for anemia due to the ↓ of iron absorption	• Monitor the client's hemoglobin and iron levels. • Discontinue the medication if necessary.
Hepatoxicity with long-term use	• Check the client's baseline liver function and perform periodic liver function tests. • Discontinue the medication if elevations occur. • The client's liver function will return to normal after the medication is discontinued.

Contraindications/Precautions

    Δ   Pregnancy Risk Category B

    Δ   Contraindicated in the treatment of diabetic ketoacidosis (DKA)

    Δ   Contraindicated for clients with gastrointestinal disorders (e.g., inflammatory disease, ulceration, obstruction)

Medication/Food Interactions, Nursing Interventions, and Client Education

Medication/Food Interactions	Nursing Interventions/Client Education
Sulfonylureas or insulin – ↑ the risk for hypoglycemia with concurrent use	• If acarbose is combined with a sulfonylurea or insulin, monitor the client carefully for hypoglycemia.
Metformin – additive gastrointestinal effects and risk for hypoglycemia with concurrent use	• If acarbose is combined with metformin, monitor the client carefully for gastrointestinal symptoms and hypoglycemia.

Therapeutic Nursing Interventions and Client Education

Δ   Instruct the client to take medication with **first bite** of each main meal.

Δ   Encourage the client to consistently exercise and to follow appropriate dietary guidelines.

Δ   Encourage the client to maintain a log of glucose levels and to note patterns that impact glucose levels (e.g., ↑ dietary intake, infection).

Δ   Consider referring the client to a dietician and/or diabetes educator.

Nursing Evaluation of Medication Effectiveness

Δ   Reduction in postprandial glucose levels (e.g., < 180 mg/dL)

Δ   HgA1c < 7%

Key Points

Medication Classification: For Insulin Overdose

Select Prototype Medication: **Glucagon**

Other Medications: None

Expected Pharmacological Action

Δ For an insulin overdose, glucagon ↑ glucose levels by:

- Increasing the breakdown of glycogen into glucose.

- Decreasing glycogen synthesis (↓ storage of glucose).

- Stimulating synthesis of glucose.

Therapeutic Uses

Δ Hypoglycemia secondary to insulin overdose in clients (not conscious and not able to take oral glucose or to receive IV glucose)

Δ ↓ in gastrointestinal motility in clients undergoing radiological procedures of the stomach and intestines

Side/Adverse Effects: Nursing Interventions and Client Education

Side/Adverse Effects	Nursing Interventions/Client Education
GI distress (e.g., nausea, vomiting)	• Turn the client onto the left side following administration to reduce risk of aspiration if emesis occurs

Contraindications/Precautions

Δ Ineffective for hypoglycemia due to starvation (no glycogen stores)

Δ Contraindicated for clients with pheochromocytoma due to catecholamine stimulating effects

Therapeutic Nursing Interventions and Client Education

Δ   Administer glucagon SC, IM, or IV immediately following reconstitution parameters.

Δ   Provide food as soon as the client regains full consciousness and is able to swallow.

Δ   Instruct the client to maintain access to a source of glucose and glucagon kit at all times.

Nursing Evaluation of Medication Effectiveness

Δ   Elevation in blood glucose level to greater than 50 mg/dL

Key Points

Medication Classification: Thyroid Hormones

Select Prototype Medication:	**levothyroxine (Synthroid, Levothroid)**
Other Medications:	liothyronine (Cytomel), liotrix (Thyrolar), Thyroid (Thyroid USP)

Expected Pharmacological Action

Δ Thyroid hormones are a synthetic form of thyroxine (T_4) that ↑ metabolic rate, protein synthesis, cardiac output, renal perfusion, oxygen use, body temperature, blood volume, and growth processes.

Therapeutic Uses

Δ Thyroid hormone replacement is used for treatment of **hypothyroidism** (all ages, all forms).

Δ Thyroid hormones **are used for the emergency treatment of myxedema coma** (IV route).

Side/Adverse Effects: Nursing Interventions and Client Education

Side/Adverse Effects	Nursing Interventions/Client Education
Overmedication – can result in signs of hyperthyroidism (e.g., anxiety, tachycardia, palpitations, ↑ appetite, abdominal cramping, heat intolerance, fever, diaphoresis, weight loss, menstrual irregularities)	• Instruct the client to report signs of overmedication to the primary care provider.

Contraindications/Precautions

Δ Pregnancy Risk Category A

Δ Use cautiously in pregnancy and lactation.

Δ Use is contraindicated for clients with thyrotoxicosis

Δ Because of cardiac stimulant effects, use is contraindicated following a MI

Δ Use cautiously in clients with cardiovascular problems (e.g., hypertension, angina pectoris, ischemic heart disease) because of cardiac stimulant effects.

Δ Thyroid hormone replacement is **not** for use in the treatment of obesity.

Medication/Food Interactions, Nursing Interventions, and Client Education

Medication/Food Interactions	Nursing Interventions/Client Education
Binding agents (e.g., cholestyramine, antacids, iron and calcium supplements) and sucralfate (Carafate) – ↓ levothyroxine absorption with concurrent use	• Separate medication administration by at least 3 hr.
Many antiseizure and antidepressant medications, including carbamazepine (Tegretol), phenytoin (Dilantin), phenobarbital, and sertraline (Zoloft) – these medications can ↑ levothyroxine metabolism	• Monitor the client for therapeutic effects of levothyroxine. The client's dosages of levothyroxine may need to be ↑.
Warfarin (Coumadin) – levothyroxine can ↑ the anticoagulant effects of warfarin by breaking down vitamin K.	• Monitor the client's prothrombin time (PT) and international normalized ratio (INR). • Instruct the client to report signs of bleeding (e.g., bruising, petechia). • ↓ dosages of warfarin may be needed.

Therapeutic Nursing Interventions and Client Education

Δ   Obtain the client's baseline vital signs, weight, and height, and monitor periodically throughout treatment.

Δ   Monitor and report signs of cardiac excitability (e.g., angina, chest pain, palpitations, dysrhythmias).

Δ   Monitor the client's T_4 and TSH levels.

Δ   Instruct the client to take daily on an empty stomach (e.g., before breakfast daily).

Δ   Provide client education regarding the importance of lifelong replacement (even after improvement of symptoms), and to not discontinue without checking with primary care provider.

Δ   Instruct the client to check with primary care provider before switching to another brand of levothyroxine as some concerns regarding interchangeability of brands has been raised.

Nursing Evaluation of Medication Effectiveness

Δ   ↓ in TSH levels

Δ   Normal T_4 levels

Δ   **Absence** of hypothyroidism symptoms (e.g., depression, weight gain, bradycardia, anorexia, cold intolerance, dry skin, menorrhagia)

Key Points

Medication Classification: Antithyroid Medications

Select Prototype Medication:	**propylthiouracil (PTU)**
Other Medications:	methimazole (Tapazole)

Expected Pharmacological Action

Δ   Antithyroid medications:

- Block the synthesis of thyroid hormones.
- Prevent the oxidation of iodide.
- Block conversion of T_4 into T_3.

Therapeutic Uses

Δ   Antithyroid medications are used:

- To treat Graves' disease.
- To produce a euthyroid state prior to thyroid removal surgery.
- As an adjunct to irradiation of the thyroid gland.
- In the emergency treatment of thyrotoxicosis.

Side/Adverse Effects: Nursing Interventions and Client Education

Side/Adverse Effects	Nursing Interventions/Client Education
Overmedication – can result in signs of hypothyroidism (e.g., drowsiness, depression, weight gain, edema, bradycardia, anorexia, cold intolerance, dry skin, menorrhagia)	• Instruct the client to report signs of overmedication to the primary care provider. • Reduced dosages and/or temporary administration of thyroid supplements may be needed.
Agranulocytosis	• Monitor the client for early signs of agranulocytosis (e.g., sore throat, fever), and instruct the client to report them promptly to primary care provider. • Monitor the client's blood counts at baseline and periodically. • If agranulocytosis occurs, stop treatment and monitor the client for reversal of agranulocytosis. • Neupogen may be indicated to treat agranulocytosis.

Contraindications/Precautions

> Δ   Use is contraindicated in pregnancy (Pregnancy Risk Category D) due to the risk of neonatal hypothyroidism and during lactation

> Δ   Use cautiously in clients with bone marrow depression and/or immunosuppression.

Medication/Food Interactions, Nursing Interventions, and Client Education

Medication/Food Interactions	Nursing Interventions/Client Education
↑ anticoagulant effects	• Monitor the client's PT, INR, and activated partial thromboplastin time (aPTT), and adjust dosages of anticoagulants accordingly.

Therapeutic Nursing Interventions and Client Education

> Δ   Advise the client that therapeutic effects may take 1 to 2 weeks to be evident. Propylthiouracil does not destroy the thyroid hormone that is present, but rather prevents continued synthesis of TH.

> Δ   Monitor the client's vital signs, weight, I&O at baseline and periodically.

> Δ   Instruct the client to take medication at consistent times each day and with meals to maintain consistent therapeutic level and ↓ gastric distress.

> Δ   Instruct the client not to discontinue the medication abruptly (risk of thyroid crisis due to stress response).

> Δ   Monitor the client for signs of hyperthyroidism (indicating inadequate medication).

> Δ   Clients with hyperthyroidism may be given a beta-adrenergic antagonist, such as propranolol (Inderal), to ↓ tremors and tachycardia.

Nursing Evaluation of Medication Effectiveness

> Δ   Weight gain

> Δ   Normal vital signs

> Δ   ↓ T_4 levels

> Δ   Absence of signs of hyperthyroidism (e.g., anxiety, tachycardia, palpitations, ↑ appetite, abdominal cramping, heat intolerance, fever, diaphoresis, weight loss, menstrual irregularities)

Key Points

Medication Classification: Thyroid-Radioactive Iodine

Select Prototype Medication: **Radioactive Iodine** (^{131}I)

Other Medications: None

Expected Pharmacological Action

Δ   At high doses, thyroid-radioactive iodine destroys thyroid cells.

Therapeutic Uses

Δ   At high doses, thyroid-radioactive iodine is used for:

- Hyperthyroidism.

- Thyroid cancer.

Δ   At low doses, thyroid-radioactive iodine is used for:

- Thyroid function studies (e.g., visualization of the degree of iodine uptake by the thyroid gland is helpful in the diagnosis of thyroid disorders).

Side/Adverse Effects: Nursing Interventions and Client Education

Side/Adverse Effects	Nursing Interventions/Client Education
Radiation sickness	• Monitor the client for symptoms of radiation sickness (e.g., hematemesis, epistaxis, intense nausea, vomiting). • Stop treatment and notify the primary care provider.
Bone marrow depression	• Monitor the client for anemia, leukopenia, and thrombocytopenia.

Contraindications/Precautions

Δ   Because of irradiating effects, use is contraindicated in pregnancy (Pregnancy Risk Category X), clients of childbearing age/intent, and during lactation.

Medication/Food Interactions, Nursing Interventions, and Client Education

Medication/Food Interactions	Nursing Interventions/Client Education
Antithyroid medications – reduced uptake with concurrent use of other antithyroid medications	• Discontinue use of other antithyroid medications for a week prior to therapy.

Therapeutic Nursing Interventions and Client Education

Δ   Instruct the client to take in the morning on an empty stomach.

Δ   Instruct the client regarding radioactivity precautions.

- Encourage the client to void frequently to avoid irradiation of gonads.

- Limit contact with client to one half hour/day/person.

- Encourage the client to ↑ fluid intake.

- Instruct the client to dispose of body wastes per protocol.

- Instruct the client to avoid coughing and expectoration (source of radioactive iodine).

Nursing Evaluation of Medication Effectiveness

Δ   Weight gain

Δ   Normal vital signs

Δ   ↓ T_4 levels

Δ   Reduction in size of thyroid gland

Key Points

Medication Classification: Thyroid-Nonradioactive Iodine

Select Prototype Medication:	**strong iodine solution (Lugol's Solution)**
Other Medications:	sodium iodide, potassium iodide

Expected Pharmacological Action

Δ   Thyroid-nonradioactive iodine **creates high levels of iodide** that will reduce iodine uptake (by thyroid gland), inhibit thyroid hormone production, and block the release of thyroid hormones into the bloodstream.

Therapeutic Uses

Δ   Thyroid-nonradioactive iodine is used for the development of euthyroid state and reduction of thyroid gland size prior to thyroid removal surgery.

Δ   Thyroid-nonradioactive iodine is used for the emergency treatment of thyrotoxicosis.

Side/Adverse Effects: Nursing Interventions and Client Education

Side/Adverse Effects	Nursing Interventions/Client Education
Iodism symptoms due to corrosive property (e.g., metallic taste, stomatitis, sore teeth and gums, gastric distress, small bowel lesions)	• Take measures to prevent overdosage. • Instruct the client to drink through a straw to prevent tooth discoloration. • Instruct the client to take the medication with meals to reduce gastrointestinal distress.

Contraindications/Precautions

Δ   Use in pregnancy is contraindicated (Pregnancy Risk Category D).

Medication/Food Interactions, Nursing Interventions, and Client Education

Medication/Food Interactions	Nursing Interventions/Client Education
Foods high in iodine (e.g., iodized salt, seafood) – risk for iodism with concurrent intake of these foods	• Monitor the client for signs of iodism (e.g., brassy taste in mouth, burning sensation in mouth, sore teeth). • Instruct the client regarding foods high in iodine.

Therapeutic Nursing Interventions and Client Education

Δ   Thyroid-nonradioactive iodine can be used in conjunction with other therapy as effects are not usually complete or permanent.

Δ   Obtain the client's baseline vital signs, weight, and I&O and monitor periodically.

Δ   Instruct the client to dilute strong iodine solution (Lugol's Solution) with juice to improve taste.

Δ   Instruct the client to take at the same time each day to maintain therapeutic levels.

Δ   Encourage client to ↑ fluid intake, unless contraindicated.

Nursing Evaluation of Medication Effectiveness

Δ   Weight gain

Δ   Normal vital signs

Δ   ↓ T_4 levels

Δ   Reduction in size of thyroid gland

Key Points

Medication Classification: Anterior Pituitary Hormones/Growth Hormones

Select Prototype Medication:	**somatropin**
Other Medications:	somatrem (Protropin)

Expected Pharmacological Action

Δ   Anterior pituitary hormones/growth hormones stimulate overall growth, the production of protein, and ↓ use of glucose.

Therapeutic Uses

Δ   Anterior pituitary hormones/growth hormones are used to treat growth hormone deficiencies (e.g., pediatric and adult growth hormone deficiencies, Turner's syndrome, Prader-Willi syndrome).

Side/Adverse Effects: Nursing Interventions and Client Education

Side/Adverse Effects	Nursing Interventions/Client Education
Hyperglycemia	• Observe clients for signs of hyperglycemia (e.g., polyphagia, polydipsia, polyuria).

Contraindications/Precautions

Δ   Pregnancy Risk Category C

Δ   Use is contraindicated in clients who are severely obese or have severe respiratory impairment (e.g., sleep apnea) due to higher risk of fatality

Δ   Use cautiously in clients with diabetes due to the risk of hyperglycemia.

Δ   Treatment should be stopped prior to epiphyseal closure.

Medication/Food Interactions, Nursing Interventions, and Client Education

Medication/Food Interactions	Nursing Interventions/Client Education
Glucocorticoids – concurrent use can counteract growth-promoting effects	• Avoid concurrent use of glucocorticoids and somatrem if possible.

Therapeutic Nursing Interventions and Client Education

Δ   Obtain the client's baseline height and weight.

Δ   Monitor growth patterns during medication administration, usually monthly.

Δ   Reconstitute medication per directions. Rotate gently, and do not shake, prior to administration.

Δ   Administer the medication IM or SC (less painful).

Nursing Evaluation of Medication Effectiveness

Δ   ↑ in height

Key Points

Medication Classification: Posterior Pituitary Hormones/Antidiuretic Hormone

Select Prototype Medication: **vasopressin (Pitressin Synthetic)**

Other Medications: desmopressin (DDAVP, Stimate)

Expected Pharmacological Action

Δ   Posterior pituitary hormones/antidiuretic hormone promotes reabsorption of water within the kidneys (Desmopressin preferred).

Δ   Posterior pituitary hormones/antidiuretic hormone causes vasoconstriction due to the contraction of vascular smooth muscle (Vasopressin).

Therapeutic Uses

Δ   Posterior pituitary hormones/antidiuretic hormones are used to treat diabetes insipidus.

Δ   Posterior pituitary hormones/antidiuretic hormones are used during cardiac arrest.

Side/Adverse Effects: Nursing Interventions and Client Education

Side/Adverse Effects	Nursing Interventions/Client Education
Reabsorption of too much water	• Monitor the client for symptoms of water overhydration (e.g., sleepiness, pounding headache). • In general, clients should be instructed to reduce fluid intake during therapy. • The client should use the smallest effective dose of desmopressin.

Contraindications/Precautions

Δ   Pregnancy Risk Category X

Δ   Use of vasopressin is contraindicated in clients with coronary artery disease (risk for angina, MI) or with ↓ peripheral circulation (risk for gangrene).

Therapeutic Nursing Interventions and Client Education

Δ   Instruct the client to administer medication by prescribed route. Routes include oral, subcutaneous, and intramuscular.

Δ   Monitor the client's I&O.

Δ   Monitor the client's serum and urine electrolytes and osmolality.

Δ   With IV administration of vasopressin, monitor the client's IV site carefully as extravasation can lead to gangrene.

Nursing Evaluation of Medication Effectiveness

Δ   Depending on therapeutic intent, evidence of effectiveness may include:

- A reduction in the large volumes of urine output associated with diabetes insipidus to normal levels of urine output.
- Cardiac arrest survival.

Primary Reference:

Lehne, R. A. (2007). *Pharmacology for nursing care* (6ᵗʰ ed.). St. Louis, MO: Saunders.

Additional Resources:

Linton, A. D. & Harris, J. A. (2000). *Pharmacology companion for introductory nursing care of adults* (2ⁿᵈ ed.). Philadelphia: Saunders.

Wilson, B. A., Shannon, M., Shields, K., Stang, C. (2007). *Nurse's drug guide.* Upper Saddle River, NJ: Prentice Hall.

Unit 11 Medications Affecting the Endocrine System

Application Exercises

1. A nurse is providing teaching to a client with type 2 diabetes mellitus who is starting the oral hypoglycemic agent repaglinide (Prandin). Which of the following statements made by the client indicates understanding of the administration of this medication?

> A. "I'll take this medicine with my meals."
>
> B. "I'll take this medicine 15 minutes before I eat."
>
> C. "I'll take this medicine just before I go to bed."
>
> D. "I'll take this medicine as soon as I wake up in the morning."

2. Clients taking metformin (Glucophage) should be monitored for

> A. lactic acidosis.
>
> B. hypertension.
>
> C. hyperlipidemia.
>
> D. respiratory alkalosis.

3. A client taking lispro insulin should be instructed to eat how soon after administering the injection?

> A. 5 to 15 min
>
> B. 20 to 30 min
>
> C. 35 to 45 min
>
> D. within 1 hr

4. A client taking glipizide (Glucotrol) for control of type 2 diabetes mellitus should be cautioned against the use of

> A. magnesium hydroxide (Milk of Magnesia).
>
> B. hydrocortisone acetate cream.
>
> C. calcium supplements.
>
> D. alcohol.

5. Four clients need to receive morning insulin. Breakfast trays are due in 15 min. A nurse should first administer insulin to which of the following clients?

   A. Client with ac glucose level of 70 mg/dL, scheduled to receive aspart insulin 3 units

   B. Client with ac glucose level of 90 mg/dL, scheduled to receive 10 units of NPH insulin and 5 units of Regular insulin

   C. Client with ac glucose level of 120 mg/dL, scheduled to receive 15 units of NPH insulin and 6 units of Regular insulin

   D. Client with ac glucose level of 170 mg/dL, scheduled to receive lispro insulin 5 units

6. Which of the following should be included in a teaching plan for a client newly diagnosed with diabetes? (Select all that apply.)

   _____ Only check blood glucose levels when not feeling well.

   _____ Take OTC cold medicine if symptoms of a cold occur.

   _____ Always carry a fast-acting glucose source.

   _____ Be sure to eat enough before exercising.

   _____ Inspect all feet surfaces daily.

7. A client tells a nurse that she has been taking her levothyroxine (Synthroid) every day for 9 days. She asks why there has been no improvement in her condition. The nurse's best response is

   A. "It may take several weeks for you to notice a therapeutic effect from the drug."

   B. "Your drug dose is probably too low."

   C. "Your body must be resistant to this drug."

   D. "Your doctor should be notified right away."

8. Propranolol (Inderal) may be prescribed to clients with hyperthyroidism to

   A. increase the blood flow to the thyroid gland.

   B. prevent thyroid hormone synthesis.

   C. decrease tachycardia and tremors.

   D. promote conversion of T_4 to T_3.

9. A client is starting on levothyroxine (Synthroid) for long-standing hypothyroidism. Which of the following dosage schedules can the nurse expect to administer?

   A. The client will start at a high dose and the dose will be tapered down as needed.

   B. The client's initial dosage will be based only on body weight.

   C. The client will have her dosage adjusted daily based on blood levels.

   D. The client will start on a low dose and dose will be gradually increased.

10. For which of the following clients would radioactive iodine (^{131}I) be contraindicated?

    A. A client who is over 40 years of age

    B. A client who is pregnant

    C. A client who is 5 kg (11 lb) underweight

    D. A client who is scheduled for thyroid surgery

Unit 11 Medications Affecting the Endocrine System

Application Exercises Answer Key

1. A nurse is providing teaching to a client with type 2 diabetes mellitus who is starting the oral hypoglycemic agent repaglinide (Prandin). Which of the following statements made by the client indicates understanding of the administration of this medication?

    A. "I'll take this medicine with my meals."

    B. "I'll take this medicine 15 minutes before I eat."

    C. "I'll take this medicine just before I go to bed."

    D. "I'll take this medicine as soon as I wake up in the morning."

    Repaglinide causes a rapid, short-lived release of insulin. The client should take this medication 15 to 30 min before each meal so that insulin is available when food is present.

2. Clients taking metformin (Glucophage) should be monitored for

    A. lactic acidosis.

    B. hypertension.

    C. hyperlipidemia.

    D. respiratory alkalosis.

    Lactic acidosis is a rare side effect, but if it occurs, it can result in 50% mortality. Hypertension, hyperlipidemia, and respiratory alkalosis are not side effects of metformin.

3. A client taking lispro insulin should be instructed to eat how soon after administering the injection?

    A. 5 to 15 min

    B. 20 to 30 min

    C. 35 to 45 min

    D. within 1 hr

    Lispro insulin is a rapid-acting insulin that has an onset of 15 to 30 min. Eating 5 to 15 min after administration will ensure that glucose is present at the time of insulin onset.

4. A client taking glipizide (Glucotrol) for control of type 2 diabetes mellitus should be cautioned against the use of

> A. magnesium hydroxide (Milk of Magnesia).
>
> B. hydrocortisone acetate cream.
>
> C. calcium supplements.
>
> **D. alcohol.**

Alcohol taken currently with a sulfonylurea hypoglycemia agent can result in a disulfiram-like reaction. The client will experience intense nausea and vomiting, flushing, and palpitations. Clients taking glipizide can use magnesium hydroxide (Milk of Magnesia), but should not take it within 1 hr of taking glipizide. Topical hydrocortisone cream will not have any systemic effects and should not interfere with glipizide. There are no contraindications of calcium supplements with the use of glipizide.

5. Four clients need to receive morning insulin. Breakfast trays are due in 15 min. A nurse should first administer insulin to which of the following clients?

> A. Client with ac glucose level of 70 mg/dL, scheduled to receive aspart insulin 3 units
>
> B. Client with ac glucose level of 90 mg/dL, scheduled to receive 10 units of NPH insulin and 5 units of Regular insulin
>
> C. Client with ac glucose level of 120 mg/dL, scheduled to receive 15 units of NPH insulin and 6 units of Regular insulin
>
> **D. Client with ac glucose level of 170 mg/dL, scheduled to receive lispro insulin 5 units**

This client's ac glucose level is already above premeal parameters. An onset of 15 min will coincide with food intake and may be helpful in avoiding postmeal hyperglycemia. The other clients' ac glucose levels are within normal range or low and a delay of a few minutes will not negatively impact their clinical outcomes.

6. Which of the following should be included in a teaching plan for a client newly diagnosed with diabetes? (Select all that apply.)

     _____   Only check blood glucose levels when not feeling well.

     _____   Take OTC cold medicine if symptoms of a cold occur.

     X   **Always carry a fast-acting glucose source.**

     X   **Be sure to eat enough before exercising.**

     X   **Inspect all feet surfaces daily.**

A client with diabetes should always carry a fast-acting glucose source to treat unexpected hypoglycemia. Active muscle cells can take in glucose without insulin, and therefore the client needs to have enough glucose available to prevent hypoglycemia. A client with diabetes should inspect his feet daily to monitor for skin breakdown and signs of infection. A client with newly diagnosed diabetes should check blood glucose levels at least before meals and at bedtime. A client with diabetes should not take any OTC medications without notifying his primary care provider. OTC cold medicines contain chemicals that can interact with hypoglycemic medications.

7. A client tells a nurse that she has been taking her levothyroxine (Synthroid) every day for 9 days. She asks why there has been no improvement in her condition. The nurse's best response is

    A. "It may take several weeks for you to notice a therapeutic effect from the drug."

    B. "Your drug dose is probably too low."

    C. "Your body must be resistant to this drug."

    D. "Your doctor should be notified right away."

It may take several weeks to months to see the therapeutic effects of thyroid replacements.

8. Propranolol (Inderal) may be prescribed to clients with hyperthyroidism to

    A. increase the blood flow to the thyroid gland.

    B. prevent thyroid hormone synthesis.

    C. decrease tachycardia and tremors.

    D. promote conversion of T_4 to T_3.

Propranolol (Inderal) is a beta-adrenergic antagonist that decreases heart rate and controls tremors. Propranolol lowers blood pressure, but does not increase blood flow to the thyroid gland. Propranolol does not have any effects on thyroid hormone synthesis.

9. A client is starting on levothyroxine (Synthroid) for long-standing hypothyroidism. Which of the following dosage schedules can the nurse expect to administer?

    A. The client will start at a high dose and the dose will be tapered down as needed.

    B. The client's initial dosage will be based only on body weight.

    C. The client will have her dosage adjusted daily based on blood levels.

    D. The client will start on a low dose and dose will be gradually increased.

This client will be very sensitive to thyroid replacement medications. Therapy should start at low doses and be increased gradually.

10. For which of the following clients would radioactive iodine (^{131}I) be contraindicated?

    A. A client who is over 40 years of age

    B. A client who is pregnant

    C. A client who is 5 kg (11 lb) underweight

    D. A client who is scheduled for thyroid surgery

Iodine (^{131}I) is in Pregnancy Risk Category X due to its irradiating effects that are harmful to the developing fetus. There are no contraindications for a client over 40 years old or a client who is 5 kg (11 lb) underweight. Radioactive iodine can be used prior to thyroid surgery to produce a euthyroid state.

Unit 12	Medications Affecting Reproduction
	Contributor: Judith A. Harris, MSN, RNC

 NCLEX® Connections:

Learning Objective: Review and apply knowledge within **"Medications Affecting Reproduction"** in readiness for performance of the following nursing activities as outlined by the NCLEX® test plans:

Δ   Assess/monitor the client for expected effects of medications.

Δ   Assess/monitor the client for side/adverse effects of medications.

Δ   Assess/monitor the client for actual/potential specific food and medication interactions.

Δ   Identify contraindications, actual/potential incompatibilities, and interactions between medications, and intervene appropriately.

Δ   Identify symptoms/evidence of an allergic reaction, and respond appropriately.

Δ   Evaluate/monitor and document the therapeutic and adverse/side effects of medications.

Δ   Provide/reinforce client teaching on actions, therapeutic effects, potential side/adverse effects, and interactions of medications.

 General Key Points

Δ   Testosterone is produced by the testes, ovaries, and adrenal cortex, and is the primary androgen in males and females.

Δ   In females, the primary estrogen is estradiol and the primary progestional hormone is progesterone. Both are endogenously produced by the ovaries and are responsible for the maturation of female reproductive organs and the development of secondary sex characteristics.

Δ   Menstruation is the result of a drop in progesterone levels toward the end of the menstrual cycle.

Δ   Menopausal symptoms are a result of a drop in estrogen levels that occur as less estrogen is produced by aging ovaries.

Δ   Clinical uses of hormone preparations include **hormone deficiencies** and **oppositional treatment of hormone dependent cancers.**

Δ **Use of hormone preparations is contraindicated during pregnancy**.

Δ Estrogen and progesterone are commonly used for **contraception. Hormone replacement therapy (HRT)** is the primary noncontraceptive use of these hormones. Progesterone counters the adverse effects of "estrogen only" therapy on the endometrium.

Δ Postmenopausal HRT has been controversial because of varying findings regarding the risk-to-benefit ratio of HRT. Benefits have included relief of **vasomotor symptoms** (e.g., hot flashes) and prevention of **osteoporosis**. Risks have included embolic events (e.g., MI, pulmonary embolism, DVT, stroke) and cancers (e.g., breast, ovarian, uterine).

Δ HRT is also used to treat **dysfunctional uterine bleeding** in adolescents and women in the period prior to menopause.

Δ Oral contraceptives (OC) **suppress ovulation**. Combination OCs contain ethinyl, estradiol, and norethindrone.

Δ The occurrence of OC risks is minimal except in women with a history of embolic disorders or women who smoke cigarettes. Clients taking OCs should be encouraged to maintain cardiovascular health and to not smoke cigarettes.

Δ OC effectiveness is reduced by the concurrent use of some antibiotics (e.g., tetracycline, ampicillin) and medications that induce hepatic metabolizing enzymes (e.g., rifampin).

Δ Long-acting OCs, such as Depo-Provera, can be a good option for clients who have difficulty maintaining compliance.

Δ **Oxytocics** (e.g., oxytocin [Pitocin], methylergonovine [Methergine]) are uterine stimulants and are used to induce postterm labor and to augment dysfunctional labor. Terbutaline (Brethine) and magnesium are **tocolytics** used to delay preterm labor.

Key Points

Medication Classification: Uterine Stimulants-Oxytocics

Select Prototype Medication: **oxytocin (Pitocin, Syntocinon)**

Other Medications: methylergonovine (Methergine)

Expected Pharmacological Action

Δ   Uterine stimulants ↑ the strength, frequency, and length of uterine contractions.

Therapeutic Uses

Δ   **Oxytocin** is used for:

- Induction of labor (e.g., postterm pregnancy, premature rupture of membranes, preeclampsia).

- Enhancement of labor, such as with dysfunctional labor.

- Delivery of afterbirth (placenta) (e.g., postpartum, miscarriage).

- The control of postpartum bleeding.

- Fetal stress testing.

- Intranasal: Promotion of milk letdown.

Δ   **Methergine** is used for:

- Emergency intervention for serious postpartum hemorrhage.

Side/Adverse Effects: Nursing Interventions and Client Education

Side/Adverse Effects	Nursing Interventions/Client Education
oxytocin (Pitocin)	
Uterine rupture	• Preassess client risk factors such as multiple deliveries. • Monitor the length, strength, and duration of contractions. • Have magnesium sulfate on standby if needed for relaxation of myometrium.
methylergonovine (Methergine)	
Hypertensive crisis	• Hypertensive crisis occurs with IV administration. • Monitor the client for symptoms of hypertensive crisis (e.g., headache, nausea, vomiting, ↑ blood pressure). • Provide emergency interventions.

Contraindications/Precautions

Δ   Contraindications of oxytocin include:

•   Maternal factors (e.g., cervix has not ripened, genital herpes, history of multiple births, uterine surgery).

•   Fetal factors (e.g., immature lungs, cephalopelvic disproportion, fetal malpresentation, prolapsed umbilical cord, fetal distress).

Δ   Methergine should not be given to clients with hypertension and used cautiously in clients with organ failure (e.g., cardiovascular, renal, or hepatic).

Medication/Food Interactions: Nursing Interventions and Client Education

Medication/Food Interactions	Nursing Interventions/Client Education
Vasopressors – can lead to hypertension	• Avoid concurrent use of oxytocin and vasopressors. • Monitor maternal blood pressure and report hypertension to the primary care provider.

Therapeutic Nursing Interventions and Client Education

Δ   **Use an infusion pump** to administer intravenously. Gradually ↑ flow rate per prescribed parameters, such as ↑ by 1 mμ/min every 30 min.

Δ   Carefully monitor uterine contractions. Generally the goal is contractions that last 1 min or less every 2 to 3 min.

Δ   Continuously monitor of the mother's blood pressure, pulse rate, and uterine contractions (frequency and duration).

Δ   Monitor for uterine hyperstimulation (e.g., **contractions lasting longer than 60 sec, occurring more frequently than every 2 to 3 min**, resting uterine pressure > 15 mm Hg). **Stop infusion and notify the primary care provider immediately.**

Δ   Continuously monitor of the fetal heart rate and rhythm. Report signs of fetal distress.

Nursing Evaluation of Medication Effectiveness

Δ   Depending on therapeutic intent, effectiveness may be evidenced by:

•   Effective contractions (lasting less than 60 sec and occurring every 2 to 3 min).

•   ↑ in uterine tone and no evidence of postpartum hemorrhage.

•   Effective milk letdown.

Key Points

Medication Classification: Tocolytic Medications

Select Prototype Medication:	**terbutaline sulfate (Brethine)**
Other Medications:	magnesium sulfate, ritodrine

Expected Pharmacological Action

Δ Terbutaline (Brethine) selectively activates beta$_2$-adrenergic receptors (beta$_2$-adrenergic agonist), resulting in uterine smooth muscle relaxation.

Therapeutic Uses

Δ IV or SC terbutaline can be used for up to 48 hr to delay preterm labor.

Side/Adverse Effects: Nursing Interventions and Client Education

Side/Adverse Effects	Nursing Interventions/Client Education
Tachycardia, palpitations, chest pain	• Monitor the client for these beta$_1$ side effects (not absolutely selective). • Intervene based on tolerance and physiological impact.
Tremors, anxiety, headache	• Monitor the client for these beta$_2$ skeletal muscle stimulant side effects, which will decline with continued use.

Contraindications/Precautions

Δ Pregnancy (near term)

Δ Lactation (enters breast milk)

Medication/Food Interactions: Nursing Interventions and Client Education

Medication/Food Interactions	Nursing Interventions/Client Education
Adrenergic agonists – concurrent use can cause additive effects.	• Monitor the client for additive adrenergic effects (e.g., tachycardia, tremors).
MAOIs – concurrent use can lead to hypertension.	• Monitor the client for hypertensive crisis.
Beta-blockers – concurrent use can blunt effect.	• Monitor the client for negation of effects.

Therapeutic Nursing Interventions and Client Education

Δ   Terbutaline should be administered IV or SC due to high first pass effect with oral administration.

Δ   Monitor the maternal pulse and blood pressure.

Δ   Monitor the frequency and duration of contractions. Notify the primary care provider if contractions persist or if contractions ↑ in frequency or duration.

Δ   Monitor the client for symptoms of fetal distress.

Nursing Evaluation of Medication Effectiveness

Δ   Cessation of preterm labor (20 to 36 weeks)

Key Points

Medication Classification: Androgens

Select Prototype Medication:	**testosterone enanthate (Delatestryl)**
Other Medications:	fluoxymesterone (Halotestin), methyl testosterone (Oreton Methyl), danazol (Danocrine)

Expected Pharmacological Action

Δ   Androgens are a hormone needed for growth and maturation of male sex organs and secondary sex characteristics. This hormone promotes skeletal muscle growth (anabolic steroid effect) in sexually mature males.

Therapeutic Uses

Δ   Androgens are used for the treatment of hypogonadism in androgen deficient men.

Δ   Androgens are used for the treatment of delayed puberty.

Δ   Androgens are used for palliative treatment of androgen-responsive breast cancer.

Side/Adverse Effects: Nursing Interventions and Client Education

Side/Adverse Effects	Nursing Interventions/Client Education
Hepatotoxicity	• Obtain baseline and periodic liver function tests. • Monitor the client for signs of hepatotoxicity (e.g., jaundice, anorexia). • Instruct the client to report signs to the primary care provider.
Cardiovascular risk – high levels of LDL cholesterol and **lower levels** of HDL cholesterol, **edema**	• Monitor the client's cholesterol levels. • Monitor the client for edema (e.g., ↑ weight gain, peripheral swelling, shortness of breath) and signs of heart failure. • A low sodium diet may become appropriate.
Virilism effects – **Males** – acne, facial hair, gynecomastia, impotence, priapism **Females** – deeper voice, unusual hair growth, clitoral enlargement, menstrual irregularities, acne	• Monitor the client for symptoms. A ↓ in dosages can lead to symptom reversal.

Side/Adverse Effects	Nursing Interventions/Client Education
Hypercalcemia – occurs with breast cancer treatment	• Monitor the client for signs of hypercalcemia (e.g., nausea, vomiting, constipation, weakness).

Contraindications/Precautions:

Δ Contraindicated in:

• Pregnancy (Pregnancy Risk Category X) and lactation.

• Clients with liver, heart, or renal failure.

• Clients with prostate cancer.

• The enhancement of athletic performance and body building.

Medication/Food Interactions: Nursing Interventions and Client Education

Medication/Food Interactions	Nursing Interventions/Client Education
Warfarin, oral hypoglycemic, and glucocorticoids – androgen effects on metabolism can ↑ medication levels of these medications	• Monitor the client's prothrombin time (PT) and International normalized ratio (INR). • Observe the client for signs of bleeding, hypoglycemia in clients with diabetes, and signs of infection.
Hepatotoxic drugs – can ↑ the risk of liver damage	• Obtain baseline and periodic liver function tests. • Monitor the client for signs of hepatotoxicity (e.g., jaundice, anorexia). • Instruct the client to report signs to the primary care provider.

Therapeutic Nursing Interventions and Client Education

Δ Instruct the client to report weight gain of more than 2 lb in a week.

Δ Follow controlled substances procedures (e.g., nandrolone [Durabolin], stanozolol [Winstrol]).

Δ Observe for and discourage androgen abuse in clients.

Δ Explain rationale for the prohibition for use in athletic strengthening (risk of serious adverse effects).

Nursing Evaluation of Medication Effectiveness

Δ Depending on therapeutic intent, effectiveness may be evidenced by:

• Resolution of the signs of androgen deficiency.

• ↓ in size/spread of breast malignancy.

Key Points

Medication Classification: Estrogens

Select Prototype Medication:	**conjugated equine estrogens (Premarin)**
Other Medications:	estradiol (Estrace), estradiol hemihydrate (Vagifem)

Expected Pharmacological Action

Δ   Estrogens are hormones needed for growth and maturation of the female reproductive tract and secondary sex characteristics. Estrogens block bone resorption and reduce low-density lipoprotein (LDL) levels. At high levels, estrogens suppress the release of a follicle stimulating hormone (FSH) needed for conception.

Therapeutic Uses

Δ   Estrogens are used for:

- Contraception.

- Relief of postmenopausal symptoms (e.g., hot flashes, mood changes).

- Prevention of postmenopausal osteoporosis.

- Treatment of dysfunctional uterine bleeding and endometriosis.

- Treatment of prostate cancer.

Side/Adverse Effects: Nursing Interventions and Client Education

Side/Adverse Effects	Nursing Interventions/Client Education
Endometrial and ovarian cancers – occur when prolonged estrogen is the only postmenopausal therapy	• Give the client progestins along with estrogen. • Instruct the client to report persistent vaginal bleeding. • Advise the client to have a endometrial biopsy every 2 years.
Potential risk for estrogen-dependent breast cancer	• Rule out estrogen-dependent breast cancer prior to starting therapy. • Encourage regular self-breast examinations and mammograms.

Side/Adverse Effects	Nursing Interventions/Client Education
Embolic events (e.g., MI, pulmonary embolism, DVT, cerebrovascular accident)	• Discourage clients from smoking. • Monitor the client for pain, swelling, warmth, or erythema of lower legs.
Feminization (gynecomastia, testicular and penile atrophy), impotence, and ↓ libido in males	• Avoid the use of estrogen vaginal creams prior to sexual intercourse. • Symptoms disappear when medication is discontinued.

Contraindications/Precautions

Δ   Contraindications include:

   • Pregnancy Risk Category X. Instruct the client to report the possibility of pregnancy immediately and to stop taking the estrogen.

   • Client or family history of heart disease.

   • Breast cancer.

   • History or risk of thromboembolic disease.

Δ   Use cautiously during breastfeeding as estrogens ↓ quantity and quality of milk and may be excreted in breast milk.

Δ   Use cautiously in prepubescent girls. If administered, monitor bone growth, and check periodically for early epiphyseal plate closure.

Medication/Food Interactions: Nursing Interventions and Client Education

Medication/Food Interactions	Nursing Interventions/Client Education
Warfarin (Coumadin) – estrogens can ↓ the effectiveness of warfarin.	• When estrogens and warfarin are used concurrently, monitor client international normalized ratio (INR) and prothrombin time (PT). • Warfarin doses may need to be adjusted.
Phenytoin (Dilantin) – use of phenytoin with estrogen can ↑ the risk of toxicity	• Monitor the client for signs of phenytoin toxicity with concurrent use of estrogen and phenytoin.

Therapeutic Nursing Interventions and Client Education

Δ   Instruct the client to take the medication at the same time each day (e.g., at bedtime).

Δ   Apply estrogen patches to the skin of the trunk.

Δ   Inject IM forms deep in a large muscle mass. Rotate injection sites.

Δ   Instruct the client to report symptoms of menstrual changes, dysmenorrhea, amenorrhea, breakthrough bleeding, and/or breast changes.

Δ   Encourage the client to perform monthly breast self-examination and schedule annual gynecologic and breast examinations with the primary care provider.

Nursing Evaluation of Medication Effectiveness

Δ   Depending on therapeutic intent, effectiveness may be evidenced by:

- No evidence of contraception.

- Relief of postmenopausal symptoms (e.g., hot flashes, mood changes).

- No evidence of postmenopausal osteoporosis.

- Reduction in dysfunctional uterine bleeding and endometriosis.

- ↓ in spread of prostate cancer.

Key Points

Medication Classification: Progesterones

Select Prototype Medication: **medroxyprogesterone acetate (Provera)**

Other Medications: norethindrone (Micronor), megestrol acetate (Megace)

Expected Pharmacological Action

Δ Progesterones induce favorable conditions for fetal growth and development and maintain pregnancy. A drop in progesterone levels results in menstruation.

Therapeutic Uses

Δ Progesterones counter adverse effects of estrogen in hormone replacement therapy for treatment of:

- Dysfunctional uterine bleeding due to hormonal imbalance.
- Amenorrhea due to hormonal imbalance.
- Endometriosis.
- Endometrial carcinoma.

Side/Adverse Effects: Nursing Interventions and Client Education

Side/Adverse Effects	Nursing Interventions/Client Education
Breast cancer	• Progesterones are contraindicated.
Thromboembolic events (e.g., MI, pulmonary embolism, thrombophlebitis, cerebrovascular accident)	• Discourage clients from smoking. • Monitor the client for pain, swelling, warmth, or erythema of lower legs.
Breakthrough bleeding, amenorrhea, breast tenderness	• Obtain baseline breast exam and Pap smear. • Instruct the client to report abnormal vaginal bleeding.
Edema	• Monitor the client's blood pressure, I&O, and weight gain.

Contraindications/Precautions

Δ   Contraindications include:

- Pregnancy Risk Category X.

- Undiagnosed vaginal bleeding.

- History of thromboembolic disease, cardiovascular, or cerebrovascular disease.

Δ   Use cautiously in clients with diabetes, seizures disorders, and migraine headaches.

Medication/Food Interactions: Nursing Interventions and Client Education

Medication/Food Interactions	Nursing Interventions/Client Education
Carbamazepine (Tegretol), Phenobarbital, phenytoin (Dilantin), and rifampin – contraceptive effectiveness ↓ with the use of these medications	• Additional contraceptive measures may be needed with concurrent use of these medications.

Therapeutic Nursing Interventions and Client Education

Δ   Instruct the client to anticipate withdrawal bleeding 3 to 7 days after stopping the medication.

Δ   Instruct the client to stop taking the medication immediately if pregnancy is suspected. Conception should be delayed for 3 months following use.

Nursing Evaluation of Medication Effectiveness

Δ   Depending on therapeutic intent, effectiveness may be evidenced by:

- Restoration of hormonal balance with control of uterine bleeding (e.g., regular menstrual periods).

- Restoration of menses.

- ↓ in endometrial hyperplasia in postmenopausal women receiving concurrent estrogen.

- Control of the spread of endometrial cancer.

Key Points

Medication Classification: Oral Contraceptives

Select Prototype Medication: **Ovcon 35**

Other Medications: Necon 1/35, ortho-novum

Expected Pharmacological Action

Δ   Oral contraceptives ↓ fertility by inhibiting ovulation, thickening cervical mucus, and making the lining of the endometrium less favorable for implantation.

Therapeutic Uses

Δ   Oral contraceptives are used to prevent pregnancy.

Side/Adverse Effects: Nursing Interventions and Client Education

Side/Adverse Effects	Nursing Interventions/Client Education
Thromboembolic events (e.g., MI, pulmonary embolism, thrombophlebitis, and cerebrovascular accident)	• Discourage the client from smoking. • Instruct the client to report warmth, edema, tenderness, and/or pain in lower legs.
Hypertension	• Monitor the client's blood pressure and take interventions to maintain normal blood pressure.
Breakthrough or abnormal uterine bleeding	• Instruct the client to record duration and frequency of breakthrough bleeding. • Evaluate the client for the possibility of pregnancy if two or more menstrual periods are missed.
Cervical cancer	• Women with the human papillomavirus are at risk for cervical cancer. • Baseline and routine Pap smear should be obtained.

Contraindications/Precautions

Δ   Contraindications include:

- Pregnancy Risk Category X, (teratogenic to fetus and carcinogenic for females exposed to them in utero).

- Client history of thrombophlebitis and cardiovascular events.

- Family history or risk factors for breast cancer.

- Client > 35 years of age who smokes.

Δ   Use cautiously in clients who are obese, who are > 35 years of age and smoke, with diabetes, and hypercholesterolemia.

Medication/Food Interactions: Nursing Interventions and Client Education

Medication/Food Interactions	Nursing Interventions/Client Education
Carbamazepine (Tegretol), Phenobarbital, phenytoin (Dilantin), rifampin, tetracyclines, and ampicillin – oral contraceptive effectiveness ↓ with concurrent use of these medications	• Additional contraceptive measures may be needed with concurrent use of these medications.
Warfarin (Coumadin) and oral hypoglycemics – oral contraceptives ↓ the effects of these medications	• Monitor the client's INR and PT levels and adjust warfarin dosages accordingly.

Therapeutic Nursing Interventions and Client Education

Δ   Instruct the client to take pills at the same time each day.

Δ   Instruct the client to take medication for 21 days followed by 7 days of no medication (or inert pill). Begin the sequence on the fifth day after the onset of menses.

Δ   For one missed dose, instruct the client to take two together at the next scheduled dose. For two missed doses, instruct the client to double-up for 2 days. For three missed doses due to an ↑ risk of ovulation and resulting pregnancy, instruct the client to use an additional form of birth control and to start a new cycle of medications after waiting 7 days.

Δ   Encourage clients who smoke to quit.

Nursing Evaluation of Medication Effectiveness

Δ   No evidence of conception

Key Points

Medication Classification: Other Antineoplastic Agents

Select Prototype Medication: leuprolide (Lupron)

Expected Pharmacological Action

Δ   Antineoplastic agents are a synthetic-luteinizing hormone that results in a ↓ in testosterone levels and a ↓ in uterine fibroid growth.

Therapeutic Uses

Δ   Leuprolide is used for palliative treatment of advanced prostate cancer.

Δ   Leuprolide is used for the treatment of uterine fibroids and endometriosis.

Side/Adverse Effects: Nursing Interventions and Client Education

Side/Adverse Effects	Nursing Interventions/Client Education
Thromboembolic events (e.g., MI, pulmonary embolism, thrombophlebitis, cerebrovascular accident)	• Discourage cigarette smoking. • Monitor the client for other risk factors. • Instruct the client to report warmth, edema, tenderness, and/or pain in lower legs.
Hot flashes	• Instruct the client of the possibility and to report if not tolerable.
Bone pain	• Monitor the client for an ↑ in bone pain and ↓ in sensory or motor function.

Contraindications/Precautions:

Δ   Pregnancy (Risk Category X) and lactation

Therapeutic Nursing Interventions and Client Education

Δ   Administer leuprolide immediately after reconstitution.

Δ   Administer leuprolide depot preparations deep IM.

Nursing Evaluation of Medication Effectiveness

Δ   Depending on therapeutic intent, effectiveness may be evidenced by:

•   ↓ spread of prostate cancer.

•   ↓ pain and growth of uterine fibroids.

Key Points

Medication Classification: Other Antineoplastic Agents

Select Prototype Medication: tamoxifen (Nolvadex) – Selective Estrogen Receptor Modulators (SERMs)

Expected Pharmacological Action

Δ   Tamoxifen (Nolvadex) competes with estrogen resulting in reduced estrogen effects.

Therapeutic Uses

Δ   Tamoxifen is used in the treatment of breast cancer.

Δ   Tamoxifen is used for breast cancer prevention (high risk clients).

Side/Adverse Effects: Nursing Interventions and Client Education

Side/Adverse Effects	Nursing Interventions/Client Education
Hot flashes	• Instruct the client to notify the primary care provider if hot flashes become intolerable.
Bone pain	• Monitor the client for an ↑ in tumor pain or bone pain, which generally is transient. • Administer analgesics.
Hypercalcemia – clients with bone metastases are at an ↑ risk for hypercalcemia	• Monitor the client's calcium levels.
Hyperlipidemia	• Monitor the client's serum cholesterol and triglyceride levels.

Contraindications/Precautions:

Δ   Contraindications include:

     •   Pregnancy Risk Category X.

     •   Lactation.

     •   History of DVT.

Medication/Food Interactions: Nursing Interventions and Client Education

Medication/Food Interactions	Nursing Interventions/Client Education
Warfarin – ↑ in anticoagulant effect with concurrent use	• Monitor the client for signs of bleeding. Monitor INR and PT and adjust warfarin dosage accordingly.
Other antineoplastic agents – ↑ antineoplastic effects (e.g., neutropenia, nausea, vomiting)	• Monitor the client for risks associated with additive antineoplastic effects, such as infection.

Therapeutic Nursing Interventions and Client Education

Δ   Administer tamoxifen with food or fluids if gastric upset occurs.

Δ   Instruct the client to omit missed doses of tamoxifen and to not double-up doses.

Δ   Monitor the client for weight gain or peripheral edema.

Δ   Instruct the client that observable effects may not be seen for several weeks.

Nursing Evaluation of Medication Effectiveness

Δ   ↓ breast cancer spread

Key Points

Medication Classification: Medications to Treat Erectile Dysfunction

Select Prototype Medication: **sildenafil (Viagra)**

Other Medications: Tadalafil (Cialis), Vardenafil (Levitra)

Expected Pharmacological Action

Δ   Sildenafil (Viagra) augments the effects of nitric oxide released during sexual stimulation resulting in enhanced blood flow to corpus cavernosum and penile erection.

Therapeutic Uses

Δ   Sildenafil is used in the treatment of erectile dysfunction.

Side/Adverse Effects: Nursing Interventions and Client Education

Side/Adverse Effects	Nursing Interventions/Client Education
MI, sudden death	• Monitor the client's risk factors and history with regard to cardiovascular health.
Priapism	• Instruct the client to notify the primary care provider if erection lasts more than 4 hr.

Contraindications/Precautions:

Δ   Contraindicated in clients taking any medications in the nitrate family, such as nitroglycerine

Δ   Use cautiously in clients with cardiovascular disease.

Medication/Food Interactions: Nursing Interventions and Client Education

Medication/Food Interactions	Nursing Interventions/Client Education
Organic nitrates, such as nitroglycerin, can lead to **fatal hypotension**	• Discourage concurrent use of organic nitrates due to the risk of possibly fatal hypotension.
Ketoconazole, erythromycin, cimetidine, ritonavir, grapefruit juice – inhibit metabolism of sildenafil thereby ↑ plasma level of medication	• Use these medications cautiously in clients taking sildenafil.

Therapeutic Nursing Interventions and Client Education

Δ   Instruct the client to take approximately 1 hr before sexual activity and to limit use to once a day.

Nursing Evaluation of Medication Effectiveness

Δ   Erection sufficient for sexual intercourse

Primary Reference:

Lehne, R. A. (2007). *Pharmacology for nursing care* (6th ed.). St. Louis, MO: Saunders.

Additional Resources:

Ignatavicius, D. D. (2006). *Medical-surgical nursing* (5th ed.). St. Louis, MO: Saunders.

Linton, A. D. & Harris, J. A. (2000). *Pharmacology companion for introductory nursing care of adults* (2nd ed.). Philadelphia: Saunders.

Skidmore-Roth, L. (2006). *Mosby's nursing drug reference*. St. Louis, MO: Elsevier.

Unit 12 Medications Affecting Reproduction

Application Exercises

1. A college student comes into the health clinic to renew her prescription for oral contraceptives. While she is there, she reports a sore throat and fever for 2 days. A throat culture for streptococcus is positive and she is placed on ampicillin and her oral contraceptive prescription is refilled. The nurse provides the following client teaching: "Take ampicillin 500 mg (1 capsule) four times a day for 10 days. Drink lots of fluid and get plenty of rest." Identify the medication error and explain your answer.

2. A woman has come to her primary care provider requesting birth control pills. Identify factors that contraindicate use of birth control pills and identify why.

3. Terbutaline (Brethine) is indicated in preterm labor to

    A. stop uterine contractions.
    B. prevent bleeding.
    C. promote placental blood flow.
    D. increase prostaglandin production.

4. Which of the following nursing interventions are indicated for a client in labor receiving oxytocin (Pitocin) to stimulate uterine contractions? (Select all that apply.)

    _____ Use an infusion pump to administer medication.
    _____ Provide continuous monitoring of maternal vital signs.
    _____ Stop infusion if uterine contractions occur every 4 min and last 45 sec.
    _____ Increase medication rapidly to assure adequate contractions.
    _____ Monitor FHR continuously.

5. A client is receiving testosterone enanthate (Delatestryl) for treatment of androgen-responsive breast cancer. Which of the following side effects should she be monitored for? (Select all that apply.)

_____ Dehydration
_____ Hypercalcemia
_____ Liver damage
_____ Increased LDL and decreased HDL levels
_____ Unusual hair growth

6. A nurse is providing teaching to a client receiving tamoxifen (Nolvadex) for breast cancer prevention. Which of the following statements indicates the client has understood the teaching?

A. "I may experience hot flashes."
B. "I will be so excited when I finally get pregnant."
C. "I should be sure to drink plenty of milk."
D. "I will eat a diet high in fat to prevent weight loss."

7. Match the following medications with their therapeutic uses.

Testosterone enanthate (Delatestryl)   A. Contraception

Conjugated equine estrogens   B. Breast cancer prevention and treatment
(Premarin)

Medroxyprogesterone acetate   C. Treatment of erectile dysfunction
(Provera)

Ovcon 35   D. Contraindicated for athletic performance
                                                  enhancement

Leuprolide (Lupron)   E. Relief of postmenopausal symptoms

Tamoxifen (Nolvadex)   F. Treatment of endometriosis

Sildenafil (Viagra)   G. Dysfunctional uterine bleeding due to
                                                  hormonal balance

Unit 12 Medications Affecting Reproduction

Application Exercises Answer Key

1. A college student comes into the health clinic to renew her prescription for oral contraceptives. While she is there, she reports a sore throat and fever for 2 days. A throat culture for streptococcus is positive and she is placed on ampicillin and her oral contraceptive prescription is refilled. The nurse provides the following client teaching: "Take ampicillin 500 mg (1 capsule) four times a day for 10 days. Drink lots of fluid and get plenty of rest." Identify the medication error and explain your answer.

   The nurse provided adequate teaching regarding the antibiotic, but did not explain the drug-drug interaction between ampicillin and oral contraceptives. Taking the medications together decreases effectiveness of the OC and could result in an unplanned pregnancy. Information regarding use of additional contraception should be given.

2. A woman has come to her primary care provider requesting birth control pills. Identify factors that contraindicate use of birth control pills and identify why.

   Factors that preclude the use of birth control pills include pregnancy, thromboembolic disorders (hypercoagulability), cancer (stimulate tumor growth), hypertension (increased angiotensin and retention of sodium and water), and women over 30 who smoke (decreased estrogenic effect and increased platelet aggregation).

3. Terbutaline (Brethine) is indicated in preterm labor to

   A. stop uterine contractions.
   B. prevent bleeding.
   C. promote placental blood flow.
   D. increase prostaglandin production.

   Terbutaline blocks beta$_2$-adrenergic receptors which causes uterine smooth muscle relaxation. Terbutaline does not have the other actions.

4. Which of the following nursing interventions are indicated for a client in labor receiving oxytocin (Pitocin) to stimulate uterine contractions? (Select all that apply.)

   X   **Use an infusion pump to administer medication.**

   X   **Provide continuous monitoring of maternal vital signs.**

   _____   Stop infusion if uterine contractions occur every 4 min and last 45 sec.

   _____   Increase medication rapidly to assure adequate contractions.

   X   **Monitor FHR continuously.**

Oxytocin must be administered by an infusion pump to ensure precise dosage. Continuous maternal and fetal monitoring is required to assess for therapeutic effects and development of adverse effects of oxytocin. Infusion should not be stopped because therapeutic effect has not been achieved. Oxytocin rate is ↑ gradually to prevent hypertonic uterine contractions.

5. A client is receiving testosterone enanthate (Delatestryl) for treatment of androgen-responsive breast cancer. Which of the following side effects should she be monitored for? (Select all that apply.)

   _____   Dehydration

   X   **Hypercalcemia**

   X   **Liver damage**

   X   **Increased LDL and decreased HDL levels**

   X   **Unusual hair growth**

Hypercalcemia, liver damage, increased LDL, decreased HDL levels, and unusual hair growth are all side effects of testosterone enanthate. This medication can lead to fluid retention rather than dehydration.

6. A nurse is providing teaching to a client receiving tamoxifen (Nolvadex) for breast cancer prevention. Which of the following statements indicates the client has understood the teaching?

   A. "I may experience hot flashes."

   B. "I will be so excited when I finally get pregnant."

   C. "I should be sure to drink plenty of milk."

   D. "I will eat a diet high in fat to prevent weight loss."

Hot flashes are a side effect of Tamoxifen. Tamoxifen is a Pregnancy Risk Category D medication that can lead to hypercalcemia, so the client should avoid dairy products. This medication can also cause hyperlipidemia, so the client should avoid a diet high in fat.

7. Match the following medications with their therapeutic uses.

Testosterone enanthate (Delatestryl)	A. Contraception
Conjugated equine estrogens (Premarin)	B. Breast cancer prevention and treatment
Medroxyprogesterone acetate (Provera)	C. Treatment of erectile dysfunction
Ovcon 35	D. Contraindicated for athletic performance enhancement
Leuprolide (Lupron)	E. Relief of postmenopausal symptoms
Tamoxifen (Nolvadex)	F. Treatment of endometriosis
Sildenafil (Viagra)	G. Dysfunctional uterine bleeding due to hormonal balance

Testosterone enanthate (Delatestryl), D.; Conjugated equine estrogens (Premarin), E.; Medroxyprogesterone acetate (Provera), G.; Ovcon 35, A.; Leuprolide (Lupron), F.; Tamoxifen (Nolvadex), B; Sildenafil (Viagra) C.